AF615204

1992
YEAR BOOK OF
OTOLARYNGOLOGY—
HEAD AND NECK SURGERY®

The 1992 Year Book® Series

Year Book of Anesthesia and Pain Management: Drs. Miller, Abram, Kirby, Ostheimer, Roizen, and Stoelting

Year Book of Cardiology®: Drs. Schlant, Collins, Engle, Frye, Kaplan, and O'Rourke

Year Book of Critical Care Medicine®: Drs. Rogers and Parrillo

Year Book of Dentistry®: Drs. Meskin, Currier, Kennedy, Leinfelder, Matukas, and Rovin

Year Book of Dermatologic Surgery: Drs. Swanson, Salasche, and Glogau

Year Book of Dermatology®: Drs. Sober and Fitzpatrick

Year Book of Diagnostic Radiology®: Drs. Federle, Clark, Gross, Madewell, Maynard, Sackett, and Young

Year Book of Digestive Diseases®: Drs. Greenberger and Moody

Year Book of Drug Therapy®: Drs. Lasagna and Weintraub

Year Book of Emergency Medicine®: Drs. Wagner, Burdick, Davidson, Roberts, and Spivey

Year Book of Endocrinology®: Drs. Bagdade, Braverman, Horton, Kannan, Landsberg, Molitch, Morley, Odell, Rogol, Ryan, and Sherwin

Year Book of Family Practice®: Drs. Berg, Bowman, Davidson, Dietrich, and Scherger

Year Book of Geriatrics and Gerontology®: Drs. Beck, Abrass, Burton, Cummings, Makinodan, and Small

Year Book of Hand Surgery®: Drs. Amadio and Hentz

Year Book of Health Care Management: Drs. Heyssel, Brock, King, and Steinberg, Ms. Avakian, and Messrs. Berman, Kues, and Rosenberg

Year Book of Hematology®: Drs. Spivak, Bell, Ness, Quesenberry, and Wiernik

Year Book of Infectious Diseases®: Drs. Wolff, Barza, Keusch, Klempner, and Snydman

Year Book of Infertility: Drs. Mishell, Paulsen, and Lobo

Year Book of Medicine®: Drs. Rogers, Bone, Cline, Braunwald, Greenberger, Utiger, Epstein, and Malawista

Year Book of Neonatal and Perinatal Medicine®: Drs. Klaus and Fanaroff

Year Book of Nephrology: Drs. Coe, Favus, Henderson, Kashgarian, Luke, Myers, and Strom

Year Book of Neurology and Neurosurgery®: Drs. Currier and Crowell

Year Book of Neuroradiology: Drs. Osborn, Harnsberger, Halbach, and Grossman

Year Book of Nuclear Medicine®: Drs. Hoffer, Gore, Gottschalk, Sostman, Zaret, and Zubal

Year Book of Obstetrics and Gynecology®: Drs. Mishell, Kirschbaum, and Morrow

Year Book of Occupational and Environmental Medicine: Drs. Emmett, Brooks, Harris and Schenker

Year Book of Oncology®: Drs. Young, Longo, Ozols, Simone, Steele, and Weichselbaum

Year Book of Ophthalmology®: Drs. Laibson, Adams, Augsburger, Benson, Cohen, Eagle, Flanagan, Nelson, Reinecke, Sergott, and Wilson

Year Book of Orthopedics®: Drs. Sledge, Poss, Cofield, Frymoyer, Griffin, Hansen, Johnson, Simmons, and Springfield

Year Book of Otolaryngology–Head and Neck Surgery®: Drs. Bailey and Paparella

Year Book of Pathology and Clinical Pathology®: Drs. Gardner, Bennett, Cousar, Garvin, and Worsham

Year Book of Pediatrics®: Dr. Stockman

Year Book of Plastic, Reconstructive, and Aesthetic Surgery: Drs. Miller, Cohen, McKinney, Robson, Ruberg, and Whitaker

Year Book of Podiatric Medicine and Surgery®: Dr. Kominsky

Year Book of Psychiatry and Applied Mental Health®: Drs. Talbott, Frances, Freedman, Meltzer, Perry, Schowalter, and Yudofsky

Year Book of Pulmonary Disease®: Drs. Bone and Petty

Year Book of Sports Medicine®: Drs. Shephard, Eichner, Sutton, and Torg, Col. Anderson, and Mr. George

Year Book of Surgery®: Drs. Schwartz, Jonasson, Robson, Shires, Spencer, and Thompson

Year Book of Transplantation: Drs. Ascher, Hansen, and Strom

Year Book of Ultrasound: Drs. Merritt, Mittelstaedt, Carroll, and Nyberg

Year Book of Urology®: Drs. Gillenwater and Howards

Year Book of Vascular Surgery®: Dr. Bergan

Roundsmanship® '92–'93: A Student's Survival Guide to Clinical Medicine Using Current Literature: Drs. Dan, Feigin, Quilligan, Schrock, Stein, and Talbott

1992

The Year Book of OTOLARYNGOLOGY—HEAD AND NECK SURGERY®

Otology

Editor

Michael M. Paparella, M.D.

Clinical Professor and Chairman Emeritus, Department of Otolaryngology, University of Minnesota; President, Minnesota Ear, Head, and Neck Clinic; Secretary, International Hearing Foundation

Head and Neck Surgery

Editor

Byron J. Bailey, M.D., F.A.C.S.

Weiss Professor and Chairman, Department of Otolaryngology, The University of Texas Medical Branch, Galveston

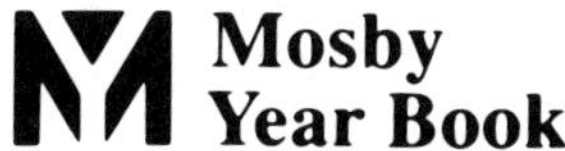

St. Louis Baltimore Boston Chicago London Philadelphia Sydney Toronto

Editor-in-Chief, Year Book Publishing: Kenneth H. Killion
Sponsoring Editor: Kristine Antens
Manager, Literature Services: Edith M. Podrazik
Senior Information Specialist: Terri Santo
Senior Medical Writer: David A. Cramer, M.D.
Assistant Director, Manuscript Services: Frances M. Perveiler
Associate Managing Editor, Year Book Editing Services: Elizabeth Fitch
Editorial Assistant: Tamara L. Smith
Senior Production/Desktop Publishing Manager: Max F. Perez
Proofroom Manager: Barbara M. Kelly

Mosby-Year Book, Inc.
11830 Westline Industrial Drive
St. Louis, MO 63146

Editorial Office:
Mosby-Year Book, Inc.
200 North LaSalle St.
Chicago, IL 60601

International Standard Serial Number: 1041-892X
International Standard Book Number: 0-8151-0536-3

Table of Contents

Journals Represented

Mosby–Year Book subscribes to and surveys nearly 900 U.S. and foreign medical and allied health journals. From these journals, the Editors select the articles to be abstracted. Journals represented in this YEAR BOOK are listed below.

ASAIO Transactions
Acta Neurologica Scandinavica
Acta Oto-Laryngologica
Aesthetic Plastic Surgery
American Journal of Epidemiology
American Journal of Neuroradiology
American Journal of Otolaryngology
American Journal of Otology
American Journal of Surgery
American Review of Respiratory Disease
American Surgeon
Annals of Allergy
Annals of Otology, Rhinology and Laryngology
Annals of Plastic Surgery
Annals of Surgery
Annals of Thoracic Surgery
Annals of the Royal College of Surgeons of England
Archives of Dermatology
Archives of Disease in Childhood
Archives of Internal Medicine
Archives of Otolaryngology—Head and Neck Surgery
Australian and New Zealand Journal of Medicine
British Journal of Plastic Surgery
British Medical Journal
Cancer
Cancer Research
Chest
Cleft Palate Journal
Clinical Otolaryngology
Clinical Pediatrics
Clinical Pharmacology and Therapeutics
Clinical and Experimental Allergy
Ear, Nose, and Throat Journal
European Archives of Oto-Rhino-Laryngology
European Journal of Plastic Surgery
European Journal of Surgery
Family Medicine
Gastroenterology
General Hospital Psychiatry
Head and Neck
Hearing Research
Human Pathology
Injury
International Journal of Cancer
International Journal of Pediatric Otorhinolaryngology
International Journal of Radiation, Oncology, Biology, and Physics
International Surgery
Journal of Clinical Endocrinology and Metabolism
Journal of Clinical Neuro-Ophthalmology
Journal of Clinical Oncology

Journal of Cranio-Maxillo-Facial Surgery
Journal of Dermatologic Surgery and Oncology
Journal of Emergency Medicine
Journal of Laryngology and Otology
Journal of Neurosurgery
Journal of Oral and Maxillofacial Surgery
Journal of Otolaryngology
Journal of Pediatric Surgery
Journal of Pediatrics
Journal of Speech and Hearing Research
Journal of Voice
Journal of the American Geriatrics Society
Journal of the National Cancer Institute
Laryngoscope
Mayo Clinic Proceedings
Neurosurgery
ORL Journal of Oto-Rhino-Laryngology and its Related Specialties
Oral Surgery, Oral Medicine, Oral Pathology
Otolaryngology—Head and Neck Surgery
Pediatric Infectious Disease Journal
Pediatric Pathology
Plastic and Reconstructive Surgery
Postgraduate Medicine
Psychosomatic Medicine
Respiratory Medicine
Seminars in Ultrasound, CT, and MR
Southern Medical Journal
Surgery

Standard Abbreviations

The following terms are abbreviated in this edition: acquired immunodeficiency syndrome (AIDS), the central nervous system (CNS), cerebrospinal fluid (CSF), computed tomography (CT), electrocardiography (ECG), human immunodeficiency virus (HIV), and magnetic resonance (MR) imaging (MRI).

Publisher's Preface

As publishers, we feel challenged to seek ways of presenting complex information in a clear and readable manner. To this end, the 1992 YEAR BOOK OF OTOLARYNGOLOGY–HEAD AND NECK SURGERY now provides structured abstracts in which the various components of a study can easily be identified through headings. These headings are not the same in all abstracts but, rather, are those that most accurately designate the content of each particular journal article. We are confident that our readers will find the information contained in our abstracts to be more accessible than ever before. We welcome your comments.

OTOLOGY

MICHAEL M. PAPARELLA, M.D.

Introduction

Some of the great names in the history of otolaryngology have served as editors of the YEAR BOOK OF OTOLARYNGOLOGY. These names include Gustavus P. Head, Albert H. Andrews, W.L. Ballenger and H.C. Ballenger, George E. Shambaugh, Sr., Samuel J. Crowe, and John R. Lindsay. I have had the distinct privilege and honor of working with some outstanding editors of the YEAR BOOK. For a short time, John Kirchner edited the Head and Neck portion with me. Stuart Strong edited the Head and Neck section for 9 years and was then succeeded by Byron J. Bailey. For this new 1992 YEAR BOOK, I would very sincerely like to extend my thanks and appreciation to Byron J. Bailey for his excellent co-editorship of the YEAR BOOK during the past 5 years. He has, at all times, been an outstanding colleague and friend, and he has done a superb job as co-editor of the YEAR BOOK.

On this occasion, I am proud to announce a new editor for the Head and Neck portion of the YEAR BOOK who, I am certain, will be an excellent representative along the continuum of the aforementioned leaders and contributors to otolaryngology. I am pleased to welcome warmly Dr. G. Richard Holt, who is a well-established educational leader in the field of otolaryngology. He currently serves as president of the American Academy of Otolaryngology—Head and Neck Surgery. Dr. Holt is well known to all members of the profession, and I am certain that he will do a superb job of selecting articles and providing editorial comments for the Head and Neck section of the YEAR BOOK OF OTOLARYNGOLOGY. In addition to extending a warm welcome to G. Richard Holt as a new co-editor of the YEAR BOOK, I want to reiterate my warmest appreciation, respect, and gratitude to Byron J. Bailey for having done such a great job and for having been such an excellent colleague throughout the years. I do think that the quality of these men has provided a useful YEAR BOOK for the readership to refer to and, we hope, to be stimulated by, to encourage their own thinking about diagnosis and treatment of otolaryngological diseases.

Michael M. Paparella, M.D.

1 Vestibular Function

Bilateral Semicircular Canal Aplasia With Near-Normal Cochlear Development: Two Case Reports
Parnes LS, Chernoff WG (Univ of Western Ontario, London, Ont, Canada)
Ann Otol Rhinol Laryngol 99:957–959, 1990 1–1

Introduction.—Explanations of congenital inner ear abnormalities have assumed that malformations result from arrested development during normal embryogenesis. Two cases of vestibular aplasia associated with normal or nearly normal cochlear development conflict with the usual assumption.

Case Report.—Woman, 27, who was retarded, was seen at the age of 5 years with hearing loss and delayed speech. An audiogram showed bilateral conductive hearing loss (Fig 1–1). A left stapedectomy was done at 8 years of age; a right-sided procedure was done at 10 years of age. In both middle ears there was a congenitally fixed footplate with a rudimentary incus. When the patient was reassessed, the physical findings were unremarkable except for a slitlike right external auditory canal. Audiometry showed a bilateral conductive hearing loss. Bithermal caloric responses were absent. A CT scan showed mild bilateral vestibular dilatation with absent semicircular canals. Although the cochleas appeared to be normal, the oval and round windows were obliterated. Binaural amplification was upgraded.

Implications.—It is difficult to explain the coexistence of aplastic vestibular labyrinths with normal or near-normal cochleas on the basis of the arrested-development view of congenital abnormalities. Developmental arrest should produce dysmorphological cochleas as well. However, a specific aberrant "place" lesion may fail to arrest the development of other structures arising from a common source.

▶ The pars superior or vestibular labyrinth is phylogenetically and embryologically older than the pars inferior, which includes the cochlea. Perhaps this helps explain this unusual aplasia of the semicircular canals. This anomaly probably represents a modified version of the so-called "Mondini deformity". Even when there are developmental abnormalities in the vestibular system and a reduction of turns in the cochlea in Mondini deformity, the sensory end organs often appear to be normal. This study describes another variation of such anomalies, and I am certain that there will be many more variations de-

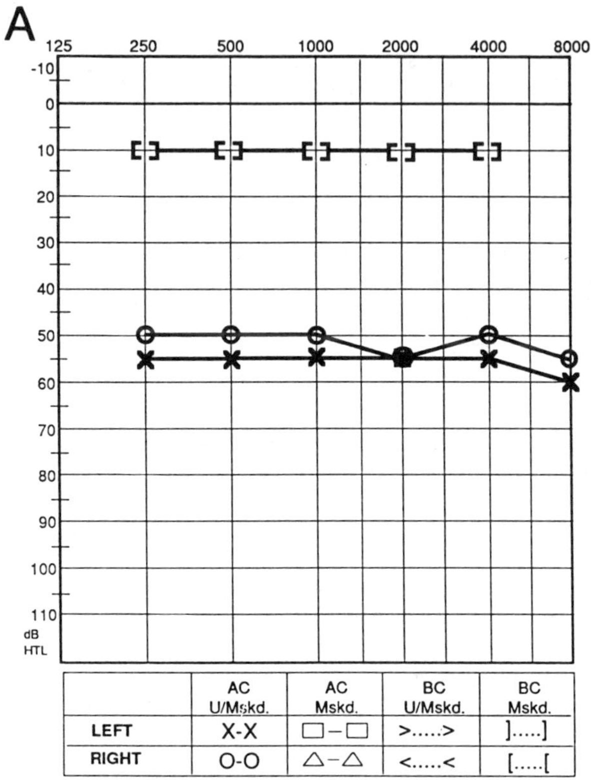

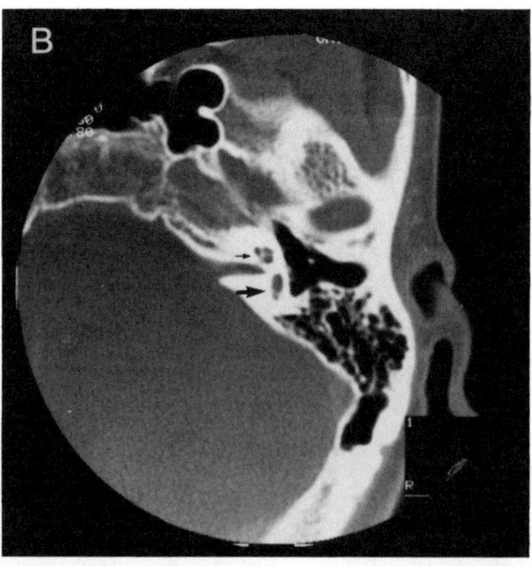

Fig 1–1.—**A,** audiogram at 5 years of age. Note the normal bone conduction thresholds in both ears; **B,** axial CT of left temporal bone. The vestibule appears mildly dilated (*large arrow*). Note the normal

scribed in the future. It is important for us to be cognizant that variations do and will occur.—M.M. Paparella, M.D.

Clinical Significance of a Dizziness History in Medical Patients With Syncope

Sloane PD, Linzer M, Pontinen M, Divine GW (Univ of North Carolina; Duke Univ)

Arch Intern Med 151:1625–1628, 1991 1–2

Background.—Although dizziness and syncope are common medical problems, their diagnosis is hampered by the limited accuracy and utility of diagnostic tests. The coexistence of these 2 problems has prognostic and diagnostic significance, but it has not been widely reported in the medical literature.

Patients.—Factors of age, race, sex, presence or absence of dizziness, character of dizziness, episodic or continuous nature of dizziness, duration of dizziness, comorbid psychiatric disease, the total number of comorbid conditions, and the results of a hyperventilation maneuver were evaluated in 121 patients referred for syncope. Associations were sought between the final diagnosis, the dependent variable, and the clinical predictor variables.

Findings.—Almost 70% of the patients with syncope had dizziness. The patients with dizziness were younger, more often female, and more likely to be assigned a psychiatric diagnosis. Multivariable logistic regression analysis identified young age and rotatory dizziness to be associated with a psychiatric diagnosis.

Conclusions.—Dizziness accompanied syncope in more than two thirds of the patients in this study. Dizziness was found more commonly in young women with a psychiatric diagnosis. Both syncope and dizziness may substantially limit patient activity. The majority of patients had presyncopal lightheadedness, a type of dizziness frequently described among patients with syncope.

▶ Of the many patients I see who have dizziness, a large number of them describe syncope or a fainting type of feeling. Recently, I have seen patients who have described actual vertigo preceded by and/or followed by syncope. Those patients with dizziness have great difficulty using terms to describe how they feel; therefore, it is important for the otologist to ask specific questions to differentiate between the various forms of dizziness and to define whether vertigo and/or syncope exists in association with possible peripheral or central labyrinthine involvement.—M.M. Paparella, M.D.

Fig 1–1 (cont).
cochlea (*small arrow*) and the complete absence of the semicircular canals. Findings were identical in the right temporal bone. (Courtesy of Parnes LS, Chernoff WG: *Ann Otol Rhinol Laryngol* 99:957–959, 1990.)

A Clinical Study of Electrocochleography in Meniere's Disease

Aso S, Watanabe Y, Mizukoshi K (Toyoma Med and Pharmaceutical Univ, Toyama, Japan)

Acta Otolaryngol (Stockh) 111:44–52, 1991 1–3

Introduction.—There are reports that an enlarged summating potential (SP) on electrocochleography is more frequent in Meniere's disease than in other types of sensorineural hearing loss. Electrocochleography was performed on 612 ears with hearing loss and on 29 normal ears. The group with hearing loss included 168 ears of 129 patients with Meniere's disease. The ratio of SP to the action potential (AP) was estimated.

Findings.—The SP/AP ratio proved to be much better than the SP amplitude in detecting endolymphatic hydrops. A ratio of .3–.4 was the upper limit of normal. The SP/AP ratio decreased significantly in 21 Meniere's ears after administration of intravenous glycerol; however, no change followed oral administration of glycerol or isosorbide. The SP/AP ratio decreased by 10% or more postoperatively in 5 patients, but 10 other patients who were followed for at least 2 years after surgery showed no significant change in either the SP/AP ratio or the pure tone threshold.

Discussion.—Repeated electrocochleography is a useful means of monitoring endolymphatic hydrops. The SP/AP ratio may have greater diagnostic value than SP amplitude.

▶ The conclusion of this study by Aso, Watanabe, and Mizukoshi reaffirms the observation that electrocochleography is a useful means of monitoring endolymphatic hydrops, thereby corroborating what is generally described in the literature. At the same time, this test—like all tests—needs to be placed in proper perspective with the history, physical, and laboratory findings, and in particular with the audiological findings.—M.M. Paparella, M.D.

Meniere's Disease: An Immune Complex-Mediated Illness?

Derebery MJ, Rao VS, Siglock TJ, Linthicum FH, Nelson RA (House Ear Clinic and House Ear Inst, Los Angeles; St Vincent Med Ctr, Los Angeles)

Laryngoscope 101:225–229, 1991 1–4

Introduction.—The etiology of Meniere's disease remains unknown; however, recent studies have suggested immune-mediated damage to the inner ear. The diagnosis of automimmune Meniere's syndrome is often based on history, clinical response to treatment with steroids or cytotoxic agents, and serological studies.

Study Design.—Using the polyethylene glycol assay, the levels of circulating immune complexes (CIC) were determined in 30 patients with Meniere's disease and in 20 controls to test the hypothesis that Meniere's disease may be associated with significant abnormalities in the cellular or humoral immune responses, or both.

Findings.—The mean levels of CIC in the patients with Meniere's disease were significantly higher than those in control patients (mean, 1,445 versus 470 absolute score/mL), even after excluding patients older than 55 years of age. In fact, 29 patients with Meniere's disease (96.6%) had significantly elevated levels of CIC.

Discussion.—These findings suggest that the humoral system may be involved in the pathogenesis of Meniere's disease. In the absence of the ability to demonstrate tissue-bound immune complexes in the inner ear (because the inner ear cannot be presently biopsied), the presence of CIC offers indirect evidence that the deposition of these complexes may account for the end-organ damage observed in Meniere's disease.

▶ Although the relationship between increased levels of CIC and Meniere's disease appears to be significant, it is hard to draw a direct cause-and-effect line in the relationship. For example, do these elevated CIC levels relate to the function or dysfunction of the endolymphatic duct and sac or of the labyrinthine portions of the inner ear?—M.M. Paparella, M.D.

Cellular Changes in Reissner's Membrane in Endolymphatic Hydrops

Yoon TH, Paparella MM, Schachern PA, Le CT (Univ of Minnesota; Ulsan Univ, Seoul, Korea)

Ann Otol Rhinol Laryngol 100:288–293, 1991 1–5

Introduction.—Reissner's membrane (RM) is consistently distended in endolymphatic hydrops associated with such disorders as Meniere's disease, otitis media, and otosclerosis. A better understanding of the cellular changes in RM might clarify the etiopathogenesis of endolymphatic hydrops and provide a means of estimating the severity of the process.

Methods.—Temporal bones were obtained from 15 individuals without a history of otopathology, 6 with unilateral endolymphatic hydrops, and 4 with bilateral endolymphatic hydrops.

Results.—The epithelial and mesothelial cells were irregularly arranged in endolymphatic hydrops. The epithelial cell layer appeared to bulge, and clusters of small cells were seen often, especially near the stretched area of the distended RM (Fig 1–2). The number of cells and the width of the RM were greater in the ears with endolymphatic hydrops than in the normal ears. Although unilateral hydrops was generally mild or moderate, hydrops were severe in patients with bilateral disease. The inner ear changes generally were not remarkable in ears with endolymphatic hydrops.

Conclusion.—The epithelial cells of the RM appear to be involved in the pathogenesis of endolymphatic hydrops. Cellular changes in the RM

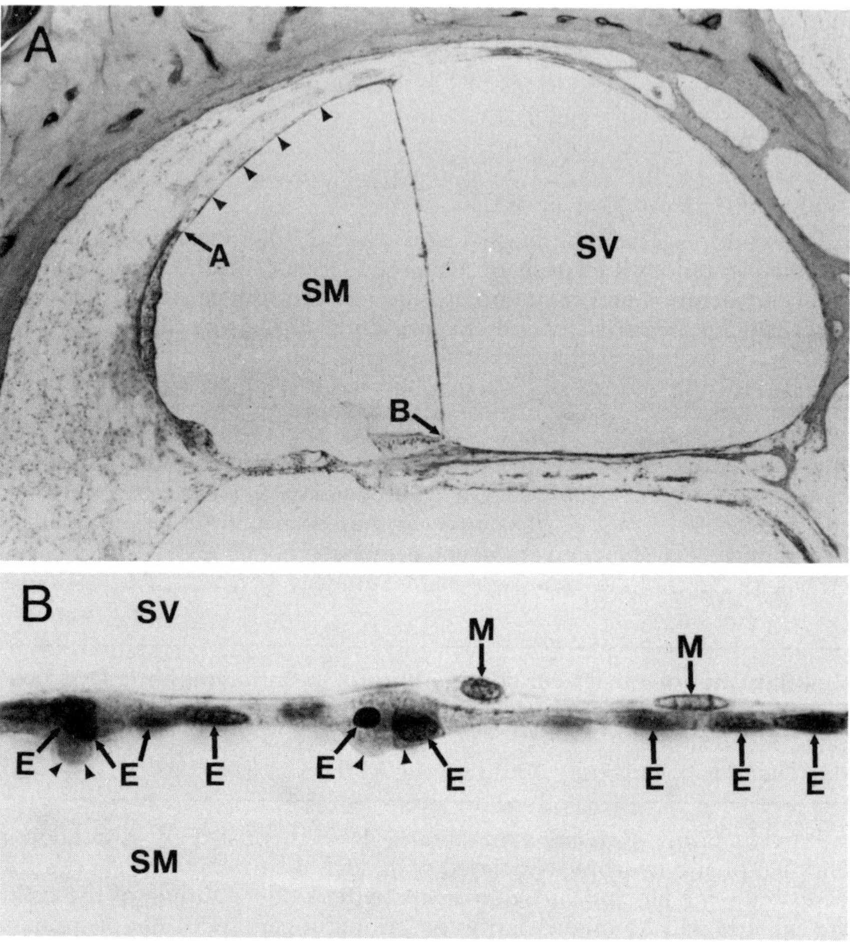

Fig 1–2.—*Abbreviations*: *SM*, scala media; *SV*, scala vestibuli. Reissner's membrane (RM) in mild degree of endolymphatic hydrops. **A,** distended RM (*arrowheads*) attached to spiral ligament (Hematoxylin-eosin; original magnification, × 90). The width of RM is from point *A* to point *B*. **B,** bulging (*arrowheads*) of epithelial cell layers and cluster formations of epithelial cells *(E)* (Hematoxylin-eosin; original magnification, × 1,270). Mesothelial cells *(M)* are occasionally seen. (Courtesy of Yoon TH, Paparella MM, Schachern PA, et al: *Ann Otol Rhinol Laryngol* 100:288–293, 1991.)

might lead to dysfunction of radial flow, a resultant ionic disturbance in the endolymph, and hearing loss.

► It is well known that RM is distended in patients with Meniere's disease and endolymphatic hydrops. This study documents the fact that there are changes in the epithelial and mesothelial cells as well. These changes suggest that, in addition to alterations in pressure, the distortion and sparsity of the cells may change the radial flow that exists between the endolymph and the perilymph of the scala vestibuli (assuming that complete hydrops does not exist). Although it is still widely believed that Meniere's disease is basically a disruption of longitudinal flow, we cannot ignore the role of radial flow.—M.M. Paparella, M.D.

Contribution of Increased Endolymphatic Pressure to Hearing Loss in Experimental Hydrops

Horner KC, Cazals Y (Pellegrin Hosp, Bordeaux, France)
Ann Otol Rhinol Laryngol 100:496–502, 1991 1–6

Background.—Ever since endolymphatic hydrops was first demonstrated in the temporal bones of patients with Meniere's disease, it has been assumed that hydrops is involved in Meniere's disease. However, it is not known whether the hydrops is the primary dysfunction or only an epiphenomenon, because hydrops is associated with other diseases as well. The contribution of increased endolymphatic pressure to hearing loss was investigated in experimental hydrops.

Methods and Findings.—Experimental hydrops was induced in guinea pigs. A strict sequence of compound action potential audiogram changes followed. A low-frequency loss occurred within days. Within weeks, a very high-frequency loss developed. Within months, the 8-kHz region was affected. The application of excess pressure to the endolymphatic spaces through a cannula placed in the endolymphatic duct resulted in a sequence of compound action potential audiogram changes unlike those observed with hydrops. First, there was a very high-frequency loss, then there was a very low-frequency loss. Finally, the 4-kHz region was affected and the thresholds for all frequencies increased even more significantly.

Conclusions.—Endolymphatic pressure may not be the crucial factor determining hearing loss at the onset of experimental hydrops. Outer hair-cell stereocilia atrophy may account for the fluctuating hearing loss. The underlying mechanisms responsible for the selective low-frequency loss, however, have yet to be determined.

▶ In this study, the conclusion indicates that endolymphatic pressure is not necessarily a crucial factor relating to hearing loss in experimentally induced endolymphatic hydrops. However, the study neglects to take into consideration the chemical changes occurring across the membranes between the endolymph, blood, and perilymph. These also could amount for dysfunction. The fluctuating nature of hearing in Meniere's disease is perhaps better explained on the basis of chemical changes rather than atrophy of stereocilia of the outer hair cells.—M.M. Paparella, M.D.

The Ionic and Electric Environment in the Endolymphatic Sac of the Chinchilla: Relevance to the Longitudinal Flow

Ikeda K, Morizono T (Tohoku Univ, Sendai, Japan; Univ of Minnesota)
Hear Res 54:118–122, 1991 1–7

Background.—Research on the function of the endolymphatic sac (ES) has focused on the role of the absorption and secretion of the endolymph as related to the longitudinal flow. Observations of dc potential and ionic concentrations have suggested physiological differences between the ES and other regions of the endolymphatic space. Because ion transport is related to water movement, the chemical gradient and electrical gradient through the cochlear duct will provide the key to understanding ES fluid transport.

Methods and Results.—The ionic composition of the endolymph in the ES of 12 healthy chinchillas was measured with double-barreled ion-selective micro-electrodes. The mean dc potential of the ES was 9.3 mV, whereas the ES concentrations of K^+, Na^+, and $C1^-$ were 13.3 mM, 129 mM, and 124.3 mM, respectively. The pressure gradient of the endolymph between the cochlea and the ES was calculated to be 71.5 mm Hg at 38°C.

Conclusions.—Accumulating evidence suggests a longitudinal flow from the cochlea to the ES. Volume flow appears to be driven primarily by an osmotic pressure.

► Both this study and its conclusions are appealing. The study not only provides additional evidence for the longitudinal flow of the endolymph from the cochlea to the ES, but it also suggests that the flow may be driven by an osmotic pressure-differential. It seems logical that osmotic or chemical alterations in pressure have as much to do with the transmission of endolymph from the apex of the cochlea to the ES as do considerations of hydrostatic pressure.—M.M. Paparella, M.D.

Structure of the Endolymphatic Sac After Instillation of Hyaluronan in the Middle Ear

Jansson B, Friberg U, Rask-Andersen H (Univ Hosp, Uppsala, Sweden)
ORL J Otorhinolaryngol Relat Spec 53:68–71, 1991 1–8

Background.—Systemic administration of hyperosmolar agents can lower hearing thresholds in patients with Meniere's disease; this is apparently related to a decline in the fluid pressure in the inner ear. The endolymphatic sac (ES) shows an increase in granule-containing light epithelial cells and filling of the luminal space with a stainable substance. Instillation of hyaluronan (HA) into the middle ear reversibly alters ABR thresholds, presumably through an osmotic effect on the inner ear via the round window membrane.

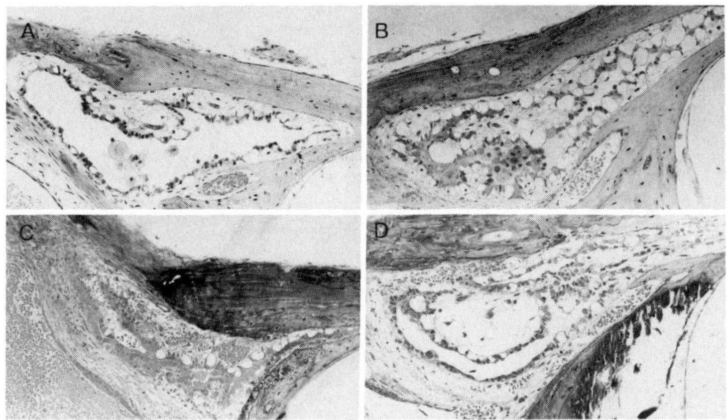

Fig 1–3.—Endolymphatic sac 2 hours after instillation of .5% HA **(A)**, 4 hours after instillation of 1.9% HA **(B)**, 6 hours after instillation of 4% HA **(C)**, and 8 hours after instillation of 4% HA **(D)** in the middle ear. Original magnification, ×220. (Courtesy of Jansson B, Friberg U, Rask-Andersen H: *ORL J Otorhinolaryngol Relat Spec* 53:68–71, 1991.)

Objective.—Whether morphological changes occur in the ES after application of increasing concentrations of HA to the round window niche was investigated in mice. Preparations of .5%, 1%, 1.9%, and 4% high-molecular-weight sodium HA were used. The control animals had a physiological saline-phosphate buffer preparation instilled.

Findings.—The proportion of ES granular cells increased slightly with instillation of 1.9% HA and markedly after 4% HA (Figs 1–3 and 1–4). At the same time, a faint luminal precipitate was noted in about half the ears treated with 4% HA.

Discussion.—Concentrated HA may have the ability to lower inner ear fluid pressure either directly through osmotic withdrawal of fluid via the round window membrane, or by passage of HA through the membrane and consequent osmotic withdrawal of fluid from the endolymphatic compartment. The clinical implications for patients having Meniere's disease remain to be determined.

▶ In an earlier study, Lim instilled tracer elements in the middle ear; they were absorbed through the round window and finally came to be deposited in the ES. Thus, it is possible that there can be changes in osmotic pressure at the level of the round window, in the labyrinth, and in the ES concomitantly. There may be a continuum of changes in osmotic pressure through the inner ear into the ES rather than only one site of change.—M.M. Paparella, M.D.

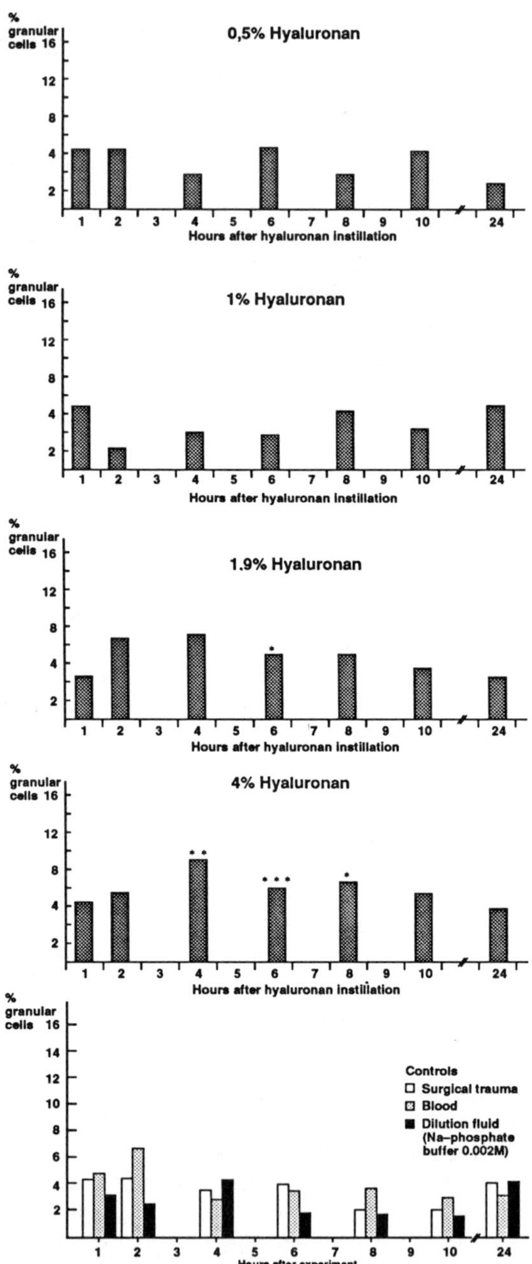

Fig 1–4.—The mean percentage of granular light cells in the epithelial lining of the ES 1-24 hours after instillation of HA in rising concentrations into the round window niche. The controls were instilled with dilution fluid and blood into the middle ear or merely underwent the surgical procedure. * *P* < .05, ** *P* < .01, *** *P* < .001. (Courtesy of Jansson B, Friberg U, Rask-Andersen H: *ORL J Otorhinolaryngol Relat Spec* 53:68–71, 1991.)

Effect of Ototoxic Drug Administration to the Endolymphatic Sac

Lee KS, Kimura RS (Korea Univ, Seoul, South Korea; Harvard Med School; Massachusetts Eye and Ear Infirmary, Boston)

Ann Otol Rhinol Laryngol 100:355–360, 1991 1–9

Background.—Various treatments have been tried to control the incapicitating vertigo and fluctuating hearing loss associated with Meniere's disease. Aminoglycosides primarily affect the inner ear sensory cells, but they also affect the structures involved with endolymph production. Whether a drug applied to the endolymphatic sac can reach the vestibular labyrinth against the flow of endolymph and what the effect would be on the inner ear sensory structures is unknown.

Methods.—Small amounts of streptomycin sulfate and gentamicin sulfate were applied to the endolymphatic sacs of 33 guinea pigs with good pinna reflexes. In group 1, about 10 μL of gentamicin sulfate was applied to the lateral surface of the endolymphatic sac. In group 2, an equal amount of gentamicin sulfate was slowly injected into the endolymphatic sac through a glass micropipette. In group 3, streptomycin sulfate was used.

Results.—The application of gentamicin in group 1 produced degeneration of the sensory cells of the macular sacculi. In group 2, gentamicin injection often produced lesions in the maculae sacculi and utriculi, the cristae of the 3 ampullae, and the organ of Corti in the basal turn. Although passive instillation of streptomycin sulfate pellets into the sac from a lateral opening in group 3 animals resulted in a similar pattern of degenerations it was less severe when compared with injection. Most of the sensory cells of the vestibular labyrinth were affected when the sensory cells of the basal turn degenerated (Fig 1–5).

Conclusions.—This study demonstrates the diffusion of drugs that occurs against the longitudinal flow of endolymph. The findings may be applicable in the treatment of Meniere's disease.

▶ This animal study by Kimura suggests that instillation of gentamicin or streptomycin causes cellular degeneration in the maculae of the otolithic organs. This may be applicable in the treatment of Meniere's disease. For the past 3 years, I have successfully used this method among the 4% of patients who are candidates for endolymphatic sac revision. Not only will a revision occur in these selected patients, but instillation of streptomycin in the endolymphatic sac region will preserve cochlear function while helping to eliminate vestibular dysfunction.—M.M. Paparella, M.D.

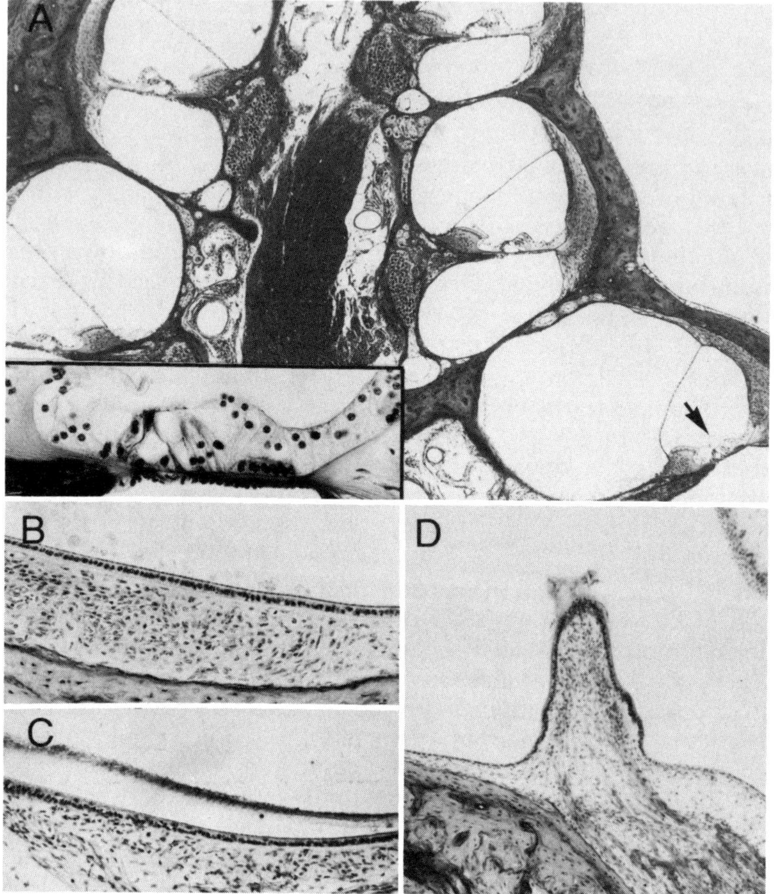

Fig 1–5.—Specimen 25, group 3. Extent of degeneration of the cochlear and vestibular sensory cells is shown 1 month after passive instillation of streptomycin sulfate into the endolymphatic sac. **A,** cochlea shows outer hair cell degeneration and slight endolymphatic hydrops in the basal turn. **Inset,** higher-power view of organ of Corti *(arrow)* shows outer hair cell degeneration. Vestibular sensory cells were degenerated in **(B)** macula sacculi, **(C)** macula utriculi, and **(D)** lateral crista ampullaris. (Courtesy of Lee KS, Kimura RS: *Ann Otol Rhinol Laryngol* 100:355–360, 1991).

Endolymphatic Sac Surgery for Refractory Luetic Vertigo

Huang T-S, Lin C-C (Chang Gung Med College, Taipei, Taiwan)

Am J Otol 12:184–187, 1991 1–10

Background.—Otitic syphilis causes symptoms that are indistinguishable from those of Meniere's disease. Although penicillin and steroids will control the symptoms in most cases, patients with refractory leutic vertigo may require surgery. Endolymphatic sac decompression, which was first reported by Shambaugh, was used to treat otosyphilis.

Patients.—Endolymphatic sac procedures were done on 37 patients with presumed leutic vertigo that was refractory to medical measures. All patients had incapacitating vertigo. A group of 21 patients had a symmetric hearing loss and 15 had asymmetric losses. The mean pure-tone average was 2.7 dB. The average period of medical treatment was approximately 6 months. A Silastic or Penrose drain sheet was utilized most often.

Outcome.—At follow-up ranging from 2 years to 9 years and 9 months, vertigo was substantially or totally controlled in 81% of the patients. Hearing, as assessed using American Academy of Otolaryngology-Head and Neck Surgery criteria, improved in 2 patients, both of whom had had a positive glycerol test or exhibited fluctuating hearing loss preoperatively. Tinnitus was lessened by surgery in about a third of the patients. Aural pressure was relieved in about half of the patients.

Conclusions.—Endolymphatic sac surgery is a reasonable approach to relieving vertigo in patients with acquired syphilis. Such surgery is definitely helpful when intensive medical treatment has failed.

▶ Refractory leutic vertigo can present a clinical picture identical to that of refractory Meniere's disease. I think it is reasonable to include leutic vertigo as a subdivision of the many clinical entities describable under the aegis of Meniere's disease. The experience described by Huang is very comparable to our own experience with these unusual selected cases.—M.M. Paparella, M.D.

Cochleosacculotomy Revisited: Long-Term Results Poorer Than Expected

Giddings NA, Shelton C, O'Leary MJ, Brackmann DE (Geisinger Med Ctr, Danville, Pa; House Ear Clinic, Los Angeles; Naval Regional Med Ctr, San Diego)

Arch Otolaryngol Head Neck Surg 117:1150–1152, 1991 1–11

Background.—In Meniere's disease, cochleosacculotomy is done for relief of vertigo in patients who have not been helped by medical therapy. It appears to reduce the number and severity of vertiginous attacks for most patients in the short term. The results in terms of hearing are more variable, but the procedure is still commonly performed. The results obtained with this procedure were examined to test their initially positive clinical impression.

Patients.—The study included 11 patients (average age, 72.8 years) who underwent cochleosacculotomy during a 7-year period and were followed for more than 6 months. The average follow-up was 17.4 months. These patients were chosen for cochleosacculotomy because of their advanced age and good vestibular function. All underwent preoperative electronystagmography, pure-tone and speech threshold testing, and speech discrimination testing. The patients were evaluated postoperatively by audiogram, chart review, and interview.

Outcome.—Vertigo was relieved immediately in all patients; however, at follow-up 5 patients still had rotary vertigo or drop attacks, 4 required a second operation, and 2 had no further vertigo. Hearing was significantly worse in 9 patients. On audiometry, significant increases were found in the pure-tone thresholds at all frequencies and in the speech reception threshold, and a significant decrease was seen in the discrimination scores.

Conclusions.—Cochleosacculotomy does not appear to offer long-term control of vertigo in patients with Meniere's disease. It is a well-tolerated procedure, but the patient will likely need a more definitive procedure to control vertigo and will probably lose significant hearing.

▶ Cochleosacculotomy is a procedure that requires direct penetration of the basal turn of the cochlea as well as the vestibule. Any time one submits the labyrinth to such a procedure, hearing losses can be expected. In this small subset of patients, some patients did not have long-term control of vertigo and required other procedures. This procedure may still have merit when performed with an appropriate technique in selected patients.—M.M. Paparella, M.D.

Retrolabyrinthine Vestibular Nerve Section: Efficacy in Disorders Other Than Meniere's Disease

Kemink JL, Telian SA, El-Kashlan H, Langman AW (Univ of Michigan Med Ctr; Alexandria Univ Med School, Egypt)

Laryngoscope 101:523–528, 1991 1–12

Objective.—Retrolabyrinthine vestibular nerve section (RVNS) is an effective means of treating intractable vertigo of peripheral vestibular origin when hearing must be preserved. Its efficacy in controlling vertigo resulting from causes other than Meniere's disease was evaluated in 42 patients with a wide variety of diagnoses.

Patients.—Of the 90 patients seen in 1983–1986 with incapacitating vertigo resistant to medical measures, 48 had a diagnosis of unilateral Meniere's disease. Twenty-three others had a diagnosis of uncompensated vestibular neuritis. The remaining 19 patients had labyrinthine dysfunction attributable to various causes. Eight of these 19 had unilateral sensorineural hearing loss. All patients underwent RVNS and were followed for at least 2 years.

Outcome.—Of the patients with uncompensated vestibular neuritis, 39% were cured and another 30% were improved at follow-up. In contrast, 94% of the patients with Meniere's disease were considered cured after RVNS and 2% were improved. Hearing improved after surgery in 10% of the patients with Meniere's disease but not in any of those with vestibular neuritis. Among the remaining patients, those with unilateral sensorineural hearing loss were consistently cured of vertigo at follow-up, although a few continued to have mild dysequilibrium. Four patients had CSF leaks after surgery; however, there were no deaths or strokes. No patient had facial paralysis or meningitis. Wound infections did not occur after the routine use of intraoperative bacitracin solution was instituted.

Conclusions.—Retrolabyrinthine vestibular nerve section is especially effective in patients with Meniere's disease, although many patients with uncompensated vestibular neuritis also have benefited. A high cure rate can be expected in those patients with sensorineural hearing loss associated with vestibular abnormality or a clear history of unilateral otitis. Vestibular rehabilitation has rendered RVNS inapplicable to most patients with uncompensated vestibular neuritis.

▶ It is certainly well known that diseases other than Meniere's disease (e.g., vestibular neuritis) can cause vertigo. This study is a bit disappointing because the small percentage of patients with vertigo resulting from other causes was not relieved of symptoms after vestibular nerve section. Apparently, better results were obtained in patients with refractory Meniere's disease. A small semantic difference exists: patients who undergo treatment for Meniere's disease are never cured because there is no cure for the disease. Only the symptoms of vertigo can be alleviated in these patients.—M.M. Paparella, M.D.

2 Hearing and Hearing Tests

The Genetics of Deafness

Reardon W, Pembrey M (Inst of Child Health, London)

Arch Dis Child 65:1196–1197, 1990 2–1

Introduction.—Hereditary deafness covers a broad spectrum from simple deafness to genetically determined syndromes. Perhaps 30% of all genetic deafness occurs in syndromic form. Many of the syndromes that include deafness are inherited in a mendelian manner, offering the possibility of accurate genetic counseling.

Problems.—When an autosomal recessive gene is affected, there is no way of knowing whether deafness in an individual case is genetic or environmental unless there are many affected siblings in a given generation. The high rate of marriage between deaf individuals can produce a complex genetic situation in which there are multiple possible causes of deafness in a given pedigree. Although as much as 85% of nonsyndromic genetic deafness is thought to result from autosomal recessive inheritance, not all autosomal recessive deafness can be explained by mutations at a single gene locus.

Gene Mapping.—Family linkage studies are based on a search for DNA probes that are reliably coinherited with the disease. Although the value of these studies is limited by genetic heterogeneity, this approach has proved important in localizing deafness-causing genes. Molecular genetic studies of collagen genes have revealed associations with deafness. Examples include osteogenesis imperfecta and the progressive sensorineural deafness seen in the Stickler-Marshall syndrome and osteogenesis imperfecta. An alternative to the family linkage approach is to isolate those genes responsible for nonsyndromic deafness in the mouse and then use them to search the human genome for genes related to deafness.

► Recently a new Institute on Deafness and other Communicative Disorders was organized by the National Institutes of Health. One of its major objectives is to better understand the genetics of deafness and the related disorders of the inner ear. In our own studies and treatment of patients, we have found a genetic predisposition to many diseases causing deafness. In addition to well-established genetic diseases such as otosclerosis, conditions of

Meniere's disease and otitis media have also been identified.—M.M. Paparella, M.D.

Adverse Perinatal Factors in the Causation of Sensorineural Hearing Impairment in Young Children

Das VK (Manchester Univ, Manchester, England)

Int J Pediatr Otorhinolaryngol 21:121–125, 1991 2–2

Background.—Hearing loss or impairment may be caused by environmental, genetic, or social factors. In children, the factors leading to prematurity or preterm birth may combine with adverse perinatal events to cause hearing loss or impairment. Various adverse perinatal causes leading to bilateral sensorineural hearing impairment were investigated in 173 children.

Patients.—A group of 22 children with a diagnosis of hearing impairment suspected to be caused by adverse perinatal factors accounted for 12.7% of the total number of hearing-impaired children studied during a 5-year period within the boundaries of Greater Manchester. The children were divided into 2 groups on the basis of a hearing loss less than 80 dB or a loss of 80 dB or more in either both ears or in the better ear.

Findings.—A detailed study of the children revealed a preterm group and a term and postterm group. Sensorineural hearing loss ≥ 80 dB affected 88% of the children in the preterm group and 100% of the term/postterm group. More than half of the children had a history of recurrent ear infections, with 40% of them having middle ear dysfunction affecting the hearing. Respiratory problems and hyperbilirubinemia were the most significant possible adverse perinatal factors affecting the newborn. The preterm group also had visual handicaps or developmental retardation.

Conclusions.—Premature infants are exposed to a number of potentially damaging events that may result in sensorineural hearing loss. Hypoxia and hyperbilirubinemia are considered common causes. Middle-ear conductive problems may also be related to poor social status, which influences preterm delivery. The high incidence of significant associated disabilities in children with hearing impairment suggests the need for attention to the problem of preterm infant morbidity as well as mortality.

► Premature infants are more susceptible to hypoxia and hyperbilirubinemia, both of which may be precursors to hearing loss. Preterm infant morbidity should be assessed further to determine possible causes of congenital hearing loss.—M.M. Paparella, M.D.

Noncongenital Hereditary Hearing Loss in Children: Prospective Documentation

Madell JR, Sculerati N (New York League for the Hard of Hearing; New York Univ School of Medicine, New York)
Arch Otolaryngol Head Neck Surg 117:332–335, 1991 2–3

Background.—Hereditary disorders are the most common single cause of sensorineural hearing loss in early childhood. Single gene mutations cause an estimated 40% of cases. Autosomal recessive inheritance reportedly accounts for at least 70% of all hereditary sensorineural hearing losses. The possibility of autosomal recessive loss in hearing-impaired children lacking a family history of hearing loss has led to recommendations for routine audiological assessment of the siblings of any child with sensorineural hearing loss, unless the loss appears to be nonhereditary in origin.

Findings.—Screening of the younger siblings of children with sensorineural hearing loss revealed 7 subjects with progressive noncongenital sensorineural losses. All the losses were bilaterally symmetrical within the limit of 10 dB. The children were from unrelated families, but 4 families were part of the Orthodox Jewish community of New York. In 5 instances the affected older sibling likely had had better hearing in early life. All the parents had normal hearing. One set of parents reportedly were second cousins.

Discussion.—Genetic sensorineural hearing loss may be noncongenital in origin and progressive. The younger siblings of children whose sensorineural loss might be hereditary in origin should have interval audiological assessment—even if normal hearing for age is documented. This is especially important when the older child's hearing loss may not have been congenital in origin.

► Hearing loss in children can be categorized as congenital or noncongenital, genetic and/or acquired. Progressive hearing loss in children may be of a nongenetic nature and is more likely to be noncongenital. Most congenital losses represent dysplasia of the sensory end organs at birth and usually do not progress subsequent to birth.—M.M. Paparella, M.D.

Hearing Screening in Children: State of the Art(s)

Haggard MP (Univ of Nottingham, England)
Arch Dis Child 65:1193–1195, 1990 2–4

Principles of Screening.—Any incidental harm resulting from screening itself or from the information acquired should be small in relation to the benefit from assessment and treatment. It is necessary to agree on guidelines for who is to know the results. Transitional counseling should be available. All screening arrangements should be reviewed periodically. A more cautious approach to screening than is presently practiced at some centers is in order. The methods used should be simple and inexpensive.

Problems in Screening.—It has proved difficult in early screening problems to ensure coverage above a level of about 95%, and the coverage in deprived areas and for older children often is much lower. Occasionally a "background" of detection by professionals and relatives makes it hard to demonstrate an appreciable further yield from screening. The high prevalence of fluctuating otitis media with effusion in young children complicates screens using a referral criterion of less than 40 dB hearing loss. As a result, a service may be overloaded with children of whom only a small minority can or should have surgery for permanent hearing loss or persistent otitis with effusion. Universal neonatal screening is not yet credible from either a logistical or a cost standpoint.

Conclusions.—Sound hearing screening requires a high degree of managerial competence to prioritize, establish, and deliver effective secondary prevention. Valid research on what is worth doing is essential.

► In general, hearing screening in children is considered to be beneficial. However, as this study suggests, even a good thing can become deleterious in some instances. This study raises some interesting questions that require further analysis.—M.M. Paparella, M.D.

The Anterior Inferior Cerebellar Artery in the Internal Auditory Canal

Reisser C, Schuknecht HF (Harvard Med School; Massachusetts Eye and Ear Infirmary, Boston)

Laryngoscope 101:761–766, 1991 2–5

Objective.—The anterior inferior cerebellar artery (AICA) runs close to the internal auditory canal where it gives rise to the labyrinthine artery, raising the question of whether it can produce dysfunction of the nearby eighth nerve trunk. A total of 1,327 temporal bones was reviewed in an attempt to relate audiovestibular symptoms with the presence of the AICA within the internal auditory canal.

Findings.—An AICA loop was found within the internal auditory canal in 12.3% of the temporal bones examined (Figs 2–1 and 2–2). This is about half the frequency found when preparations with intact brains are studied. Five individuals with a loop had unexplained hearing loss, and 3 of 8 with unexplained tinnitus had an AICA loop present. Seven (12.5%) of 56 temporal bones in 29 patients with unexplained vertigo exhibited an AICA loop in the internal auditory canal. Five of the 23 patients with unilateral Meniere's disease had a loop, 3 in the hydropic ear, 1 in both ears, and 1 in the opposite ear.

Conclusion.—In this series, no significant correlation was found between an AICA loop in the internal auditory canal and the occurrence of unexplained hearing loss, tinnitus, vertigo, or Meniere's disease.

► When in doubt, always look at the pathology. The role of the AICA in the

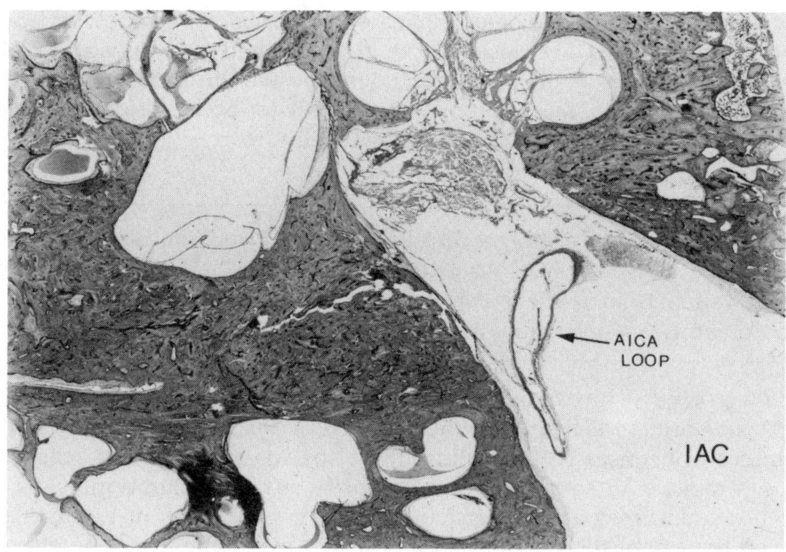

Fig 2–1.—Woman, 96, presbycusis. The AICA extends into the middle third of the internal auditory canal *(IAC)*. Lumen size = .8 mm. Hematoxylin and eosin; original magnification, × 10.1. (Courtesy of Reisser C, Schuknecht HF: *Laryngoscope* 101:761–766, 1991.)

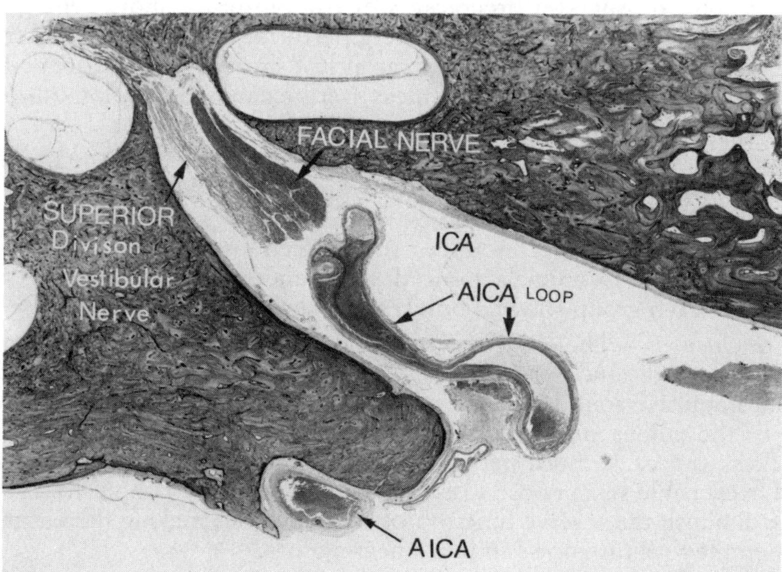

Fig 2–2.—Male, age unknown, presbycusis. The AICA lies in a groove in the posterior wall of the petrous bone and then loops into the middle third of the internal auditory canal *(ICA)*. Lumen size = .8 mm. Hematoxylin and eosin; original magnification, × 11.3. (Courtesy of Reisser C, Schuknecht HF: *Laryngoscope* 101:761–766, 1991.)

internal auditory canal has been implicated as a cause of a variety of labyrinthine symptoms and findings. This study attempted to correlate an AICA loop with peripheral pathologic conditions; however, it failed to do so. Clinical studies should continue to look to pathology for better insight into understanding these disorders.—M.M. Paparella, M.D.

Inner Ear Damage From Toy Cap Pistols and Fire-Crackers

Axelsson A, Hellström P-A, Altschuler R, Miller JM (Univ of Göteborg, Göteborg, Sweden; Univ of Michigan)

Int J Pediatr Otorhinolaryngol 21:143–148, 1991 2–6

Background.—Investigations have shown that teenage boys have a slight sensorineural high-tone hearing loss consistent with exposure to high levels of noise. Toys with impulsive sounds, such as firecrackers and toy cap guns, emit sounds of high intensity but short duration. Thus, the impulse sound may not be particularly loud even though its intensity may exceed the established damage risk criteria for hearing loss. The effect of impulsive sounds on the histopathology of the inner ear was investigated in guinea pigs.

Methods.—Seven groups of 7 guinea pigs each were exposed to 10, 50, or 100 exposures of firecrackers or toy cap pistol shots. One group served as controls. The exposures were performed at 15-second intervals at a distance of .25 m for the toy cap pistol shots and .8 m for the firecrackers. After 3 weeks, the cochleas were examined histologically and the missing outer or inner hair cells were counted.

Findings.—With 10 pistol shots or firecracker explosions, the cochleas of the experimental animals were not significantly different from those of the controls. With 50 or 100 exposures to toy cap pistol findings, 11 of 14 animals showed pronounced sensory cell loss. With 50 or 100 firecrackers, 13 of 14 animals showed pronounced sensory cell loss. One animal in each group showed only a slight sensory cell loss.

Conclusions.—The animals were exposed to a realistic number of explosions at a distance from the ear that can occur during play or holidays when impulsive sound toys are used. The dramatic changes in the cochlea of the guinea pigs show that explosions of toy cap pistols or firecrackers can cause both permanent damage to the inner ear structures and irreversible sensory cell loss. Repeated exposure to impulsive sounds may diminish the reserve function of the inner ear, making the ear more vulnerable to future noise-induced hearing loss.

▶ Children's cochleas are subject to all the same extrinsic causative problems that affect adult cochleas. These problems include infection and trauma as well as other causative possibilities.—M.M. Paparella, M.D.

Autoimmune Inner Ear Disease: A Review of Basic Mechanisms and Clinical Correlates

Ruckenstein MJ, Harrison RV (Hosp for Sick Children, Toronto; Univ of Toronto)

J Otolaryngol 20:196–203, 1991 2–7

Introduction.—Immunosuppressive therapy may result in improved auditory function in patients with autoimmune inner ear disease. The basic science and experimental and clinical data on this disorder were reviewed.

Basic Science.—Initiating, amplifying, and perpetuating factors are all involved in the complicated process of autoimmune response. In autoimmune inner ear disease, the major histocompatibility complex and the helper T (T_H) cell both play important roles. The process of an autoimmune reaction may be affected in a variety of ways by immunosuppressive drugs. Corticosteroids may inhibit the activity of the autoreactive T_H cells and all effector cells, whereas cyclophosphamide decreases the concentration and function of T and B lymphocytes and suppresses macrophage function.

Experimental Data.—Experiments in guinea pigs have shown that repeated systemic administration of the antigen keyhole-limpet hemocyanin (KLH) caused no significant increase in perilymphatic antibody titers, whereas administration of perilymphatics gave a primary and secondary response in the perilymph and serum. The immune response thus seems to be locally generated. On histological study a fibromyxoid infiltrate was found in the scala tympani, with no destruction of sensorineural structures. All the areas of the cochlea were affected in severe inflammatory reactions. Local administration of KLH reduced both local and systemic antibody response in sacculotomized guinea pigs. Although there have been several attempts to create an animal model of autoimmune ear disease, none have proved reproducible.

Clinical Data.—The diagnosis of autoimmune inner ear disease is based on arbitrary criteria that are not unique to an autoimmune process. The lymphocyte migration inhibition assay is not specific. A lymphocyte transformation test has been advocated; however, it is difficult to evaluate because of the absence of an objective mechanism of diagnosis. One group has shown an antibody directed against inner ear antigen in 35% of the patients with rapidly progressive sensorineural hearing loss. No clinical studies have addressed HLA typing; however, 57% of 1 group of patients with the criteria for autoimmune hearing loss have shown HLA Cw7, compared with only 21% of the controls.

Conclusions.—Autoimmune ear disease appears to be a true clinical entity, but its verification requires careful immunological evaluation and sensitive and specific diagnostic tests. The study of this condition has been held back by the absence of an appropriate model and the lack of clinical information. Pathologic correlates may eventually be established by temporal bone studies.

▶ It is generally accepted that there are systemic autoimmune diseases that can manifest in the inner ear. The associated difficulty comes in identifying the isolated diseases of the inner ear and their significant correlation to autoimmunity. The discussion and study continues. However, this study summarizes some of the progress to date very nicely.—M.M. Paparella, M.D.

Characterization of Severely and Profoundly Hearing Impaired Adults Attending an Audiology Clinic

McClymont LG, Browning GG (Royal Infirmary, Glasgow, Scotland)
J Laryngol Otol 105:534–538, 1991 2–8

Background.—Approximately 12% of adults visiting audiology departments will be severely hearing impaired; however, their clinical and audiometric characteristics have not been well documented.

Patients.—A group of 132 patients who visited a severe impairment clinic during an 18-month period was studied. The patients, aged 16–95 years (mean age, 68 years), had a hearing impairment of at least 70 dB HL. The female-to-male ratio was 2:1.

Findings.—In 52% of the patients the inability to provide sufficient masking made audiometric assessment of the severity of impairment uncertain. The limited bone conduction output made it almost impossible to evaluate the masked bone conduction thresholds and the air-bone gap in the poorer ear. In 67% of the better hearing ears, a mixed hearing impairment was noted. The air-bone gap in these ears was 20 dB or more. The etiology of the conductive component was otosclerosis and chronic otitis media in equal numbers of cases. Only 19% had impairments of a pure sensorineural type; 6% were acquired congenitally, 5% were caused by meningitis, and 9% had an onset in adulthood. In the remaining 14%, the impairment type could not be classified because the bone conductive thresholds were off scale.

Conclusions.—The profoundly hearing impaired are a neglected group of patients for whom much can be done. Bringing together interested clinicians at a tertiary referral clinic may improve the management of the severely hearing impaired, and the establishment of severe impairment clinics is encouraged.

▶ We all see these patients in our offices. Although they have profound hearing losses, a specific etiologic agent or pathogenesis cannot always be identified. In addition, these patients often have mixed problems, such as problems in the inner ear that are associated with problems in the middle ear. By identifying the causative and pathologic characteristics in these individuals, we can consider treatment in some and rehabilitation with the use of hearing aids in all of these patients, thereby helping them to function better in society.—M.M. Paparella, M.D.

Contrast Enhancement of the Labyrinth on MR Scans in Patients With Sudden Hearing Loss and Vertigo: Evidence of Labyrinthine Disease

Seltzer S, Mark AS (George Washington Univ; Washington Hosp Ctr, Washington, DC)

AJNR 12:13–16, 1991 2–9

Background.—The sudden onset of hearing loss with or without vertigo is a diagnostic challenge. The findings of labyrinthine enhancement on gadopentetate dimeglumine-enhanced MRI in 5 patients with sudden hearing loss or vertigo or both were reported.

Methods.—All patients were studied with T2-weighted axial images through the whole brain, contrast-enhanced 3-mm axial T1-weighted images through the temporal bone, and enhanced T1-weighted sagittal images through the whole brain. The findings on MR were correlated with audiological and electronystagmographical (ENG) studies. Three patients had recent or concurrent viral illness and 2 had leutic labyrinthitis.

Findings.—Cochlear enhancement was seen on the symptomatic side in 4 patients with unilateral hearing loss and on the side of the profoundly deaf ear in 1 patient with bilateral but asymmetric hearing loss. Of the 4 patients with vertigo, vestibular enhancement was observed only in the 3 patients with severe ENG abnormalities. In 2 patients, follow-up MR studies done 4–6 months later showed resolution of the cochlear enhancement that correlated with resolution of symptoms. In contrast, labyrinthine enhancement was not seen in 30 controls or in 6 patients with acoustic neuromas studied with contrast-enhanced MR.

Conclusions.—Enhancement of the labyrinth on contrast-enhanced MR imaging appears to be a highly specific sign of labyrinthine disease. Because abnormalities on ENG and audiograms are nonspecific and indicate only a sensorineural problem, contrast-enhanced MR scans may distinguish patients with retrocochlear lesions—such as acoustic neuromas—from those patients in whom the abnormal process is labyrinthine or intraaxial. It is important to scrutinize the structures of the membranous labyrinth carefully—in addition to the internal auditory canal, the cerebellopontine angle, and the brain stem—when evaluating a patient with sudden hearing loss or vertigo.

► The next 5 abstracts (Abstracts 2–10—2–14) are articles on the unfortunately common engima of sudden deafness and vertigo. Together, they provide insights into these disorders so that we might better determine a specific diagnosis and appropriate management plan before considering rehabilitation.

This study by Seltzer and Mark considers the importance of contrast enhancement of the labyrinth on MR scans. Although MR scanning is of interest and is certainly an expensive test, it does have limitations. Its main value is in identifying tumors of the soft tissue in the cerebellopontine angle. I have ordered many hundreds of such MR scans, and in the vast majority of the patients—practically all of them—they do not provide a specific diagnosis relating to hearing loss per se, especially in the case of sudden hearing losses. It is well known that a vestibular schwannoma will only rarely be associated with sudden deafness.—M.M. Paparella, M.D.

Sudden Hearing Loss Due to AIDS-Related Cryptococcal Meningitis: A Temporal Bone Study

Kwartler JA, Linthicum FH, Jahn AF, Hawke M (Univ of Medicine and Dentistry of New Jersey; House Ear Research Inst, Los Angeles; Univ of Toronto)
Otolaryngol Head Neck Surg 104:265–269, 1991 2–10

Introduction.—The otolaryngologist who gives steroids to a patient with AIDS who has sudden hearing loss runs the risk of potentiating undetected opportunistic infection. *Cryptococcus neoformans* has been

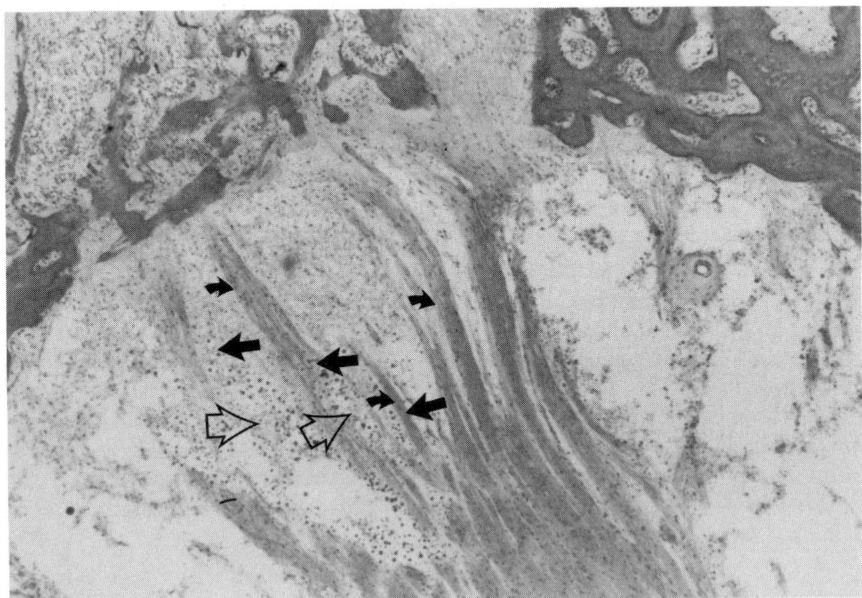

Fig 2–3.—Right ear. Cochlear nerve *(small curved arrows)* shows marked disruption of fibers, with invasion by cryptococcal organisms *(straight black arrows)* and neutrophils *(open arrows)*. Hematoxylin-eosin original magnification, × 100). (Courtesy of Kwartler JA, Linthicum FH, Jahn AF, et al: *Otolaryngol Head Neck Surg* 104:265–269, 1991.)

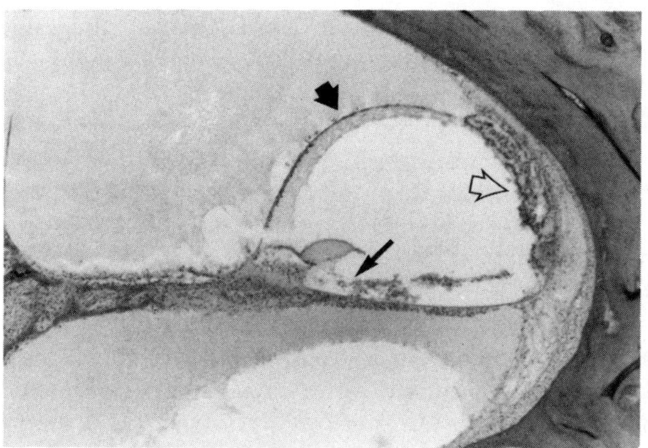

Fig 2–4.—Right ear. Posterior middle turn of the cochlea shows necrosis of the organ of Corti *(long black arrow)*. The stria vascularis is edematous *(open arrowhead)*, and Resner's membrane is mildly distended *(short black arrowhead)*. The perilymph is darkly stained, suggesting increased protein. Hematoxylin-eosin; original magnification, × 45. (Courtesy of Kwartler JA, Linthicum FH, Jahn AF, et al: *Otolaryngol Head Neck Surg* 104:265–269, 1991.)

found in 13% of patients with AIDS. Progressive and sudden hearing loss has been associated with cryptococcal infection.

Case Report.—A man, 36, reported decreasing hearing, frontal headache, and difficulty walking for 3 days. For 16 years he had used drugs intravenously; he had recently lost weight and had both diarrhea and oral candidiasis. Acoustic reflex testing was negative at 1,000 and 2,000 Hz. Auditory brain stem response studies were markedly abnormal; however, a CT study was negative. The patient's mental status deteriorated. India ink staining of the CSF revealed C. *neoformans.* Although amphotericin B and 5-fluorocytosine were given, the patient died in cardiorespiratory arrest. The internal auditory canals were invaded by cryptococci, and there was early necrosis of the cochlear and vestibular nerves. The cochlear nerve fibers were infiltrated by cryptococci, macrophages, and exudate (Fig 2–3). Organisms extended along the greater superficial pertrosal nerve to the geniculate ganglion and then invaded Scarpa's ganglion. The epithelium of the utricle, saccule, and ampullae was necrotic, and the organ of Corti was variably necrotic (Fig 2–4). The stria vascularis was edematous, and mild endolymphatic hydrops was present.

Comment.—The histopathological findings in this patient were similar to those in earlier reports of patients without AIDS. Cryptococcal infection must be considered when progressive or sudden hearing loss develops in a patient with AIDS.

▶ With the rampant increase of AIDS throughout the United States and other countries, this is a timely study. It suggests that the use of steroids in patients with AIDS may lead to potentiating an undetected opportunistic infection by the *C. neoformans* organism. This is an interesting study—one we should examine closely.—M.M. Paparella, M.D.

Idiopathic Sudden Sensorineural Hearing Loss and Postnatal Viral Labyrinthitis: A Statistical Comparison of Temporal Bone Findings

Khetarpal U, Nadol JB Jr, Glynn RJ (Harvard Med School; Massachusetts Eye and Ear Infirmary, Boston)

Ann Otol Rhinol Laryngol 99:969–976, 1990 2–11

Introduction.—The cause of idiopathic sudden sensorineural hearing loss (ISSHL) remains unknown; however, in many cases the anamnestic microbiologic and pathologic findings have suggested a viral origin. A total of 22 temporal bone specimens from 18 patients with sudden partial or complete sensorineural hearing loss was examined. The cases fell into 3 diagnostic categories.

Findings.—Six patients had ISSHL with no history of upper respiratory infection. Their ears were deaf to the limits of clinical audiometry. One patient had bilateral cochlear involvement. The ganglion cell counts did not differ appreciably between the affected and unaffected ears. Six patients had ISSHL with a history of upper respiratory tract infection, which preceded or accompanied the hearing loss. Considerable pathologic heterogeneity was present in this group (Fig 2–5). Six patients had presumed postnatal viral labyrinthitis, with profound hearing loss occurring after an attack of measles, mumps, or herpes zoster. Three of these patients had bilateral cochlear involvement. Spiral ganglion cell counts were reduced markedly for age. Pillar cell losses were greater in the cases of ISSHL that were not associated with respiratory tract infection than in those that were.

Discussion.—It appears that ISSHL may be caused by non-neurotropic viruses. The neurotropic property of cytopathic viruses such as mumps and measles viruses might account for the severe neuronal atrophy seen in postnatal viral labyrinthitis. It is possible that the involvement of different target cells in these disorders reflects the differences in routes of invasion rather than in causation or viral strain.

▶ Virus has clearly been implicated in cases of sudden deafness, the classical example being viral endolymphatic labyrinthitis resulting from mumps. These authors study the role of postnatal viral labyrinthitis and raise some interesting questions regarding the mechanisms by which viruses may or may not cause sudden deafness.—M.M. Paparella, M.D.

Bilateral Sudden Deafness and Acute Acquired Toxoplasmosis

Katholm M, Johnsen NJ, Siim C, Willumsen L (Gentofte Univ Hosp; Glostrup

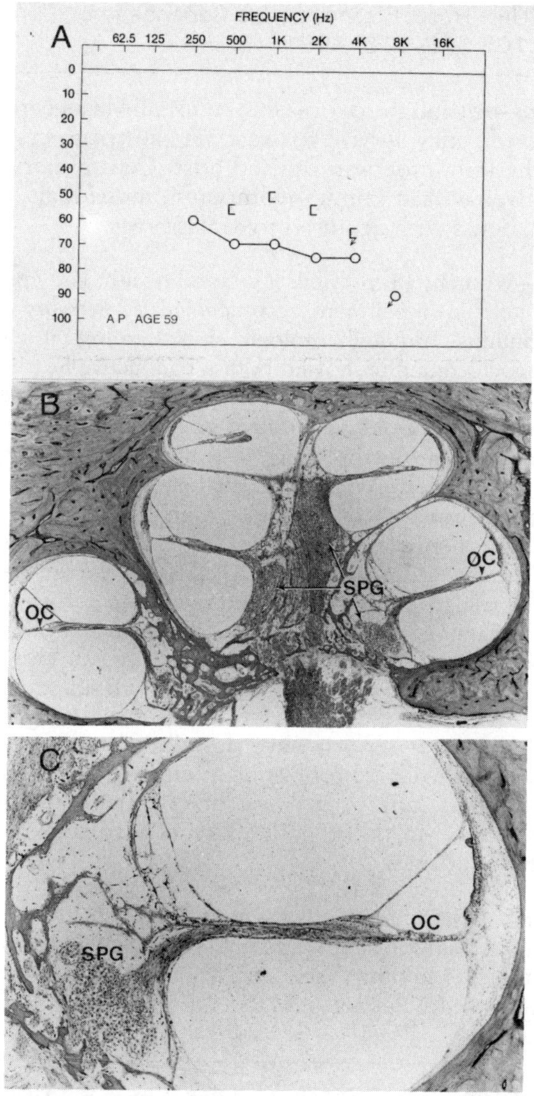

Fig 2–5.—Temporal bone histopathologic findings in an individual with idiopathic sudden sensorineural hearing loss of right ear concurrent with viral upper respiratory tract infection (group 2) 20 years before death. **A,** an audiogram done at age 59, the year of death (20 years after hearing loss on the right side). Hearing on the left side was normal. Speech discrimination was not tested. **B,** midmodiolar section of the right temporal bone. Hematoxylin-eosin; original magnification, × 29. The major histopathologic correlate of hearing loss was loss of the organ of Corti *(OC)*, whereas the spiral ganglion cell *(SPG)* population was normal. **C,** a higher-power view of basal turn showing normal SPG population and marked degeneration of OC. Hematoxylin-eosin; original magnification, × 79. (Courtesy of Khetarpal U, Nadol JB Jr, Glynn RJ: *Ann Otol Rhinol Laryngol* 99:969–976, 1990.)

Univ Hosp; and Univ Hosp, Rigshospitalet, Copenhagen)
J Laryngol Otol 105:115–118, 1991 2–12

Introduction.—Although toxoplasmosis usually lasts for a few months, *Toxoplasma gondii* may survive for years in the tissue cysts; reactivation is possible in the immunocompromised host. Central nervous system involvement is infrequent in immunocompetent individuals. Hearing rarely is affected in patients with acquired toxoplasmosis.

Case Report.—Woman, 18, previously in good health, had episodes of fluctuating left-sided hearing impairment accompanied by gyratory vertigo, nausea-vomiting, and tinnitus. Although otologic and neurological assessments were negative, electrocochleography showed both a conductive hearing loss of 30 dB at 2 kHz and a high-frequency sensorineural hearing loss. Eighteen months after presentation, anacusis occurred on the right side; vestibular function was absent on this side. The cochlear microphonics were markedly reduced, and no action potential was noted on electrocochleography. Left-sided anacusis occurred a few months later, with extinction of vestibular function. A nut-sized swelling appeared in the neck between the attacks of anacusis, and histological study showed typical changes of toxoplasmosis. The Sabin-Feldman-Dye test and fluorescence antibody test gave positive results. Steroid therapy was replaced by sulfadiazine, pyrimethamine, and folinic acid. Serviceable hearing gradually returned; the patient was able to communicate using a body-worn aid and lip-reading. Vestibular function became normal on both sides.

Discussion.—Previous reports have described cochleovestibular symptoms in association with toxoplasmic meningoencephalitis. Acute acquired toxoplasmosis may be a cause of cochleovestibular disease and should be considered in those patients who have sensorineural hearing loss of an unknown origin.

▶ A toxoplasmic meningoencephalitis may occur in immunocompromised patients, leading to bilateral sudden deafness. Tragically this happened in this patient. Thus there is another mechanism and causative consideration for sudden deafness.—M.M. Paparella, M.D.

Sudden Sensorineural Hearing Loss as a Complication of Non-Otologic Surgery

Journeaux SF, Master B, Greenhalgh RM, Bull TR (London)
J Laryngol Otol 104:711–712, 1990 2–13

Introduction.—In 21 cases of sudden sensorineural hearing loss after nonotologic surgery, 70% involved heart-lung bypass procedures. An embolic phenomenon or a localized perfusion deficit are 2 theories suggested to explain the etiology of a hearing loss after a bypass procedure.

Causes.—In a less common case, sudden sensorineural hearing loss was seen after a left adrenalectomy. It was the first documented case after a general anesthetic in a patient with a previously stapedectomized ear. Microemboli have been investigated as a possible cause of sensorineural deafness in nonbypass patients. Sensorineural deafness may be caused by the formation of a perilymph fistula. Another possible cause is the use of nitrous oxide to maintain anesthesia. Nitrous oxide can affect middle ear pressures, and the stapedectomized ear may be more susceptible to insult. Altering the anesthesia to a mixture of air and oxygen instead of using the highly diffusable nitrous oxide may protect such patients.

▶ We have all seen these patients in whom sudden sensorineural deafness has resulted from nonotologic surgery. I have seen this happen after cardiac surgery, one of the surgeries discussed in this article. However, it can also occur in other forms of surgery. The possible causative mechanisms include embolisms and perilymphatic fistulae.

The preceding 5 abstracts (Abstracts 2–8—2–12) are of interest because each one describes a different cause of sudden deafness. Other well-established causes of sudden deafness are tympanogenic middle ear infection, bacterial meningitis, trauma, tumors, and other metabolic conditions (including certain forms of Meniere's disease). Because there are many causes of sudden deafness, it is important for the diagnostician to create a differential diagnosis before considering appropriate forms of treatment. The majority of causes will probably be related to viral etiologic agents, as described earlier by Schuknecht.—M.M. Paparella, M.D.

Tinnitus Severity Measured by a Subjective Scale, Audiometry and Clinical Judgement

Halford JBS, Anderson SD (Cromwell Hosp, London)

J Laryngol Otol 105:89–93, 1991 2–14

Background.—Physicians in all areas of medicine encounter patients with tinnitus. A simple questionnaire that could accurately classify the severity of tinnitus would be most helpful.

Methods.—A severity scale was developed on the assumption that meaningful estimates require an assessment of how tinnitus affects an individual. A Subjective Tinnitus Severity Scale (STSS) was created using data from 112 members of a tinnitus self-help group, most of whom had had tinnitus for 4 years or longer. The scale consisted of 16 yes-or-no items dealing with awareness of tinnitus and its effects on concentration, relating to others, and other aspects of daily function.

Validity.—A coefficient alpha of .84 indicated that the STSS had a high degree of internal consistency, measuring aspects of a single dimension. In a distinct sample of 30 individuals attending the tinnitus clinic, the mean STSS scores correlated with 2 independent clinical ratings of severity at levels of .76 and .73. In addition, the STSS scores correlated significantly with several audiometric variables.

Discussion.—The STSS may well prove to be a reliable, simple, and useful means of determining the severity of tinnitus in individual patients. More normative data are needed before the scale can serve as an aid to diagnostic classification.

► Tinnitus is an important problem that frustrates many otologists attempting to treat their patients. The following 3 abstracts (Abstracts 2–15—2–17) discuss different aspects of the problem of tinnitus.

It is interesting to consider the role and usefulness of the STSS. Halford and Anderson have used this method of categorization and gradation of tinnitus that has proven both interesting and useful for diagnostic and therapeutic reasons. Perhaps the rest of us should try this method.—M.M. Paparella, M.D.

Tinnitus Reaction Questionnaire: Psychometric Properties of a Measure of Distress Associated With Tinnitus

Wilson PH, Henry J, Bowen M, Haralambous G (Univ of Sydney, New South Wales , Australia)

J Speech Hear Res 34:197–201, 1991 2–15

Introduction.—Tinnitus may be accompanied by substantial psychological distress; however, the psychological aspects of tinnitus have not received much systematic study. Although symptoms usually appear to be a result of tinnitus, awareness of tinnitus may increase during environmental stress, and stress may exacerbate tinnitus in some individuals.

Methods.—The data from 156 subjects were used to assess a scale designed to reflect the psychological distress associated with tinnitus, the Tinnitus Reaction Questionnaire (TRQ). The items came chiefly from the symptom categories described by Tyler and Baker. The sample included subjects participating in a study of electromyographic biofeedback therapy and relaxation training; referrals to an audiology department; and subjects volunteering for a psychological treatment program for tinnitus. Most had bilateral tinnitus. The mean duration of tinnitus was nearly 10 years.

Findings.—A high degree of internal consistency and very good test-retest reliability were observed. There was moderate to high correlation between the TRQ results and both clinician ratings and self-report measures of anxiety and depression. However, correlation with neuroticism was low.

Conclusions.—The TRQ is a psychometrically sound measure of the impact of tinnitus on psychological function. It may well be useful in assessing patients with tinnitus and in gauging the degree of psychological distress before and after treatment.

▶ Although individuals with tinnitus will have a psychological reaction to tinnitus, how they deal with it from a cognitive and psychological point of view will determine how disturbing the symptoms will actually be. I always counsel the patient from a psychological-educational point of view so that they know how to deal with tinnitus in terms of listening behavior. The automatic use of a form of biofeedback to diminish rather than enhance the tinnitus is the most critical part of the management of tinnitus.—M.M. Paparella, M.D.

Idiopathic Subjective Tinnitus Treated by Biofeedback, Acupuncture and Drug Therapy

Podoshin L, Ben-David Y, Fradis M, Gerstel R, Felner H (Bnai Zion Med Ctr, Technion-Israel Inst of Technology, Haifa, Israel)

Ear Nose Throat J 70:284–289, 1991 2–16

Background.—The high incidence of subjective tinnitus and the severe reactions to it have prompted many types of treatment. However, most treatment modalities have had little to moderate success rates. The efficacy of 3 treatments of idiopathic-subjective tinnitus (IST)-acupuncture, biofeedback, and Cinnarizine-was compared.

Methods and Results.—Fifty-eight patients with IST were randomly divided into 5 treatment groups. At the end of treatment, 50% of the patients in the biofeedback group had some improvement in the level of tinnitus, compared with 30% in the acupuncture group and 10% in the Cinnarizine group. Biofeedback caused a significant easing in the degree of discomfort from tinnitus when patients were resting.

Conclusions.—Biofeedback and general relaxation appear to be of real benefit to patients with severe tinnitus, especially during rest. However, none of the treatments available is ideal. Other modes of treatment for tinnitus need to be investigated.

▶ One can assume that biofeedback and general relaxation help the patient to deal with tinnitus by encouraging cerebral control over the cochlear focus of irritation. Every patient's symptoms or problems will be defined by the brain's ability to interpret and deal with the problem. I think that this is an important part of the management of tinnitus.—M.M. Paparella, M.D.

Electromagnetic Semi-Implantable Hearing Device: Phase I. Clinical Trials

McGee TM, Kartush JM, Heide JC, Bojrab DI, Clemis JD, Kulick KC (Michigan Ear Inst, Farmington Hills; Smith and Nephew Richards Inc, Memphis; Ear Consultants of Michigan, Southfield; Chicago)

Laryngoscope 101:355–360, 1991 2–17

Introduction.—Although more than 24 million individuals in the United States are hearing impaired, less than 3 are currently using hearing aids. The drawbacks of available hearing aids include poor sound fidelity, acoustic feedback, poor performance in noisy environments, and the perceived stigma of wearing a visible hearing aid. The results of a clinical phase I trial of a new electromagnetic hearing device (EMHD) that uses low-consumption electronic circuitry and strong rare-earth magnets were evaluated.

Device.—With the EMHD, incoming sound energy is amplified, compressed, and frequency spectrum shaped to fit a patient's residual hearing before entering the output stage where sound energy is converted into analogue magnetic forces that vibrate a target magnet coupled to the middle ear (Fig 2–6). For this phase I study, an electromagnetic driver was coupled with a target magnet that was temporarily affixed onto the lateral surface of the malleus. Six hearing aid patients with pure sensorineural loss participated in the study. Each patient underwent audiometric testing at baseline, with the current hearing aid, and with the EMHD. Speech discrimination comparisons for these 3 conditions were also carried out.

Results.—Pure-tone testing confirmed that all 6 patients had significant amounts of functional gain with the EMHD. The average amount of functional gain improvement compared with the current hearing aids at speech frequencies of 500, 1,000, and 2,000 Hz was 17.5 dB. However, the patients' existing hearing aids produced more functional gain at 4,000 Hz. Speech sensitivity with the EMHD was improved by an aver-

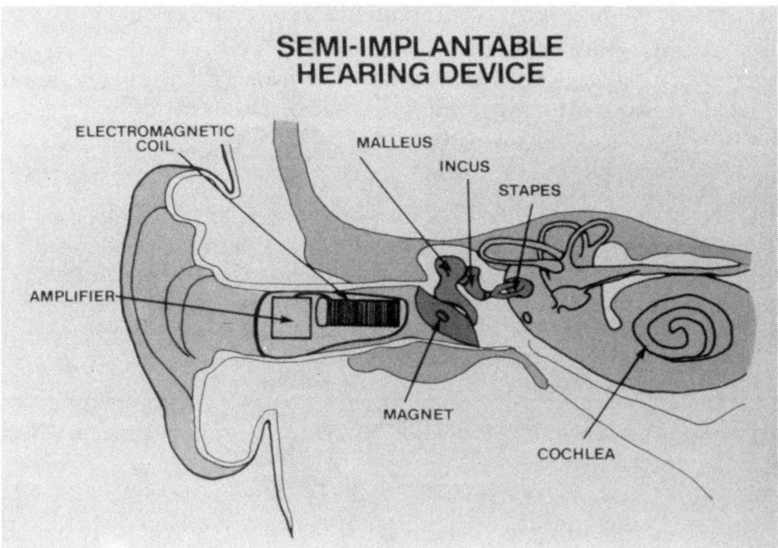

Fig 2–6.—Phase I investigation of semi-implantable electromagnetic hearing device in which target magnet is temporarily affixed to tympanic membrane. (Courtesy of McGee TM, Kartush JM, Heide JC, et al: *Laryngoscope* 101:355–360, 1991.)

age of 10.8 dB. Speech discrimination was not noticeably improved by the use of the EMHD. Only 1 patient scored significantly better with the EMHD than with the existing hearing aid on speech discrimination testing. None of the patients had problems with acoustic feedback, and 5 patients found the EMHD to work significantly better in noisy environments. All patients felt that the EMHD provided a quiet, more natural type of sound than their traditional hearing aids.

Conclusion.—The EMHD provides sufficient gain and output characteristics to benefit individuals with sensorineural hearing loss.

▶ It is hoped that someday the field of otology will be revolutionized by the availability and efficacy of an implantable hearing aid. There are "sound" reasons that this can happen. These clinical studies by McGee and colleagues are an important first step toward this goal. The studies to date would suggest that conduction of sound and elimination of interference are more ideal with an implanted hearing aid. The inability to provide a source of energy without external involvement will continue to be a problem.—M.M. Paparella, M.D.

Hearing Aid Prescribing: Is the Specialist Opinion Necessary?

Campbell JB, Nigam A (Birmingham and Midland Ear, Nose, and Throat Hosp, Birmingham, England)

Clin Otolaryngol 16:124–127, 1991 2–18

Background.—The current system of dispensing hearing aids in England has been called inadequate because patients have to wait for long periods. The Royal National Institute for the Deaf (RNID) proposes that ear, nose, and throat (ENT) surgeons do not need to be involved in dispensing hearing aids because very little significant ear disease passes through a typical hearing aid clinic. If ENT surgeons could be bypassed, then the process would be expedited. Therefore, whether a specialist opinion is necessary in dispensing hearing aids was investigated.

Methods and Results.—The case notes of 200 consecutive patients referred to a hearing aid clinic were reviewed. Without a specialist opinion, only half of these patients would have been prescribed a hearing aid. The rest either did not need a hearing aid or needed further examination and surgical or medical treatment. The general practitioners showed a lack of expertise in recognizing ear disorders.

Conclusions.—Patients referred to a hearing aid clinic can have significant incidences of ear disease requiring examination and treatment. In addition, patients with deafness should be seen by an ENT specialist before being fitted with a hearing aid so that curable deafness can be treated and serious disease can be detected.

▶ The answer to the question raised in the title of this paper is a clearcut "yes." Every single hearing loss is a symptom (as defined by the patient) or a finding (as documented by the audiologist) of some disease process that is either genetic or nongenetic, congenital or acquired. Therefore, every single patient with a hearing loss first requires a medical diagnosis, followed by considerations of medical management and considerations of rehabilitation through the use of amplification or hearing aids.—M.M. Paparella, M.D.

Use of Hearing Aids in Infancy

Wood S, McCormick B (Gen Hosp, Nottingham, England)

Arch Dis Child 65:919–920, 1990 2–19

Introduction.—Severe and profound hearing loss may now be detected in the first year of life, and congenital sensorineural hearing loss will be diagnosed in a significant number of infants before age 6 months. The earlier rehabilitation begins, the better the outcome is likely to be.

Recommendations.—Accurate information on hearing sensitivity in a very young infant usually requires electric response audiometry. Initial fitting of an aid is often based on limited information. Amplification is generally recommended for hearing losses averaging greater than 30 dB; however, this is only a guideline. As much speech information as possible is provided by amplifying speech to fit within the listener's dynamic range of hearing. The amount of speech frequency information available to the child may be estimated by obtaining sound field thresholds with the infant wearing an aid.

Aids.—Many hearing aids deliver acoustic signals through air conduction deep into the external meatus. It also is possible to use a bone conduction hearing aid based on a head-worn vibrator. Generally, a postaural aid is preferred to a body-worn instrument, except for a child with low-frequency residual hearing only. The problem of a poor signal-to-noise ratio may be overcome by using a remote microphone system.

General Management.—A full developmental assessment is necessary for the hearing-impaired infant. These infants and their families require educational and rehabilitative support. Close liaison with a specialist teacher of the deaf and a specialist speech therapist may be very helpful.

▶ Any deaf or hard-of-hearing infant requires the use of a hearing aid to receive the sound cues that lead to the development of speech and speech perception. This is a critical part of the origin and development of the communicative process and should be considered in every infant with a significant hearing loss, assuming that medical treatment has already been tried or is not applicable.—M.M. Paparella, M.D.

Cochlear Implant Histopathology

Linthicum FH Jr, Fayad J, Otto SR, Galey FR, House WF (House Ear Inst, Los

Angeles; Univ of Southern California, Los Angeles)
Am J Otolaryngol 12:245–311, 1991 2–20

Background.—Approximately 3,000 adults have received cochlear implants since they were approved for clinical use in 1984. The acquisition of 22 temporal bones and 1 brainstem from 13 cochlear implant patients provided an opportunity to examine the effects of implantation on inner ear and central structures. These findings were then related to the patients' auditory perception.

Patients.—Ten of the 13 patients had unilateral implants, and 3 had bilateral implants. Five underwent revision surgery because of either a failed internal device or poor patient performance. The mean duration of stimulation was 5 years (range, 1–14 years), and the mean age of patients at death was 60 years.

Methods.—Sections of the temporal bone were studied for the number of spiral ganglion cells, the number of dendrites in both ears, and the number of hair cells representing rows of hair cells in the organ of Corti. The anatomical location and extent of fibrosis and the amount of ossification in the cochlea were also recorded. Perceptual performance was evaluated using the Monosyllable-Trochee-Spondee (MTS) word test, the MTS stress test, the House Ear Institute Environmental Sounds Test, and the dynamic range.

Findings.—In all 16 implanted bones, the ganglion cells and their axons were the only sensorineural structures present. Only 2 bones had surviving hair cells, but this population was less than 25% of normal. The average number of ganglion cells in the implanted bones was 12,522 (range, 3,212–21,340 cells). There was no correlation between the number of ganglion cells and perceptual performance. All implanted bones exhibited varying amounts of damage to the inner ear structures, including disruption of the basilar membrane and organ of Corti, and fibrosis and ossification of the perilymph. The damage extended for the length of the electrodes insertion, but it did not affect the ganglion cell population. The duration of electrical stimulation did not effect the ganglion cell population, and prolonged electrical stimulation had no effect on ganglion cell survival in 3 patients or on the cochlear nuclei in 1 patient. There was no difficulty with electrode insertion in the 5 patients who had revision surgery. In these patients, there were no histopathological cochlear changes that could be attributed to the second electrode insertion.

Conclusion.—The ganglion cells and their axons are the elements in the inner ear that respond to electrical stimulation, and useful auditory sensation can result from as as few as 3,212 cells. Traumatic changes and prolonged stimulation do not affect the ganglion cell population.

▶ This very comprehensive study provides the largest collection to date of cases assessed histopathologically after cochlear implantation. These studies are important, and future studies like them will be of value. As always, they should be correlated with functional information from the clinical chart, as was done in this study.—M.M. Paparella, M.D.

The Output Characteristics of an Implanted Bone Conduction Prosthesis

Gatehouse S, Browning GG (Royal Infirmary, Glasgow, Scotland)
Clin Otolaryngol 15:503–513, 1990 2–21

Background.—Most bone-conduction hearing aids have not been well accepted by patients because of discomfort, a poor appearance, and high distortion. The Xomed Audiant device uses an implanted cobalt-samarium permanent magnet and an external electromagnetic coil secured by a second permanent magnet, which is attached to either a body-worn or an ear-level amplifier. The guidelines for selecting patients to receive the Audiant have come from clinical trial. Whether frequency-specific guidelines are necessary was determined.

Methods.—The manufacturers of the Audiant device provided a curve of maximal output for both the body-worn and ear-level amplifiers (Fig 2–7). Two independent measures of the maximum output of the Audiant were acquired from 2 subjects whose audiometric findings are shown in Fig 2–8.

Findings.—The maximum output values ranged from 15 dB HL at 250 Hz to 60.5 dB HL at 6,000 Hz for the body-worn amplifier. The esti-

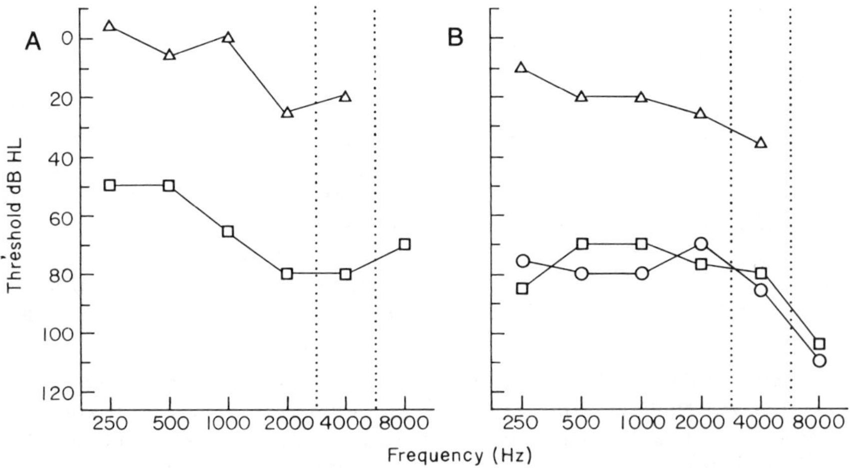

Fig 2–7.—Audiometric thresholds for air and bone conduction for subject 1 **(A)** and subject 2 **(B)**. *Circle* indicates right ear air conduction; *square*, left ear air conduction; *triangle*, not masked bone conduction. (Courtesy of Gatehouse S, Browning GG: *Clin Otolaryngol* 15:503–513, 1990.)

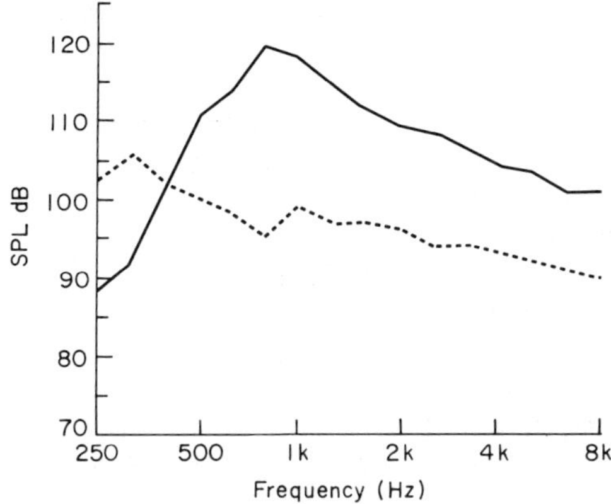

Fig 2–8.—The maximum output levels of the Audiant device using the body-worn *(solid line)* and ear-level amplifiers *(dotted line)*, from the manufacturer's literature. (Courtesy of Gatehouse S, Browning GG: *Clin Otolaryngol* 15:503–513, 1990.)

mates for the ear-level amplifier ranged from 6.5 dB HL at 250 Hz to 42 dB HL at 6,000 Hz.

Discussion.—The ear-level amplifier appears to be suitable only for patients with essentially normal bone-conduction thresholds at 1,000 Hz or lower. Modifications to increase magnet strength in both the amplifier and the implant will improve output by less than 5 dB.

▶ This study suggests that the implanted bone conduction prosthesis is useful in a more select group of patients than was formerly considered to be the case. It also suggests that patients should have essentially normal bone conduction thresholds "at 1000 Hz and below."—M.M. Paparella, M.D.

Cochlear Implants in Children: Past and Present Perspectives
House WF (Univ of Southern California, Los Angeles)
Am J Otol 12 [Suppl]:1–2, 1991 2–22

Background.—The cochlear implant program is, after 20 years, still in its infancy. In 1973, the experts predicted that, based on animal studies, cochlear implant users could expect deterioration of the remaining neural elements of the eighth nerve complex. The predicted deterioration has not occurred in the 3,000 cochlear implant users in the United States and worldwide.

Findings.—The concepts based on animal studies have been proven false by temporal bone studies of patients who have had cochlear implants. The dendrites of the eighth nerve do not exist, and if the electric current passes through the modiolus from active to ground electrodes, the lowest thresholds are experienced. Cochlear implant patients also have been found to have timing and intensity differences; this is contrary to the predictions of neurophysiologists. The most important feature in the processing of cochlear implant stimulation is the CNS. The brain can receive 2 very different signals and integrate them into more meaning than either 1 separately. These findings negate the predictive value of animal models and conventional cochlear neurophysiology and suggest an empirical approach.

Conclusion.—The large expected market of deaf people has not materialized. Future expansion is predicted in the childrens' program with an emphasis on simpler, smaller analog systems patterned after present day digitally programmed hearing aid technology. Emphasis on the development of the less expensive analog systems (instead of the expensive digital processing systems) will benefit a much larger segment of the deaf population.

▶ The role of cochlear implants in children continues to be worthy of great study. This study is a sober assessment by a pioneer contributor of cochlear implants: WF House. However, hope and optimism is expressed for both future studies and for possible applications of cochlear implantation in children.—Michael M. Paparella, M.D.

3 Interactions of the Middle and Inner Ear

Microfissures of the Temporal Bone: Do They Have Any Clinical Significance?

El Shazly MAR, Linthicum FH Jr (House Ear Inst, Los Angeles; Univ of Southern California School of Medicine, Los Angeles)

Am J Otol 12:169–171, 1991 3–1

Introduction.—Microfissures of the temporal bone occur most often between the ampulla of the posterior canal and the middle ear. They also are found anterior to the oval window between the labyrinth and the middle ear and extending from the vestibule to the middle ear mucosa. They have been implicated as a possible cause of sudden sensorineural hearing loss.

Findings.—Fissures were found in 79.4% of the 34 temporal bones examined—in the oval or round window or in both (Figs 3–1, 3–2, and 3–3). Twelve patients had had sudden sensorineural hearing loss. Neither the presence or absence of fissures nor the presence of fissures with or without collagen could be related to sudden sensorineural hearing loss.

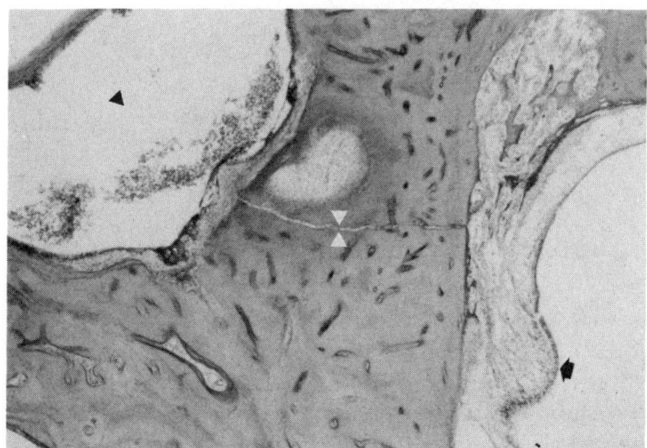

Fig 3–1.—Fissure *(white arrowheads)* extending from the posterior canal ampulla *(black arrow)* to the round window niche *(black arrowhead)*. Hematoxylin-eosin; original magnification, ×39. (Courtesy of El Shazly MAR, Linthicum FH Jr: *Am J Otol* 12:169–171, 1991.)

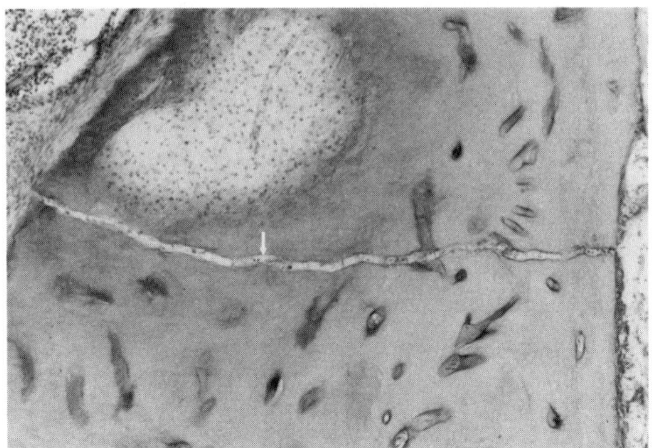

Fig 3–2.—Same fissure as in Figure 3-1, with higher magnification. The *white arrow* shows cells within the fissure. Hematoxylin-eosin; original magnification, ×103. (Courtesy of El Shazly MAR, Linthicum FH Jr: *Am J Otol* 12:169–171, 1991.)

Conclusion.—Microfissures in the cochlear capsule between the inner ear and the middle ear have no clinical significance.

► Microfissures in the cochlear capsule between the inner ear and middle ear were studied in 34 human temporal bones. All patients had unknown sensorineural hearing loss; 12 had sudden deafness. This study does not indicate a significant correlation between this common finding of microfissures in the temporal bones and the clinical problem of sudden deafness. In our studies of temporal bones, the presence of microfissures is most common

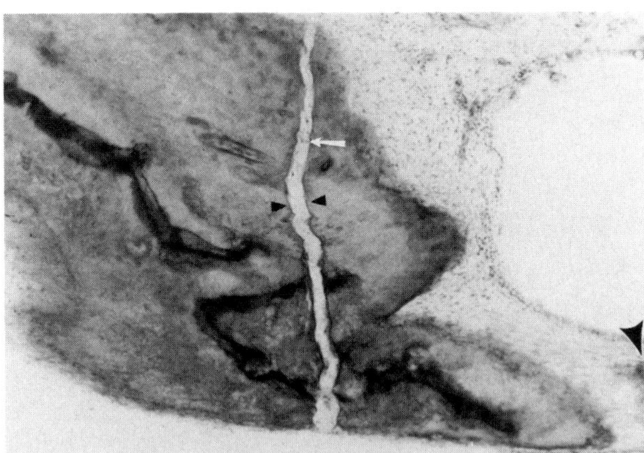

Fig 3–3.—Fissure *(small black arrows)* extending from the vestibule to the middle ear. The *white arrow* shows a cell within the fissure. *Large black arrowhead* points to the stapes footplate. Hematoxyline-eosin; original magnification, ×103. (Courtesy of El Shazly MAR, Linthicum FH Jr: *Am J Otol* 12:169–171, 1991.)

between the round window niche and the ampulla of the posterior inferior semicircular canal, and it is generally considered an innocuous coincidental finding.—M.M. Paparella, M.D.

Identification of Perilymph Proteins by Two-Dimensional Gel Electrophoresis

Paugh DR, Telian SA, Disher MJ (Univ of Michigan)
Otolaryngol Head Neck Surg 104:517–525, 1991 3–2

Introduction.—The diagnosis of perilymph fistula (PLF) remains controversial because there are no reliable clinical diagnostic criteria for PLF. The definitive diagnosis of PLF is currently made during operation. Whether perilymph contains any unique protein constituents that could distinguish it from serum or CSF was determined.

Methods.—Uncontaminated serum, CSF, and perilymph samples were obtained from 18 healthy guinea pigs and 7 patients undergoing translabyrinthine resection of acoustic neuromas, cochlear implantation for sensorineural deafness, or transmastoid labyrinthectomy for Meniere's disease. The protein concentration of all samples was measured using the Bio-Rad Protein Assay. The purity of each sample was then confirmed by comparing the protein concentration with known normal values for serum, CSF, and perilymph. Each sample was then subjected to 2-dimensional gel electrophoresis. The gels were stained with a diamine silver stain. Plasma samples were obtained from all guinea pigs and patients. Cerebrospinal fluid was obtained only from the guinea pigs.

Findings.—The perilymph samples of the guinea pigs and patients contained a group of acidic proteins with molecular weights of about 30,000 daltons that were not seen in plasma and that occurred in extremely low concentrations in the CSF of guinea pigs. The fact that the prominent spots were found on all of the gels—independent of pathology—strongly suggests that these proteins are normal constituents of perilymph.

Conclusion.—Perilymph contains proteins that are distinct from those found in plasma. Further studies are now being planned to create a clean sample collection technique and a simple, clinically applicable marker system to be used in the diagnosis of PLF.

▶ It is of interest to study the chemical characteristics of perilymph if one is to collect perilymph from the round window niche. Although this may be of benefit from the point of view of scienitific research, one wonders about its usefulness in the clinical condition. Only a couple of drops of perilymph exist in the inner ear. Therefore, unless there is a patent communication with the CSF in the subarachnoid space, one cannot expect this perilymph to drain continuously. A few drops could easily drain and be absorbed, or such leakage could be intermittent. The absence of an identification of perilymph does not mean that it may not have existed recently or that it might not recur in the future.—M.M. Paparella, M.D.

Perilymph Fistulas: The House Ear Clinic Experience

Rizer FM, House JW (House Ear Clinic, Los Angeles)

Otolaryngol Head Neck Surg 104:239–243, 1991 3–3

Introduction.—Perilymph fistulas are often diagnosed from the patient's history alone. Whereas sudden hearing loss was formerly considered to result from the formation of a perilymph fistula, none of 50 consecutive patients with sudden hearing loss who were explored had a fistula. The causes of perilymph fistulas in 86 patients undergoing exploration in 1974–1985 were reviewed.

Patients.—Approximately half of the patients had hearing loss, whereas nearly half had dizziness—many in association with hearing loss. Of the 58 patients tested, 33 (56.9%) had positive clinical fistula test results, and 12 (29%) of 41 patients had positive electronystagmography-enhanced fistula test results. A fistula was found at surgery in 35 (41%) of 86 patients, including 19 (42%) of those with hearing loss as their chief symptom.

Results.—Of the 31 patients followed after repair with fat, fascia, or perichondrium, 21 (67.7%) were subjectively improved. Only 14 (28.6%) of the 49 patients without a fistula were subjectively improved, for a significant difference (Fig 3–4). A prophylactic patch was applied in 26 patients without a fistula, and 6 (24%) of 25 who were available for follow-up were improved. Of the 24 patients who were not patched, 8

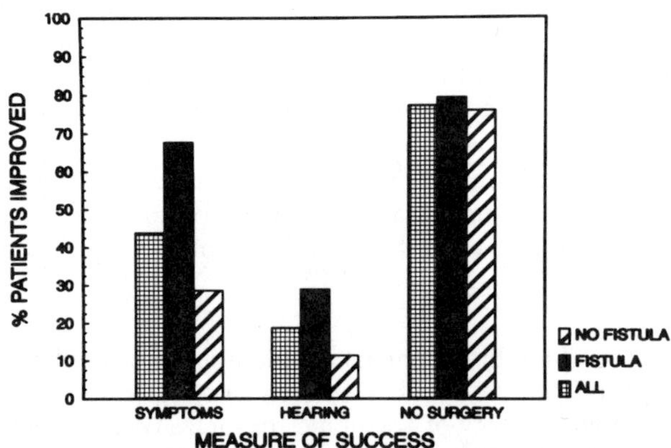

Fig 3–4.—The percentage of patients who had a successful outcome after surgery for perilymph fistula is shown for 3 measures of success: subjective evaluation of improvement in symptoms (*Symptoms*); audiometrically confirmed improvement in hearing (*Hearing*); and lack of need for subsequent surgery (*No Surgery*). The results are shown for all patients and for those with and without surgical evidence of perilymph fistula. (Courtesy of Rizer FM, House JW: *Otolaryngol Head Neck Surg* 104:239-243, 1991.)

(33.3%) also reported improvement at follow-up. The postoperative pure-tone threshold average values did not change significantly overall; however, the discrimination scores did improve. Further surgery was necessary in 19 patients; 7 of these patients required surgery for perilymph fistula.

Conclusion.—Discovery of a perilymph fistula at exploration was the best predictor of improvement. Surgeons must still rely on their clinical judgment in deciding which patients to explore.

▶ The authors of this very nice comprehensive study found what most of us have found to be the case: in spite of all the sophisticated diagnostic tests, the only test that has really stood the test of time is exploration of the middle ear. Such exploration can reveal not only a fistula, but also evidence of a fistula having occurred (such as a tent of adhesions, found between the round window niche and the incus). The patient's history continues to be the most important consideration in the diagnostic workup to date.—M.M. Paparella, M.D.

4 Otosclerosis and Stapedial Surgery

Further Studies on the Effects of Magnetic Resonance Imaging Fields on Middle Ear Implants
Applebaum EL, Valvassori GE (Univ of Illinois, Chicago)
Ann Otol Rhinol Laryngol 99:801–804, 1990 4–1

Background.—Magnetic resonance imaging is now an indispensable diagnostic imaging modality for the head and neck region. However, there may be potential hazards to patients undergoing MRI who have a middle ear or cochlear implant. The effects of MRI fields on middle ear implants were studied.

Methods and Findings.—A group of 21 stapedectomy prostheses and other middle ear implants and 2 different receiver-stimulator modules from 22-channel cochlear implants were studied. The magnetic field did not displace any of the middle ear implants except for 1 platinum stainless steel stapedectomy piston. This implant was suddenly, rapidly impelled against the edge of the Petri dish when brought within 1 m of the MRI unit opening. Prolonged exposure to the MRI scanner did not induce magnetism in any of the middle ear implants.

Conclusions.—Magnetic resonance imaging may be hazardous to patients who have had stapedectomy using certain platinum stainless steel piston prostheses. Patients with cochlear implants may also be at risk. However, MRI should not be a hazard to patients with the other middle ear implants tested in this study.

▶ In this study, MRI was considered a possible hazard to patients who had undergone earlier insertion of stapedectomy protheses of a certain substance. The numbers are too small to determine a conclusion one way or the other. It has been a general clinical observation that many patients who have had stapedectomy prostheses, including those prostheses that contain a stainless steel wire, have managed to go through MRI studies without any difficulty. In this study, only one platinum stainless steel piston was apparently visibly dislocated. Nevertheless, this assessment should continue.—M.M. Paparella, M.D.

Metallic Otologic Implants: In Vitro Assessment of Ferromagnetism at 1.5 T

Shellock FG, Schatz CJ (Cedars-Sinai Med Ctr, Los Angeles)
AJNR 12:279–291, 1991 4–2

Introduction.—Patients with certain ferromagnetic implants may be unable to undergo MRI because of the possibility of injury if the object is moved or dislodged. However, many metallic implants are nonferromagnetic or have an insignificant degree of ferromagnetism. To determine the ferromagnetism of metallic otologic implants, 35 different implants were exposed to a 1.5-T MRI system.

Methods.—The implants chosen were commonly used in the United States and were likely to be seen in the MRI setting. The otologic implants were placed inside a plastic Petri dish that had a millimeter scale on the underside. The dish was then placed on the MRI scanner table 2 mm from the bore. The implants were closely observed to detect any visible displacement along the scale.

Results.—The testing process was repeated 3 times for each implant. Because none of the implants moved during the evaluation, those particular otologic implants were judged to be made from nonferromagnetic materials and were considered safe for MRI at 1.5 T.

Conclusion.—The manufacturers of metallic biomedical implants do not routinely test their devices or guarantee the implants to be nonferromagnetic. Some older otologic implants may not be safe in MRI. Patients with cochlear implants that use electronic and/or magnetic components should not undergo MRI because of the danger of injury and the possibility of damage to the implant.

▶ This in vitro study determined that nonferromagnetic prostheses are safe and cannot be disturbed by MRI. Other implants, however, might be displaced or damaged during such a diagnostic assessment.—M.M. Paparella, M.D.

Effect of Sodium Fluoride on Early Stages of Otosclerosis

Colletti V, Fiorino FG (Univ of Verona, Italy)
Am J Otol 12:195–198, 1991 4–3

Objective.—Clinical otosclerosis follows a relatively long "silent" phase when severe stapes fixation is absent. Assessment of the stapedius reflex is the only audiometric measure of disease at this stage. Whether sodium fluoride (NaF) treatment can modify the course of early otosclerosis (as monitored by the stapedius reflex) was investigated.

Study Design.—The study included 128 relatives of patients with surgically confirmed footplate otosclerosis. Some of the subjects received NaF in doses of 6–16 mg plus vitamin D and calcium for 2 years. The treated and control subjects were matched for age and stapedius reflex findings. Subclinical otosclerosis was diagnosed from the on-off effect.

Outcome.—Initially, 72% of the ears in the NaF-treated group had partial on-off, whereas 28% had complete on-off. No marked changes occurred after 1 and 2 years. At 5 years, 56.3% of the ears had a partial on-off reflex and 35.2% had a complete on-off reflex; 8.5% had no reflex. Progressive worsening of the stapedius reflex was noted in the controls, 2.8% of whom exhibited no reflex at 5 years. In no patient in either group did the reflex findings improve. More control ears had a conductive hearing loss at 5 years compared with treated ears.

Conclusions.—Treatment of early otosclerosis with NaF for 2 years appears to be effective during the medium term; however, the long-term behavior of the disease is unpredictable. Stapedius reflex measurements make it possible to detect otosclerosis at an early stage and implement secondary preventive measures.

▶ The observation by these authors mirrors what I have seen. Even though we use NaF and calcium gluconate in certain patients, we have found that the long-term use in many patients does not seem to make any difference. Nevertheless, administration of NaF should be tried in these patients, and a serial follow-up must be done to determine whether there is any change of cochlear function over time and whether NaF should subsequently be reinstituted.—M.M. Paparella, M.D.

Surgery for Congenital Stapes Ankylosis With an Associated Congenital Ossicular Chain Anomaly

Teunissen B, Cremers CWRJ (Univ Hosp of Nijmegen, The Netherlands)

Int J Pediatr Otorhinolaryngol 21:217–226, 1991 4–4

Background.—Conductive hearing loss in young children is rarely caused by a congenital ear anomaly. A series of 32 patients with congenital stapes ankylosis and an associated congenital anomaly of the ossicular chain was reviewed.

Patients.—All 32 patients had a history of hearing loss since early childhood without any evidence of long-term middle ear pathology. One third of the patients had a syndromal diagnosis.

Outcomes.—Stapedectomy was performed in 26 ears. In another 2 ears, stapes ankylosis to the bony facial canal was successfully mobilized. In the remaining 4 ears, surgery had to be limited to an exploratory tympanotomy. The 28 ears on which stapes surgery was done had an average hearing gain of 23 dB. Of these ears 68% had a substantial hearing gain of at least 15 dB (Fig 4–1). The outcomes were somewhat limited by an average preoperative sensorineural component of 16 dB in the hearing loss.

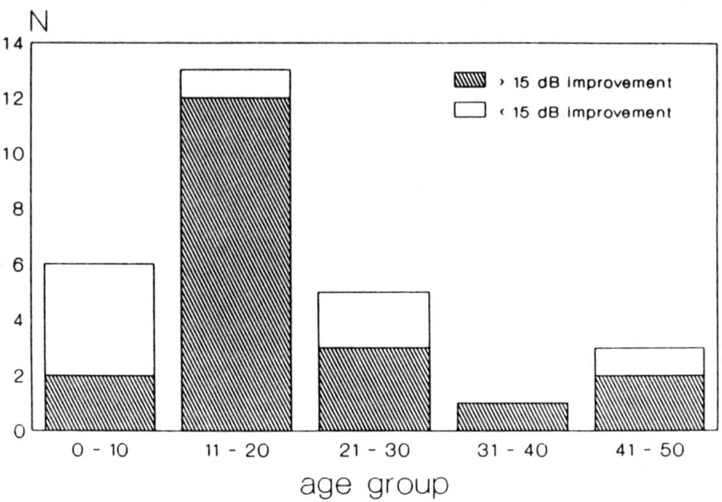

Fig 4–1.—Improvement in hearing per age group. *Shaded areas* show the ears in which the hearing level improved by 15 dB or more. (Courtesy of Teunissen B, Cremers CWRJ: *Int J Pediatr Otorhinolaryngol* 21:217–226, 1991.)

Conclusions.—In experienced hands, reconstructive middle ear surgery generally results in a marked improvement in hearing in ears with congenital stapes ankylosis and an associated deformity of the ossicular chain. There was a low incidence of total failures in this series.

▶ Otosclerosis does not mean stapedial fixation. The stapes can be fixed on the basis of congenital causes such as those described in this abstract. Tympanosclerosis and osteoneogenesis resulting from otitis media or trauma may also result in fixation of the stapes. One frequently finds the stapes bent and attached to the promontory although no histological otosclerosis exists. The stapes also may be fixed to the facial nerve, the facial nerve canal, the fallopian canal, or a dehiscent facial nerve. This series of stapedectomies for congenital ankylosis is of interest and represents a fairly sizable series.—M.M. Paparella, M.D.

Stapes Surgery: Complications and Airway Infection

Pedersen CB, Felding JU (Aarhus Univ Hosp, Aarhus, Denmark)

Ann Otol Rhinol Laryngol 100:607–611, 1991 4–5

Background.—Stapedectomy or stapedotomy performed with either a small or large fenestra approach has produced good hearing results in patients with otosclerosis. Partial sensorineural hearing losses or anacusis may occur postoperatively; however, the causes of these complications are not always clear. In a group of 1,111 patients undergoing stapedectomy, the causes of sensorineural hearing loss were evaluated.

Patients.—During a 10-year period, 1,111 stapedectomies were performed, and the results in 1,091 ears were evaluated for at least 1 year postoperatively. More than 99% of the surgeries were performed with the use of local anesthesia.

Findings.—After surgery, 11 patients with total hearing loss and 8 patients with a partial sensorineural hearing loss were evaluated in detail. A reasonable explanation of damage was found in 2 of the 8 patients with partial sensorineural hearing loss. In the 11 patients with dead ears, 1 granuloma and 1 surgical complication were found; however, the other 9 cases were unexplained. By plotting the cases of anacusis and partial sensorineural hearing loss on a diagram of influenza epidemics in Denmark, an increase in the side effects during 1 influenza epidemic was noted. In 1 case, a patient returned home after surgery to find her entire family had been affected by influenza. She later returned to the hospital with dizziness and anacusis in the surgically treated ear.

Conclusions.—Although it is reasonable to believe that infection with influenza virus is a dominating factor for the development of sensorineural hearing loss after stapedectomy, it cannot be proved that viral infection was the cause of hearing loss. However, the association between the postoperative complications of stapes surgery and influenza epidemics should be considered in scheduling stapes surgery.

▶ These authors had a very large study group of more than 1,000 patients with stapedectomy. The causes of sensorineural hearing loss were assessed. There are many causes for post-stapedectomy sensorineural deafness. This paper raises another possibility that should be considered by those of us who deal with post-stapedectomy concerns: influenza.—M.M. Paparella, M.D.

5 Facial Nerves and Tumors

Facial Nerve Regeneration Through Autologous Nerve Grafts: A Clinical and Experimental Study

Spector JG, Lee P, Peterein J, Roufa D (Washington Univ School of Medicine and CNSDR, Searle R&D, St Louis; Univ of Chicago; Gliatech, Inc, Beachwood, Ohio)

Laryngoscope 101:537–554, 1991 5–1

Introduction.—Facial nerve defects ideally are repaired by primary anastomosis, but longer defects necessitate repair with autologous neural (cable) grafts from nonessential sensory nerves. Although gross motor and facial tone is routinely recovered, recovery of fine motor activity and selective neural function is a considerable problem.

Experimental Study.—Rabbits received 8-mm neural cable grafts to repair the buccal division of the facial nerve. Assessment after 5 weeks showed that, although more unmyelinated axons were present than in normal nerves there was an equal number of myelinated axons. Myelin debris was seen in the graft repairs, as well as in both the extrafascicular

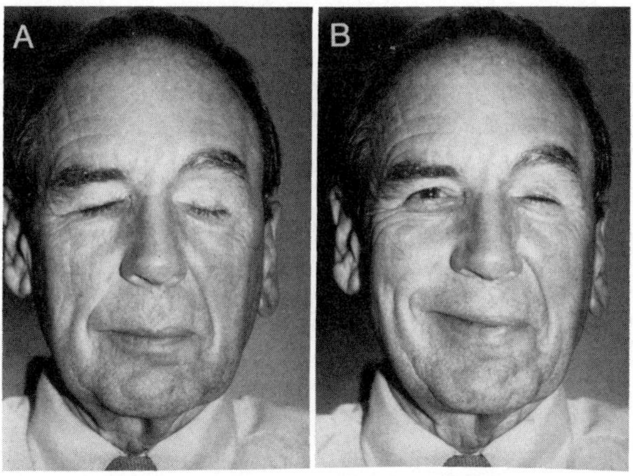

Fig 5–1.—Total neural transposition with sural autologous cable graft repair. The left upper lid was repaired with gold weight implant (temporary) and brow lift. **A,** the face at rest demonstrates good facial symmetry and tone; **B,** during voluntary motion, note severe synkinesis on the left; postoperative result at 18 months. (Courtesy of Spector JG, Lee P, Peterein J, et al: *Laryngoscope* 101:537–554, 1991.)

and intrafascicular axons. The extrafascicular axons comprised a majority of major neurite regenerates, whereas the intrafascicular axons were the chief reinnervators of the distal nerve stump. Increased coinduction velocity related to both the number and the size of the myelinated axonal regenerates.

Clinical Study.—A group of 56 patients received autologous neural cable grafts; 34 others underwent direct end-to-end anastomosis. All the patients had improved facial tone and symmetery at rest. Those patients with direct total-nerve anastomoses generally produced better voluntary functional movements than those whose neural stumps were rerouted before direct anastomosis. The latter patients had better overall results than those having neural cable graft repairs. Selective anastomosis of facial nerve divisions resulted in incomplete functional recovery and synkinesis. Voluntary functional recovery was slightly better after neural transposition with direct anastomosis than with autologous selective cable graft repair (Fig 5–1). The results of cable graft repair deteriorated over time as synkinesis progressed.

Summary.—Immediate facial nerve end-to-end anastomosis unquestionably produces the best overall results. When necessary, the cable grafts are best taken from the sural nerve, the dorsal cutaneous nerve of the foot, or the greater auricular nerve.

► This experimental study in rabbits confirms a clinical observation: when the facial nerve is injured, particularly as a result of trauma within the temporal bone, a better histological and clinical result in terms of recovery will happen with an end-to-end anastomosis compared with the use of a cable graft.—M.M. Paparella, M.D.

Bilateral Facial Nerve Palsies: Groote Schuur Hospital Experience

Wormald PJ, Sellars SL, de Villiers JC (Groote Schuur Hosp, Cape Town, South Africa)

J Laryngol Otol 105:625–627, 1991 5–2

Background.—Bilateral synchronous facial nerve palsies (BSFNP) are rare in otolaryngology practice. The most frequent cause of facial nerve palsies is Bell's palsy. Skull trauma and sclerosteosis, which is autosomal recessive in inheritance in the Afrikaner population of South Africa, may also cause these palsies.

Patients.—During a 20-year period, 24 patients with BSFNP were seen. There were 15 males and 9 females with a mean age of 23.7 years. The palsy was incomplete on 1 side in 7 patients. Eight cases were idiopathic. Seven cases were caused by sclerosteosis. All 7 occurred in Afrikaners, 6 of whom underwent craniocervical decompression for increased intracranial pressure. In addition, 6 cases resulted from fracture of the temporal bone, and 1 each was associated with bilateral tuberculous mastoiditis, lymphosarcoma, and Guillain-Barré syndrome. In the idiopathic group, 7 patients achieved complete recovery and 1 had partial recovery. None of the patients with sclerosteosis showed recovery. In the temporal bone fracture group, 2 patients recovered completely; 2 recovered partially, including 1 patient who had reanastomosis of the nerve; 1 had no recovery; and 1 was lost to follow-up. The other 3 patients have all recovered at least partially.

Discussion.—A definite cause should always be sought in BSFNP because two thirds of all patients have such a cause. Those associated with head injury typically result from a longitudinal petrous fracture across the skull base. Sclerosteosis is rare outside of the Afrikaner community; its management consists mainly of craniotomy or craniocervical decompression.

► A patient with BSFNP is a rarity; usually, however, it is possible to identify a cause for it. Sclerosteosis, one of the 3 main disorders in which BSFNP is found, should be included in our differential diagnosis.—M.M. Paparella, M.D.

Primary Tumors of the Facial (Extracranial) Nerve

Sneige N, Batsakis JG (Univ of Texas MD Anderson Cancer Ctr)

Ann Otol Rhinol Laryngol 100:604–606, 1991 5–3

Background.—Primary neoplasms of the seventh cranial (facial) nerve can be classified according to their site of origin along the course of the nerve as either intratemporal or extracranial. The primary tumors of the facial extracranial nerve were reviewed.

Discussion.—Almost one fourth of all primary neurogenous tumors arise from the peripheral nerves in the head and neck. However, the extracranial parts of the facial nerve are uncommon sites. When they do occur, these tumors are difficult to diagnose and manage. Intraparotid facial nerve neurogenic tumors are rarely diagnosed before surgery (Fig 5–2). These tumors are usually seen as mass lesions accompanied by various degrees of facial weakness in one third of the patients. Except for the peculiar predilection of childhood plexiform neurofibromas to afflict the facial nerve, most of the tumors are neurilemomas. After the neurilemomas and neurofibromas are surgically removed, recurrences are unusual. Sarcomas of the facial nerve are rare high-grade malignancies.

Conclusions.—Surgical removal is the only effective treatment for neurogenic tumors of the facial nerve. Such surgery can require sacrificing the nerve, and it is then followed by nerve grafting. In any of the histological forms, identifying the nerve can be difficult because nerve fibers are often splayed over the surface of the tumor.

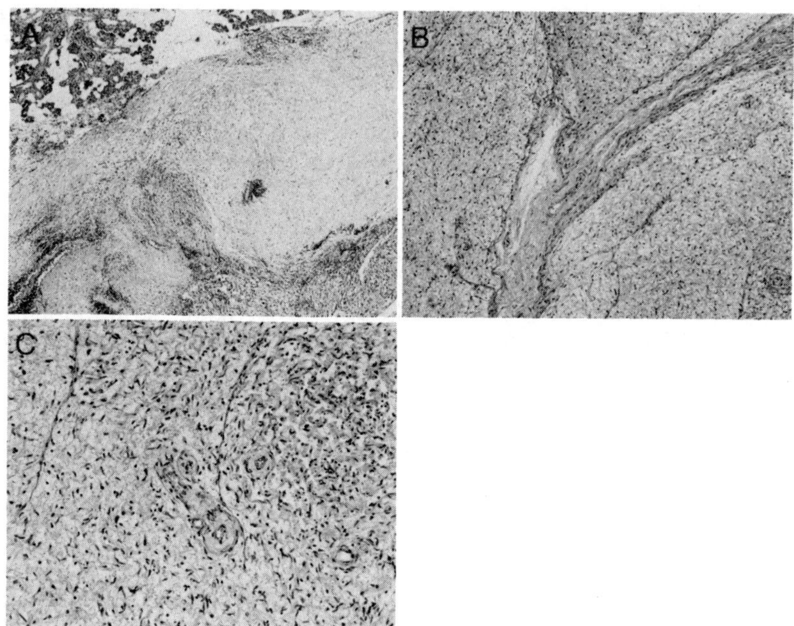

Fig 5–2.—Primary tumors of the facial nerve. **A,** intraparotid neurilemoma. Hematoxylin-eosin; original magnification, ×40. Note the thick capsule separating the neoplasm **(bottom left)** from the gland's parenchyma. **B,** plexiform neurofibroma in a 12-year-old girl. Hematoxylin-eosin; original magnification, ×40. **C,** higher magnification of the neurofibroma in **B.** Hematoxylin-eosin; original magnification, ×200. (Courtesy of Sneige N, Batsakis JG: *Ann Otol Rhinol Laryngol* 100:604–606, 1991.)

▶ Most of the extracranial facial nerve tumors are neurilemomas. Other types of tumor may also exist. These authors correctly surmise that surgical removal followed by nerve grafting is the only effective treatment for neurogenic tumors.—M.M. Paparella, M.D.

New Aspects of Facial Nerve Pathology in Temporal Bone Fractures

Felix H, Eby TL, Fisch U (University Hosp, Zürich; Univ of Alabama, Birmingham)

Acta Otolaryngol (Stockh) 111:332–336, 1991 5–4

Background.—Longitudinal temporal bone fractures usually injure the facial nerve in the labyrinthine segment next to the geniculate ganglion. Facial nerve regeneration often, but not always, produces some recovery of function. The exact pathology in those cases where function does not recover has not been established.

Methods.—Surgical specimens were removed from 12 patients in whom the repair of a facial nerve lesion after temporal bone trauma necessitated end-to-end anastomosis or grafting. The speciments were then

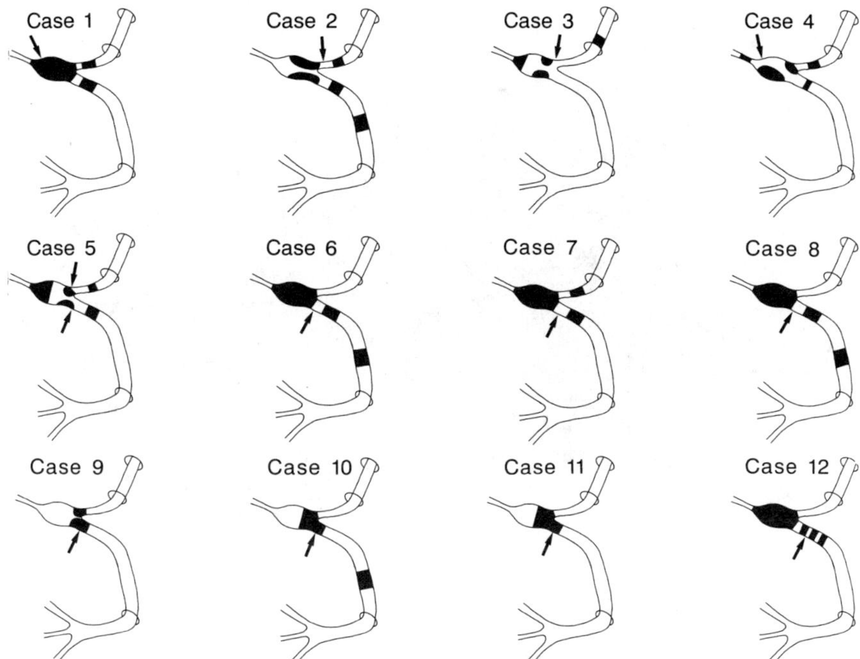

Fig 5–3.—A diagram showing the location of the main lesion (*arrows*) and the extent of neural resection for each case. (Courtesy of Felix H, Eby TL, Fisch U: *Acta Otolaryngol (Stockh)* 111:332–336, 1991.)

analyzed by light and electron microscopy. All patients had persisting facial paralysis.

Findings.—A pronounced retrograde degeneration of myelinated fibers was noted in the facial nerve proximal to the geniculate ganglion. In the 6 labyrinthine and 1 meatal segments studied, 95% to 100% of the myelinated fibers had degenerated. In the proximal nerve segments, regeneration and degeneration coexisted. Many regenerating axons were noted in Büngner's bundles in all labyrinthine and 1 meatal nerve specimen. All specimens showed some endoneural fibrosis. In 2 specimens, regenerating axons were surrounded by a thick scar. This fibrosis occurred early and late after injury. The regenerating myelinated fibers were blocked by fibrosis in the distal labyrinthine or proximal tympanic segment of the facial nerve in all specimens (Figs 5–3 and 5–4).

Conclusions.—Histological assessment of intratemporal facial nerve biopsy specimens from patients with no recovery of function after temporal bone fractures indicated that the extent of retrograde degeneration is larger than expected. Also, degeneration is accompanied by fibrosis that prevents regeneration. Intraneural fibrosis can occur as early as 5 weeks after injury. Prolonged denervation can induce extensive atrophy of the distal nerve trunk and endoneurial tube shrinkage.

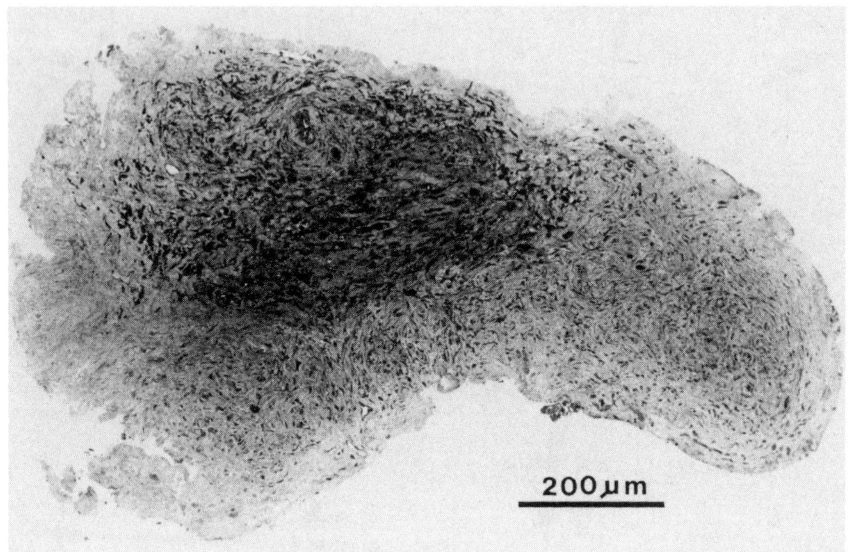

Fig 5–4.—Transverse section through the distal labyrinthine segment from a patient with extensive fibrosis (semithin section, toluidine blue stained). (Courtesy of Felix H, Eby TL, Fisch U: *Acta Otolaryngol (Stockh)* 111:332-336, 1991.)

▶ The results of this study are interesting and, to my mind, new. I was not aware of the extent of the degeneration of facial nerve lesions in fractures of the temporal bone. These findings should help to guide us in the diagnosis and management of such lesions.—M.M. Paparella, M.D.

Predicting Recovery of Facial Nerve Function Following Injury from a Basilar Skull Fracture

Adegbite AB, Khan MI, Tan L (Univ of Saskatchewan, Saskatoon, Canada)
J Neurosurg 75:759–762, 1991 5–5

Background.—The facial nerve is likely to be injured in individuals who sustain basilar skull fractures. Historically, it has been believed that recovery of function is most likely with nonsurgical treatment in the case of incomplete or delayed facial nerve paralysis. The ability of the time of onset of palsy to predict recovery was evaluated in 25 patients with posttraumatic facial nerve palsies.

Patients.—The subjects were 16 males and 9 females (mean age, 34 years) selected from about 2,000 patients who had sustained closed head injuries during a 12-year period. Most were injured in motor vehicle accidents and falls. All patients were followed as outpatients for a mean of 34 weeks. The recovery of function was assessed by electromyography and clinical examination at first; however, it was later assessed by clinical means only.

Findings.—At 18 months, 95% of the patients had achieved at least partial recovery. At 5 months, 92.5% of the patients with a partial lesion showed some recovery, compared with 10% of those with a complete lesion. At 10 months, 53.5% of the patients had achieved complete recovery. Of the patients with partial lesions, 62% recovered by 4 months, compared with none of those with complete lesions. Immediate or delayed onset of palsy had no effect on the recovery of function.

Conclusions.—In patients with facial nerve injury after basilar skull fracture, the degree of palsy appears to have a significant effect on the recovery of function; however, time of onset does not. Therefore, such patients should be approached conservatively; surgery should be considered for those patients who still have complete facial palsy 12–18 months after the injury.

▶ According to this study, if the facial nerve palsy lasts more than 1 year after injury, then decompression should be considered. It seems reasonable that basilar skull fractures do not always cause exactly the same type of lesion in the course of the facial nerve through the temporal bone. Thus site-of-lesion testing and specific attention to temporal bone findings will not only help understand the site of the lesion but also guide the method of management.—M.M. Paparella, M.D.

Acute Peripheral Facial Palsy: CSF Findings and Etiology

Roberg M, Ernerudh J, Forsberg P, Fridell E, Frydén A, Hydén D, Linde A, Ödkvist L (Linköping Univ, Linköping, Sweden; Natl Bacteriological Lab, Stockholm)

Acta Neurol Scand 83:55–60, 1991 5–6

Background.—Recent findings indicate that facial palsy is not only a mononeuritis, but is also a part of a polyneuropathy with CNS involvement. *Borrelia burgdorferi* is emerging as a major causative agent of facial palsy. An antibody study of CSF and serum was done over the course of acute idiopathic peripheral facial palsy. Based on the annual incidence figures of facial palsy in Sweden, most patients with the disease were included in this study.

Methods.—Cerebrospinal fluid protein analysis and viral and *Borrelia* serology were performed in 56 consecutive patients. A substantial number of antimicrobial antibodies were analyzed, and CSF was examined with serum in both the acute phase and convalescence.

Findings.—Evidence for viral or bacterial infection was found in 27% of the patients. A total of 16% was associated with *Borrelia* infection. There was an obvious seasonal variation, with all cases occurring from June to December when the vector *Ixodes ricinus* is present. *Borrelia* was also associated with reactivation of the Epstein-Barr virus and was the most common pathogen in patients with pleocytosis. Of the 6 patients with viral infections, 3 viruses were in the herpes virus group. This finding does not support the hypothesis that herpes simplex virus is significant in the etiology of facial palsy.

Conclusion.—In patients with acute idiopathic peripheral facial palsy, viral infection was found infrequently. *Borrelia burgdorferi* was the most common infectious cause of facial palsy. The reactivated Epstein-Barr virus infection that was frequently associated with *Borrelia* may have been an aberrant immune response. Half of the patients with *Borrelia* infection had signs of intrathecal antibody synthesis. Facial palsy can probably occur either in the form of an isolated mononeuritis or as part of a generalized CNS infection.

▶ Bell's palsy refers to idiopathic acute peripheral facial palsy. Earlier studies have indicated that lesions of the vasonervorum can cause constriction and death of the neurons, thereby resulting in paralysis. More recent studies have suggested that a viral etiologic agent was most often found with histological changes in the nerve characteristic of viral involvement with round cell invasion. This study examines other possible causes. The etiology of Bell's palsy continues to present a dilemma.—M.M. Paparella, M.D.

Malignant Tumours of the Middle Ear

Savić DLJ, Djerić DR (Univ Clinical Ctr, Belgrade, Yugoslavia)
Clin Otolaryngol 16:87–89, 1991 5–7

Introduction.—Malignant tumors of the middle ear are rare.

Patients.—Between 1971 and 1988, 15 patients with a malignant tumor of the middle ear were admitted to the Clinic of Otorhirolaryngology at the University Clinical Center in Belgrade, Yugoslavia. Thirteen patients (age, 42–77 years) had squamous cell carcinomas; of these 13, 11 had long-standing chronic suppurative otitis media before the malignant tumor occurred. The other 2 patients did not have a history of chronic ear infection. Five patients with squamous cell carcinomas had undergone surgery for suspected chronic otitis 1–2 years before referral to the clinic. All were totally deaf, and 3 had peripheral facial nerve paralysis. In all 5 patients, the malignant tumor involved the pyramid of the temporal bone. In 4 patients, the tumor had also invaded the endocranium. None of the patients had received postoperative radiation therapy. Two patients died soon after admission before receiving any therapy. The other 3 patients were given radiation therapy because their tumors were inoperable; however, all 3 died within the first 2 years after treatment. Eight patients with squamous cell carcinomas received their initial diagnosis at the clinic, and 7 of them were treated. One patient was admitted with partial destruction of the occipital bone and lung metastases. This patient died soon after admission—without receiving any treatment. Of the remaining 7 patients, 3 were totally deaf and 4 had a peripheral facial nerve paralysis. All 7 patients underwent radical excision of the temporal bone, and 4 of them also received postoperative radiation therapy. Four patients died of their disease, and 3 patients were still alive without signs of tumor more than 5 years after treatment. One patient with an embryonal rhabdomyosarcoma of the middle ear and 1 patient with a malignant lymphoma of the middle ear received the diagnosis at an advanced stage. Both patients died soon after admission without being treated.

Conclusion.—Squamous cell carcinoma of the middle ear usually occurs as a complication of chronic suppurative otitis media. Early diagnosis is rare because the exact timing of a malignant change is very difficult to determine. A malignant tumor should be suspected whenever there is a change in the patient's symptoms.

▶ In this study, squamous cell carcinoma of the middle ear cleft usually occurs as a complication of chronic otitis media. This would assume that the epithelial cells of the mucoperiosteum in the middle ear undergo metaplasia to become cancer cells. I think a more likely explanation is that infection in such patients is accompanied by infection and irritation of the adjacent skin of the external auditory canal. It has been my observation from past clinical experience—as well as from past studies by others—that a lesion of the skin in the adjacent canal often silently invades the middle ear and causes a squamous cell carcinoma. Differential diagnosis of the histology of a tumor is always essential to its management when a patient is seen with such a clinical problem.—M.M. Paparella, M.D.

Adenomas of the Mastoid and Middle Ear

Noel FL, Benecke JE Jr, Carberry JN, House JW, Patterson M (St Louis Univ; St Vincent Med Ctr, Los Angeles)

Otolaryngol Head Neck Surg 104:133–134, 1991 5–8

Introduction.—Approximately 100 cases of adenomatous tumor of the temporal bone have been evaluated. Sixteen cases seen by an otologic group between 1961 and 1990 were studied.

Histology.—Ten patients had mixed tumors with variable proportions of acinar, solid, and trabecular components, as well as cords and ribbons of cells. Mitoses were rare. Dense secretory inclusions were observed. Six patients had papillary tumors with gland formation and ultrastructural features of exocrine glandular epithelium. The apical cytoplasm contained a secretory product.

Clinical.—Mixed tumors occurred most often in males, who were seen with imaging findings of a soft tissue density in the middle ear and mastoid. No patient had otic capsule involvement or intracranial invasion. Tympanoplasty was done using mastoidectomy techniques, but 4 of the 10 patients required further surgery for residual or recurrent disease. The papillary tumors tended to occur in females, who most often were seen with sensorineural hearing loss and facial paralysis. Vestibular abnormalities were frequent, and there were extensive bone destruction and intracranial involvement in all cases. The patients were managed aggressively by transtemporal and infratemporal approaches; 2 patients received postoperative radiotherapy. One of the 5 patients followed had persistent disease.

Recommendations.—Adenomatous tumors of the mastoid and middle ear must be removed with a wide margin of normal tissue, even when overt malignancy is absent. Mixed tumors may be managed by tympanoplasty, whereas papillary tumors require more extensive temporal bone surgery—often in conjunction with intracranial surgery.

▶ Although pleomorphic adenomas can occur in the mastoid or middle ear, adenomas and adenocarcinomas can also occur in the middle ear cleft. I recently treated a patient who indicated that he had a sense of fullness and normal hearing. A wide excision and partial removal of the temporal bone was indicated for adenocarcinoma. The patient should be advised that a hearing loss will result after treatment. In this patient, the hearing loss amounted to nearly a 30 dB conductive loss, which is certainly a small price to pay for treatment of a large adenocarcinoma that filled the middle ear cleft.—M.M. Paparella, M.D.

Histopathology of Metastatic Temporal Bone Tumors

Nelson EG, Hinojosa R (Univ of Chicago)

Arch Otolaryngol Head Neck Surg 117:189–193, 1991 5–9

Introduction.—Temporal bone metastases are being reported more frequently. Data on 60 temporal bones from 33 patients with metastatic malignancy were reviewed, excluding those bones with lymphoma and leukemia. Specimens were collected for more than 50 years. Of the 19 different primary malignancies represented, breast cancer occurred most frequently.

Results.—The metastases were bilateral in 27 patients. Those metastases secondary to hematogenous spread were present in the petrous apex. Tumors that metastasized to the meninges and involved the temporal bone secondarily were found in the internal auditory canal. Head-neck tumors extending directly to the temporal bone most often involved the petrous apex and foramen lacerum. Only 10 patients had a history of otologic symptoms, most often hearing loss. Diffuse metastases were present throughout the body in all patients with hematogenous or meningeal spread. In 1 patient with hematogenous metastases, a vascular otosclerotic focus was involved by metastatic tumor (Fig 5–5).

Conclusion.—These findings represent an end-stage process. Temporal bone metastases often do not produce symptoms—even in patients with advanced disease.

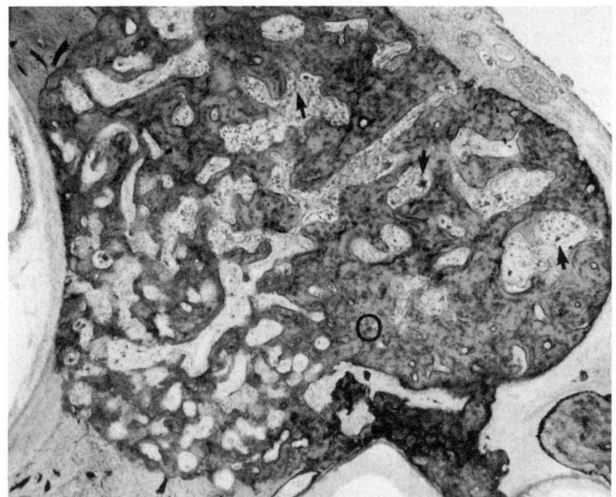

Fig 5–5.—Invasion of an otosclerotic focus *(O)* in the anterior oval window in a 56-year-old woman with metastatic adenocarcinoma of the breast. Hematoxylin-eosin, original magnification, ×48. (Courtesy of Nelson EG, Hinojosa R: *Arch Otolaryngol Head Neck Surg* 117:189–193, 1991.)

▶ This study reflects our earlier finding that the metastatic spread of tumors to the temporal bone is far more common than most of us realize. Hematogenous tumors frequently show cellular infiltration of the bone marrow of the petrous apex. Although metastatic spread to the temporal bone can be quite common histologically, patients often show little or nothing in the way of otologic symptoms or findings.—M.M. Paparella, M.D.

6 External Ear, Exploratory Tympanotomy, Middle Ear, and Mastoid

Surfer's Ear: Exostoses of the External Auditory Canal

Turetsky DB, Vines FS, Clayman DA (Univ of Florida Health Science Ctr, Jacksonville)

AJNR 11:1217–1218, 1990 6–1

Background.—Exostosis of the external auditory canal is found only in humans. Typical clinical and CT findings allow definitive diagnosis in most cases.

Case Report.—Man, 56, a physician, had had recurrent hearing loss for 5 years. The loss was becoming more frequent and was interfering with his auscultatory proficiency. Hearing returned temporarily when carbamide peroxide drops were applied. There was no history of ear infection; however, the patient reported prolonged exposure to cold sea water when swimming and body surfing. He had practiced this activity for 12–15 years. Both external auditory canals were severely stenosed, and impacted cerumen occluded the right canal. Audiologic testing was normal after the cerumen was removed. A CT scan showed a multinodular bony mass arising from the anterior and posterior walls of the right external canal. The remaining lumen was 1 mm in diameter on that side and 2 mm on the left. The right-sided exostosis was excised, leaving a 3-mm to 4-mm canal lumen.

Discussion.—Exostoses of the external auditory canal are a result of chronic irritation of physical, chemical, or thermal origin. Today they are more often a result of prolonged exposure to cold sea water than of infection. The lesions occur most often in the anterior area of the tympanosquamous suture and near the tympanomastoid suture posteriorly. The symptoms may include hearing loss, aural infection, pain, and tinnitus. Computed tomography characteristically shows bilateral bony proliferation in the external auditory canal.

► We have seen many patients with exostoses of the ear canal. As this study suggests, many of these patients will have a history of swimming, not always in salt water but sometimes in fresh water. However, I was surprised to find that exostoses developed in some patients without a history of swimming. Most of the time these bony growths can be managed in the office; however, if they become symptomatic and cause severe intractable infection or obstruction of hearing, then they must be treated. A patient I treated eventually had severe complete obstruction resulting from exostoses; this was followed by otitis media and the beginning signs of meningeal complications. If patients are symptomatic they should be treated; if they are asymptomatic, they can be managed in the office.—M.M. Paparella, M.D.

The Validity of Questionnaire Reports of a History of Acute Otitis Media

Alho OP (Univ of Oulu, Oulu, Finland)
Am J Epidemiol 132:1164–1170, 1990 6–2

Introduction.—Because many epidemiological surveys of acute otitis media are based on questionnaires, the accuracy of questionnaire data was examined in a random sample of 2,512 children who were monitored to 2 years of age using a questionnaire dealing with infection. There were 6,510 visits by children who had 3 or more episodes of acute otitis media and 3,833 visits by children who had few or no episodes of acute otitis.

Results.—The cumulative incidence of acute otitis to 2 years of age (based on questionnaire data) was 48%, compared with a rate of 71% from medical records. The questionnaire data suggested 1.3 episodes of acute otitis per child per year, compared with a rate of .9 per child per year from the medical records. The incidence rates of acute otitis demonstrated by tympanocentesis were the same for the 2 data sets. Acute otitis was definitely more prevalent in children of nonrespondent parents.

Conclusion.—The discrepancies between the questionnaire and medical records data on acute otitis may reflect inadequate or overly complicated information given to parents by the physician when the child is treated. A recall period of 2 years may produce recall bias, especially in a large family. The effect of how the data are sampled must be considered when interpreting questionnaire-based surveys of acute otitis media in childhood.

▶ When a questionnaire and/or statistical methodology is applied, the results of a study on any form of otologic disease will depend upon the bias of the input. In this instance, the results were influenced by the questionnaire and the way it was structured.—M.M. Paparella, M.D.

Chronic Middle Ear Effusion: A Possible Cause of Protracted Vomiting and Failure to Thrive in Infancy

Granot E, Matoth I, Feinmesser R (Hadassah Hebrew Univ, Jerusalem)
Clin Pediatr 29:722–724, 1990 6–3

Introduction.—Although protracted vomiting in infancy may be caused by a range of disorders, chronic otitis media with effusion has not previously been considered among its causes.

Patients.—Three infants (aged 8–10 months) were admitted to the Hadassah Hebrew University Medical Center in Jerusalem for persistent vomiting and failure to thrive. Two infants had previously undergone lengthy and extensive in-hospital evaluation elsewhere. Although middle ear effusion was evident in all 3 infants, it had not been associated with protracted vomiting. However, myringotomy and insertion of ventilating tubes resulted in the immediate cessation of vomiting, and all 3 children showed a steady, progressive weight gain.

Conclusion.—Chronic otitis media with effusion in infants may cause protracted vomiting and failure to thrive. Physicians should be aware of this previously unreported association.

▶ We have recently described how the spread of otitis media through the round window can cause cochleitis and sensorineural hearing losses in children and adults. This has been substantiated histologically. It seems reasonable that infection can travel to the vestibular labyrinth, thereby causing irritation of both the vestibular and the cochlear portion of the inner ear. Perhaps this is the mechanism in this newly defined relationship in children. We should be alert to this possibility in children who are seen with chronic otitis media with effusion.—M.M. Paparella, M.D.

Dysequilibrium and Otitis Media With Effusion: What is the Association?

Grace ARH, Pfleiderer AG (Addenbrookes Hosp, Cambridge, England)
J Laryngol Otol 104:628–684, 1990 6–4

Background.—The association between nonsuppurative otitis media (NOSM) and a disturbance of balance in the pediatric age group has been described but not quantified in studies. The incidence of balance-related problems in 154 children with surgically proven glue ear and 51 children with normal ear function was compared.

Methods.—The findings were based on subjective evidence obtained from the parents on a written questionnaire relating to balance, personal interview, and physical examinations of each child. The children with surgically proven secretory otitis media were anesthetized, and either 1 or 2 grommets were inserted depending on whether a unilateral or bilateral condition existed. The children were followed for 4 months after surgery, and balance was rated as returned to normal, unchanged, or worse.

Findings.—Nearly one quarter of the children with NOSM had some degree of dysequilibrium or vestibular-like disturbance, compared with no symptoms in the control group. A disturbance of balance occurred as frequently in the children with unilateral effusions as in those with bilateral effusions. This important aspect of otitis media with effusion may have been frequently overlooked by the clinicians because the parents rarely volunteered information. Otalgia was common during episodes of dysequilibrium, indicating that infection may have played a role in the pathogenesis of the vestibular disturbances. There was a complete resolution of symptoms after grommet insertion in 85% of the children.

Conclusion.—A history of balance-related symptoms should be more actively sought in all children with otitis media with effusion.

▶ This abstract and Abstract 6–3 bring a new diagnostic possibility to the otologist's workshop: children with otitis media with effusion may be seen with vestibular symptoms. This is a very elegant study because a large number of children were followed. It is interesting that one fourth of the children who had otitis media with effusion of a nonsuppurative type also had some degree of disequilibrium or vestibular-like symptoms. No symptoms were found in the control group. Most of the children were benefited by the use of a ventilation tube in treatment. These 2 studies suggest that research should attempt to discover the mechanism of involvement. As clinicians, we should consider vestibular studies when a child is seen with otitis media with effusion and symptoms of a vestibular nature.—M.M. Paparella, M.D.

Passive Smoking and Otitis Media With Effusion

Barr GS, Coatesworth AP (Queen Elizabeth Hosp, Birmingham, England)

Br Med J 303:1032–1033, 1991 6–5

Background.—Parental smoking may be a risk factor for otitis media with effusion. This possible relationship was further explored in a case-control study.

Methods.—A group of 115 children, aged 17 months–11 years, had otitis media with effusion confirmed by myringotomy. They were matched by age, sex, race, and social class to healthy children. The control group had no history of ear problems. The parents of the children in the 2 groups were then asked about their smoking habits.

Findings.—The parental smoking habits were not significantly different between the 2 groups. The median number of ciagarettes smoked by mothers alone and by all adults in the household was also comparable in the 2 groups.

Conclusions.—Otitis media with effusion is more prevalent among the poorer socioeconomic classes. The children of nonmanual workers have been found to have significantly better hearing than those of manual workers. Although cigarette smoking is more common among the lower classes, it is not likely to be a risk factor for otitis media effusion.

► Although this study is not necessarily definitive, it is of interest. Smoking is considered to be a possible etiological factor in otitis media. In this study the conclusion is logical: otitis media seems to be more prevalent among the poorer socioeconomic classes, where cigarette smoking is more common. Therefore, socioeconomic class may be a more important factor than smoking.—M.M. Paparella, M.D.

Middle Ear Fluid Lysozyme Source in Experimental Pneumococcal Otitis Media

Nonomura N, Giebink GS, Zelterman D, Harada T, Juhn SK (Univ of Minnesota)

Ann Otol Rhinol Laryngol 100:593–596, 1991 6–6

Background.—Lysozymes (α-1,4 glycan hydrolases with a range of biological functions) are found in the middle ear fluid (MEF) and are important inflammatory mediators in pneumococcal middle ear infection. It was hypothesized that MEF lysozyme is derived from the MEF inflammatory cells and from the middle ear epithelium, and that inflammatory responses are generated by inflammatory cells, humoral factors, and mediators released from the mucosa. To determine the source of MEF lysozyme, experimental pneumococcal otitis media was induced in chinchillas.

Methods.—Eighteen chinchillas were irradiated, and their middle ears were inoculated with heat-killed, encapsulated pneumococci. The number of inflammatory cells and the lysozyme concentration were measured in the MEF between 6 and 72 hours after inoculation. The findings were compared with those in a control group of 90 pneumococcal-inoculated, nonirradiated chinchillas.

Findings.—In the pneumococcus-inoculated ears, the mean number of inflammatory cells was virtually nil at 6 hours in the irradiated animals. In contrast, the MEF from the nonirradiated animals showed significant cell influx as early as 6 hours. At 24–72 hours, the mean number of inflammatory cells in the MEF from the irradiated animals was similar to the level in the MEF from the nonirradiated animals. This result suggests that killed pneumococci are strong chemoattractants for inflammatory cells. There was no significant difference in the mean lysozyme concentrations in the MEF between the pneumococcal-inoculated irradiated and nonirradiated animals.

Conclusions.—Pneumococci in the middle ear space may directly stimulate the middle ear epithelial cells to release lysozymes. Lysozymes are found in high concentrations in the MEF of patients with chronic otitis media with effusion and in animal models of otitis media; they appear to be important inflammatory mediators. Future therapeutic interventions for the middle ear inflammation of otitis media must take into account the direct inflammatory action of pneumococci on middle ear epithelium.

▶ This study states again what has been demonstrated in earlier studies: lysozyme appears to be an important enzyme mediator in otitis media and a mechanistic factor in its pathogenesis as well. Whether pneumococci in the middle ear space may stimulate middle ear epithelial cells to release this important enzyme and whether other markers can be considered causative mechanistic factors in the pathogenesis of otitis media require further study.—M.M. Paparella, M.D.

In Search of Missing Links in Otology. II. Development of an Implantable Middle Ear Drug Delivery System: Initial Studies of Sustained Ampicillin Release for the Treatment of Otitis Media

Goycoolea MV, Muchow DC, Sirvio LM, Winandy RM (Minnesota Ear, Head and Neck Clinic; Univ of Minnesota; 3M Company, Minneapolis)

Laryngoscope 101:727–732, 1991 6–7

Objective.—A method of safely delivering effective levels of antimicrobial drugs directly to the middle ear for a prolonged period would be very useful. A device was developed that could be inserted via a myringotomy incision; it could expand toward its original shape to contact the middle ear walls without substantially occluding the middle ear space. This expanded device should provide extended release of an active drug by diffusion into middle ear effusions.

Methods.—A Poly-L-lactic acid film incorporating antibiotic was inserted into the middle ears of chinchillas via a transtympanic approach. Films plasticized with triethyl citrate were prepared to decrease their brittleness. The efficacy of this approach was examined in chinchillas with *Streptococcus pneumoniae* instilled into the middle ear.

Results.—Ampicillin-containing film was readily inserted into the middle ear cavity. The device unrolled totally and contacted the middle ear walls. The drug was effectively released from the material. In vivo studies demonstrated sterile middle ear effusions in animals with an ampicillin-containing device in place. Prophylactic placement of the device also was effective in preventing infection.

Implications.—Devices such as this could become an important means of treating otitis media and other middle and/or inner ear syndromes. The possible ototoxic effects of these devices require further study before they are adopted for clinical use.

► Time will tell whether an implantable system for delivery of drugs to the middle ear could be a breakthrough for the management of otitis media. Such a system provides an opportunity for the sustained release of medication over time and may even help obviate more radical surgical treatment for these patients. One has to consider the foreign body effect of the implantable device and then weigh that effect against the ability to treat soft tissue inflammatory disease. Another problem, of course, is that no treatment device in the middle ear will circumvent eustachian tubal obstruction or obstructive sites, which are commonly identified throughout the middle ear cleft. Nevertheless, this is an important new method, and we are looking forward to clinical trials with this new device.—M.M. Paparella, M.D.

Antimicrobial Treatment of Acute Otitis Media

Giebink GS, Canafax DM, Kempthorne J (Univ of Minnesota; Hennepin County Med Ctr, Minneapolis)

J Pediatr 119:495–500, 1991 6–8

Background.—There are many types of antimicrobial treatment available for children with acute otitis media (AOM). Although the newer drugs may be preferred because of their broader spectrums of activity, they are expensive and their clinical efficacy is not substantially better. The issues related to antimicrobial treatment for acute otitis media were studied.

Choice of Treatment.—Spontaneous resolution of AOM often confounds studies seeking to compare drug treatments; however, antimicrobials have a profound effect on the morbidity of the condition. Semisynthetic β-lactam drugs, cephalosporins, and drug combinations have comparable clinical effectiveness, but they vary in their ability to eradicate infection. Acute otitis media represents a pathologic continuum, and its varying manifestations complicate management. The diagnosis is not easily made in about half of the patients, and the distinction between asymptomatic otitis media with effusion and AOM is important in choosing therapy. In neonates, ampicillin and gentamicin are generally used for neonates with intensive care exposure, whereas ampicillin and cefotaxime are used for those without. Older children can generally be treated as outpatients, most commonly with amoxicillin and trimethoprim-sulfamethoxazole (TMP-SMZ). Second-line drugs are used in those patients with persistent or recurrent AOM.

Related Issues.—Among the many factors affecting drug choice are age, associated illnesses, history of otitis media, and drug hypersensitivity. When symptoms persist, another antibiotic should not be chosen without culture of effusion fluid. Switching from amoxicillin to TMP-SMZ, or vice versa, is often successful. Hypersensitivity is usually a contraindication; however, if the drug is essential, an experienced physician may perform desensitization. The use of ear drops rarely adds to the activity of systemic antibiotics in patients with AOM and otorrhea of recent onset. Most current dosing guidelines are based on clinical studies—the pharmacokinetics have just recently begun to be evaluated. Although the traditional duration of treatment has been 10–14 days, some studies have shown success with shorter durations of treatment. According to the pharmacokinetic data, treatment need not be the same for every patient.

Discussion.—Although no antimicrobial drug is best for all patients with AOM, amoxicillin and TMP-SMZ remain the mainstays of treatment. Otherwise, drugs should be selected in accordance with the patient's characteristics. Further pharmacokinetic studies of treatment for AOM are needed to make more precise recommendations.

▶ Clinical experience will always influence the physician's choice of drug in the treatment of AOM. Factors such as age, associated illness, history of otitis media, and hypersensitivities to drugs should be considered. According to this study, amoxicillin and TMP-SMZ continue to be important drugs to consider when treating such problems.—M.M. Paparella, M.D.

Systemic Steroids for Otitis Media With Effusion in Children
Rosenfeld RM, Mandel EM, Bluestone CD (Children's Hosp of Pittsburgh)
Arch Otolaryngol Head Neck Surg 117:984–989, 1991 6–9

Background.—The role of oral steroids continues to be debated in the treatment of otitis media. The existing evidence was assessed on both sides of this debate.

Methods.—A combined computer and manual search identified 14 articles and abstracts published through September 1990. Six randomized clinical trials involving a total of 264 children were selected from these 14 for formal meta-analysis.

Findings.—Those children given steroids for 7–14 days were 3.6 times more likely to have both ears free of effusion at the end of treatment than the children given placebo. Weighting studies by a quality score or stratifying them by use of concurrent antibiotic had essentially no effect on this finding. The studies analyzed were very heterogeneous.

Conclusions.—The heterogeneity of the studies analyzed suggests a need for additional trials to identify the specific subsets of children most likely to benefit from steroid treatment.

▶ Earlier studies have indicated that systemic steroids are not effective in treating otitis media with effusion in children. The conclusion of this study suggests that there might be some treatment effect after using steroids for 1 to 2 weeks. Children receiving the steroid were compared with those receiving a placebo. Once again, clinical judgment is needed, and we look forward to more definitive studies in the future.—M.M. Paparella, M.D.

Adenoidectomy in Otitis Media: A Review

Sadé J, Luntz M (Meir Gen Hosp, Kfar Saba, Israel; Tel Aviv Univ, Israel)

Ann Otol Rhinol Laryngol 100:226–231, 1991 6–10

Background.—For years clinicians believed that adenoids adversely affected middle ear (ME) aeration by obstructing the eustachian tube opening, thereby resulting in ME infections and effusions. Therefore, children with ME diseases often had their adenoids removed. Adenoidectomy is still performed on millions of children around the world every year. The relationship of adenoids to the ME and the effect of adenoidectomy on ME effusions and infections were reviewed.

Discussion.—Most patients with acute otitis media (AOM) or secretory otitis media (SOM) recover without adenoid removal. Even in extremely chronic and refractory cases, adenoidectomy is often of no benefit. However, when considering the entire population of such patients, adenoidectomy seems to reduce AOM and SOM relapse rates by approximately a factor of 2, depending on the type of population studied. It has not been established which patients are likely to benefit from surgery. The central question at issue is whether adenoidectomy or ventilation tube (VT) insertion should be done in SOM. However, the question should be whether an adenoidectomy should be done when VTs are inserted.

Conclusions.—Adenoids do not appear to play a major pathogenetic role in either AOM or SOM. When clinicians wish to clear the ME of effusion to restore hearing, they usually place a VT in the tympanic membrane—even if they are ardent advocates of adenoidectomy.

▶ Previous studies in the literature have suggested that adenoidectomy is more important than insertion of a VT in children who have a middle ear full of fluid. This study indicates that the use of the tube to provide ventilation and drainage is a more important priority than consideration of adenoidectomy. As clinicians we can certainly agree with this study and selectively choose the appropriate technique for patients on the basis of clinical findings.—M.M. Paparella, M.D.

Topical Ophthalmologics in Otology

Hoffman RA, Goldofsky E (New York Univ, New York)

Ear Nose Throat J 70:201–205, 1991 6–11

Background.—In June 1988, the American Medical Association reaffirmed its policy that "a physician may lawfully use a Food and Drug Administration (FDA) approved drug product for an unlabeled indication when such use is based upon sound scientific evidence and sound medical opinion." The use of topical ophthalmologics in otology was evaluated.

Discussion.—Most available topical otologic preparations contain a combination of antibiotic/antibiotics and steroid in a medium of acidic pH. However, these preparations are often ineffective because of the limited selection of antibiotic and the potential adverse effect of acidic pH antibiotic activity. In addition, the potential for ototoxicity exists when these agents are applied in the presence of a tympanic membrane perforation or tympanostomy tube. Topical otologic drops are often painful when applied in these conditions, and they may hinder patient compliance. As an alternative, ophthalmic drops increase the spectrum of available antibiotics at a more comfortable and effective pH, with a higher concentration of steroids. They also offer safe alternatives in the choice of nonototoxic antibiotics for patients with a tympanic membrane perforation or tympanostomy tube. Topical ophthalmologic drops are effective in the treatment of postintubation otorrhea, and the higher-dose topical steroid in the ophthalmologic drops is particularly effective in treating the inflammatory component of external ear and chronic middle ear disease.

Implications.—Topical ophthalmologics are often effective when topical otologics have failed. Although topical otologics should be reevaluated, their use appears to be justified in the mean time.

▶ Hoffman and Goldofsky discussed a practice we are observing increasingly often in the clinic: when otologic topical medication fails, ophthalmologic preparations are used. This applies to patients who have chronic otitis media and to those who have severe external otitis. It would be helpful if the drug companies would initiate double-blind controlled studies that could help the otolaryngologist determine when it is safe and efficacious to use ophthalmologic drops in the ear. This study is very timely.—M.M. Paparella, M.D.

Distribution of Ear Drops Using a Non-Aerosol Spray Delivery System

Wilson PS, Dingle A, Grocutt M, Reid AP (Selly Oak Hosp, Birmingham, England)

J Laryngol Otol 105:651–652, 1991 6–12

Background.—There is marked variation in the distribution of both water- and oil-based ear drops, with the least viscous drops being most successful in reaching and covering the tympanic membrane. The new dexamethasone and neomycin ear spray Otomize, which has a nonaerosol spray mist delivery system, was evaluated for distribution in normal subjects.

Methods.—The study sample comprised 20 normal ears that were cleared of wax and liberally dusted with povidone powder. With the subjects lying on their sides, a single dose of Otomize was administered. After 1 minute, the tympanic membrane was reinspected and the position of any residual powder was noted. In addition, the spray was tried both with the subjects sitting upright and with 2 doses.

Results.—The spray always reached the tympanic membrane, covering it completely in 9 ears and covering it by less than half in only 4. These results were significantly better than those achieved in an earlier study of ear drops. Two doses always provided complete coverage, and dosing in the upright position provided complete coverage half of the time.

Conclusions.—The nonaerosol spray mist delivery system for ear drops is easier, more acceptable to patients, and provides better distribution than the standard drop delivery method. The Otomize product compares favorably in cost; however, distribution in diseased ears remains to be determined.

► This method of treating the ear with a spray mist seems logical, has clinical appeal, and should work.—M.M. Paparella, M.D.

Evaluation of Ventilating Tubes and Myringotomy in the Treatment of Recurrent or Persistent Otitis Media

Le CT, Freeman DW, Fireman BH (Kaiser Permanente Med Ctr, Sacramento; Kaiser Permanente Med Care Program, Oakland, Calif)

Pediatr Infect Dis J 10:2–11, 1991 6–13

Objective.—One third of all pediatric practice in the first 5 years of life results from middle ear infection. The treatment of acute otitis media is especially urgent because of the possible adverse effects on both speech and language development and behavior. An estimated 1 million children in the United States receive ventilating tubes (VT) each year. The efficacy of VTs was studied prospectively, the risk factors for persistence of middle ear problems were identified.

Patients.—A total of 44 children with more than 6 episodes of bilateral acute otitis media per year had a VT inserted in 1 ear. Thirteen children with bilateral middle ear effusion for longer than 3 months were similarly treated. The contralateral ear was randomized either to myringotomy alone or no treatment. The children were followed for 3 years. Medical treatment and antibiotic prophylaxis were used as required.

Observations.—The episodes of acute otitis media decreased markedly in the ventilated ears during the first year, and they decreased gradually but significantly in myringotomized ears and in unoperated ears (Fig 6–1). Intubated ears continued to have less otitis and greater hearing improvement as long as the tube remained functional. The surgically treated ears tended to have more otitis and worse hearing after extrusion of the tube, but not to a significant degree. Tympanosclerosis, retraction, and atrophy all were more common in the intubated ears. Most medically treated ears also improved. Tube placement did not provide long-term benefit for most children with recurrent otitis.

Conclusions.—Although VTs do lower the incidence of otitis media and improve hearing, ongoing medical treatment may also be effective in

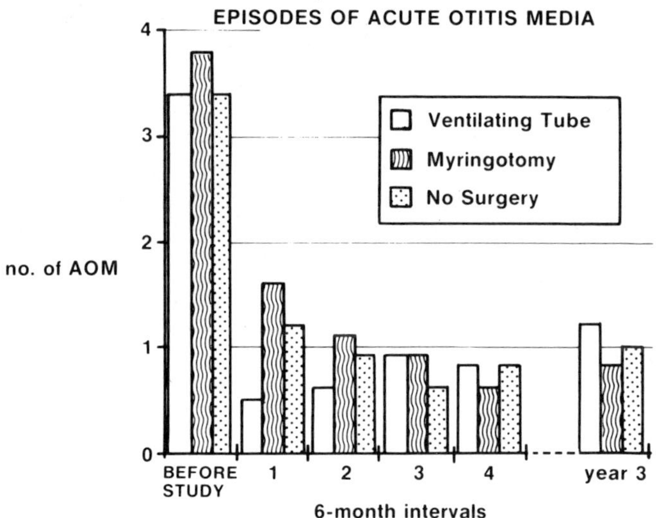

Fig 6–1.—The effect of ventilating tubes, myringotomy and medical therapy alone (no surgery) on the number of episodes of acute otitis media (AOM), per 6-month intervals before study enrollment and for the first 2 years of the study. The numbers of AOM episodes for year 3 are for the whole year. (Courtesy of Le CT, Freeman DW, Fireman BH: *Pediatr Infect Dis J* 10:2–11, 1991.)

many children. Significant adverse sequelae are a problem with VT placement. Ventilating tubes should be used more selectively and cautiously.

▶ I believe that I was the first to publish the results of using a a VT in children with recurrent, frequent bouts of acute otitis media who were receiving cyclical and almost constant antibiotic therapy. There have been very few studies since then to document what has become a common clinical treatment in the United States. I think there should be more documented studies of this type so that we can show evidence not only to our own profession but also to pediatricians. They need to understand the importance of treating these children without the constant use of drugs—the alternative for such children. Based on laboratory and clinical data, it is our observation that the use of VTs actually helps prevent sequelae in a very significant way, both in the middle ear and in the tympanic membrane itself.—M.M. Paparella, M.D.

Radial Versus Circumferential Incision in Myringotomy and Tube Placement

Guttenplan MD, Tom LWC, DeVito MA, Handler SD, Wetmore RF, Potsic WP (Children's Hosp of Philadelphia; Univ of Pennsylvania)

Int J Pediatr Otorhinolaryngol 21:211–215, 1991 6–14

Background.—Pressure equalization tubes are well established as a treatment for persistent otitis media with effusion and recurrent acute

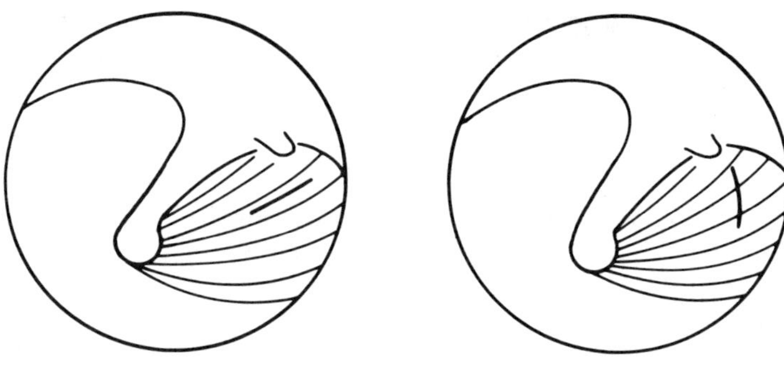

Fig 6–2.—Radial and circumferential incisions in the anterior-superior quadrant of the right tympanic membrane. (Courtesy of Guttenplan MD, Tom LWC, DeVito MA, et al: *Int J Pediatr Otorhinolaryngol* 21:211–215, 1991.)

otitis media. Ideally, the tube remains in place until the return of eustachian tube function. Attempts to improve the functional life expectancy of the tubes have focused on tube design; however, little attention has been directed to modifying surgical technique. Some studies suggest that a radial incision offers theoretical advantages over a circumferential incision. Therefore, radial and circumferential incisions in myringotomy with tube placement were compared.

Methods.—A group of 228 patients with no prior history of ear surgery was studied. Of the patients, 95 were girls and 133 were boys (aged 8 months - 9 years). The incisions were performed in the anterior-superior quadrant (Fig 6–2), and Paparella 1-mm inner diameter tubes were used.

Results.—Adequate follow-up data were available on 125 patients. In 37 of the patients, the tube placed through the circumferential incision extruded earlier, whereas in 26 patients the tube placed through the radial incision extruded first. According to the sign test, the extrusion rates of the 2 groups were not significantly different.

Conclusions.—Theoretically, the radial incision would seem to have some advantages; however, there was no significant difference in the average time of tube extrusion between radial and circumferential incisions in this series. Other factors, such as tube material and design, incision location, and status of the tympanic membrane, may also affect the extrusion rates of pressure equalization tubes.

▶ This study suggests that it doesn's matter whether the incision is radial or circumferential when placing the myringotomy tube. If a very large incision is placed and a relatively small inner flange of a tube is inserted, then these tubes are apt to extrude in a short period of time. However, if the tympanic membrane is taut, the incision is small, and the inner flange is carefully seated with a space below the tympanic membrane (such as in the anterior mesotympanum adjacent to the umbo), then these tubes are apt to stay in place. Therefore, I think that the size of the incision is more important than whether it is radial or circumferential.—M.M. Paparella, M.D.

Ventilation Tube Insertion Under Local Anesthesia

Hickey SA, Buckley JG, O'Connor AFF (Guy's and St Thomas' Hosps, Univ of London, England)

Am J Otol 12:142–143, 1991 6–15

Background.—It is often desirable to perform myringotomy and tympanocentesis and insert a ventilation tube without the use of a general anesthesia. Attempts to anesthetize the external canal and tympanic membrane with topical lignocaine solution or gel have proved ineffective. The use of local irritants such as a phenol-based carrier solution is more effective; however, it can cause external otitis and discolor the meatal skin. Directly infiltrating anesthetic into the meatus and tympanic membrane often is too painful.

New Technique.—After removing meatal wax, EMLA cream (a mixture of 2.5% lignocaine and 2.5% prilocaine in an oil-water emulsion) is instilled to completely fill the meatus, using an aural suction cannula mounted on a syringe (Fig 6–3). The anterior recess is filled first, and the cannula is withdrawn as filling continues (Fig 6–4). The cream is removed by suction after 30 minutes again using the microscope. Myringotomy is then performed in the usual manner. The effusion is suctioned away, and a ventilation tube is inserted when indicated.

Discussion.—This method can be readily used in patients older than 12 years of age, and it has been performed in those as young as 5 years of age. Excellent tympanic membrane anesthesia and adequate meatal analgesia are obtained without the need for local infiltration.

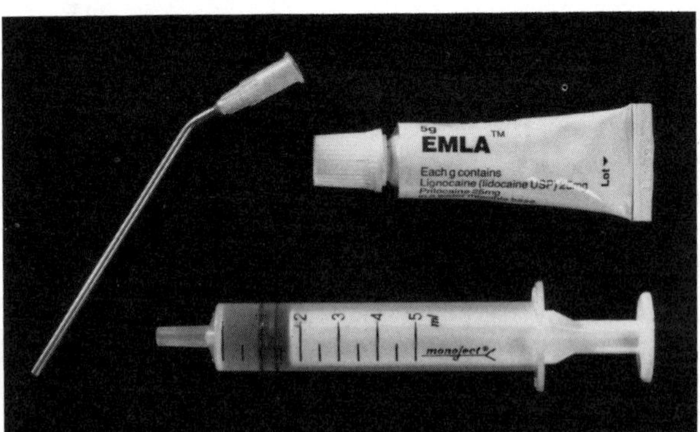

Fig 6–3.—Equipment required to anesthetize the external meatus. (Courtesy of Hickey SA, Buckley JG, O'Connor AFF: *Am J Otol* 12:142–143, 1991.)

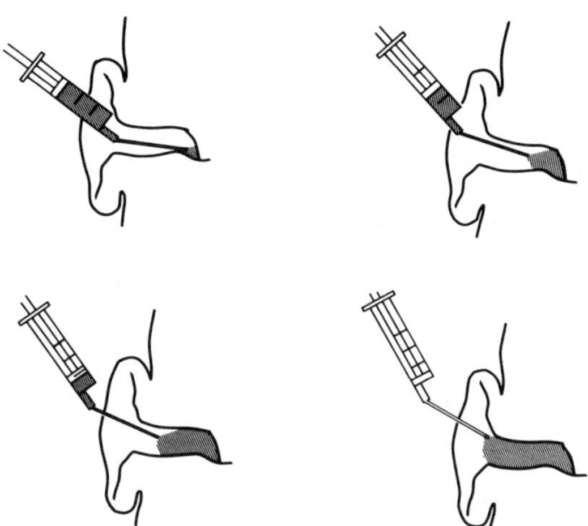

Fig 6–4.—The method used to instill EMLA cream into the external meatus. (Courtesy of Hickey SA, Buckley JG, O'Connor AFF: *Am J Otol* 12:142–143, 1991.)

▶ Clinicians have much to learn from this article. The cost of insertion of a ventilation tube is significant when hospital costs and general anesthesia, are considered. If we could perform more ventilation tubal insertions with local anesthesia, using the method described herein, we could cut costs and morbidity by a considerable extent. This might help provide not only quality care but also cost-effective care to children and adults who have these relatively common problems.—M.M. Paparella, M.D.

Complications Following Ventilation of the Middle Ear Using Goode T Tubes

Bulkley WJ, Bowes AK, Marlowe JF (Univ of Texas Health Science Ctr; San Antonio)

Arch Otolaryngol Head Neck Surg 117:895–898, 1991 6–16

Background.—Maintaining aeration of the middle ear during eustachian tube dysfunction and recurrent otitis media is one of the most frequently encountered problems in pediatric otology. There have been few objective reports on the use of temporary T tubes for this purpose, and conclusions have differed as to the frequency of complications. The complications associated with the use of Goode T tubes were studied.

Patients.—A group of 93 patients treated during a 4-year period was evaluated. The patients all had recurrent acute or chronic otitis media that had not responded to conservative therapy. Overall, 210 Goode T tubes were placed in 182 ears of patients receiving general anesthesia on an outpatient basis. The mean age was 5 years, and the median age was 4 years; only 12% were older than 10 years of age. At follow-up, 23% of the tubes remained in situ.

Complications.—The mean functional period was 35 months. Postoperatively, 35.2% of the ears had otorrhea. In 7% of the cases, this drainage lasted at least 4 months. Twenty-eight tubes were replaced after extrusion. After removal or extrusion of the tubes, perforations were seen in 18.7% of the ears; 7.1% of the ears had chronic perforations requiring tympanoplasty. The physicians reviewed the literature to find other studies of the complications of tympanoplasty tubes. The rate of perforation of the Goode T tube was significantly higher than that of conventional tubes.

Conclusions.—Tympanic membrane perforation appears to be more common as a complication of Goode T-tube placement than was previously reported. This complication occurs despite immediate placement of paper patches over the ostomy site. New methods of maintaining middle ear aeration are needed in these patients.

▶ The Goode T tube has proven useful in treating long-term, intractable forms of chronic otitis media with effusion. Many of us have also seen a relatively high incidence of perforations after the use of this tube. This study documents a rate of perforations of almost 19%, with 7% of the patients requiring tympanoplasty subsequent to the use of this tube.—M.M. Paparella, M.D.

Incidence of Perforation With Goode T-Tube

Matt BH, Miller RP, Meyers RM, Campbell JM, Cotton RT (Univ of Cincinnati; Des Plaines, Ill)

Int J Pediatr Otorhinolaryngol 21:1–6, 1991 6–17

Objective.—Different regimens were compared in groups of children seen in the same years with chronic or recurrent otitis media who underwent T-tube placement. A total of 75 patients underwent myringotomy with insertion of a standard silicone T-shaped ventilating tube. Seventy-one other patients had myringotomy and insertion of a small grommet (Donaldson) tube, whereas 93 children received a Goode T-style tube.

Outcome.—The incidence of perforation in patients given a standard T tube was 13.6%. For those given a Donaldson grommet the rate was 1.8%, a significant difference. Children given a Goode T-style tube had an 18.8% rate of persistent perforation after 12 months. The overall rate of persistent perforation was 16.7% in 300 treated ears.

Recommendations.—Caution is suggested when using T tubes to treat middle ear disorders. Use of the Sheehy collar button tube for patients requiring prolonged middle ear ventilation is recommended. Alternately, the standard Armstrong tube is placed with its flange near the Eustachian tube entrance.

▶ This study, which is similar to the study outlined in Abstract 6–16, shows an incidence of perforation of almost 14% after use of this tube. Any tube—not only the Goode tube—has a potential for causing a perforation. I am reminded of Wullstein's former method of treating obstinate forms of intractable otitis media with effusion. He would create a large perforation on purpose to obviate the otherwise serious sequelae, such as chronic otitis media and chronic mastoiditis, that can result from otitis media with effusion. Certainly, perforations after the use of this and/or other tubes are to be avoided; however, it is more important to avoid serious long-term chronic disease with its sequelae or potential complications.—M.M. Paparella, M.D.

Development of Tympanosclerosis in Children With Otitis Media With Effusion and Ventilation Tubes

Maw AR (Bristol Royal Infirmary, Bristol, England)

J Laryngol Otol 105:614–617, 1991 6–18

Background.—Ventilation tube (VT) placement is the most frequent surgical indication for hospital admission of children. Several reports have related VT insertion in patients having otitis media with effusion to the later development of tympanosclerosis.

Series.—A group of 185 children, aged 3 to 9 years, with established bilateral otitis media with effusion underwent unilateral myringotomy with VT insertion. They were then followed prospectively for 5 years.

Findings.—The cumulative frequency of tympanosclerotic changes increased from 4.5% at 6 weeks to 40% at 2 years after VT insertion, and to 49% at 5 years (Fig 6–5). After 5 years, tympanosclerosis of some degree was present in 38.7% of the patients given only 1 VT (Fig 6–6). More severe changes were not seen in patients given more than 1 VT. After 5 years, tympanosclerotic change was evident in 2.8% of the contralateral ears not receiving treatment.

Conclusions.—As many as half of all ears with otitis media effusion treated with 1 or more ventilating tubes eventually may develop tympanosclerotic changes. No definite resolution of sclerotic change has been observed over time.

Recommendation.—Children with bilateral involvement might undergo bilateral myringotomy with aspiration of middle ear fluid, with a VT placed only in the ear with worse hearing. This would be especially appropriate for children who are to have adenoidectomy.

▶ This study and other studies have suggested that VTs cause tympanosclerosis of the tympanic membrane. My observation is that many patients with extensive tympanosclerosis have never had a VT inserted. Thus, it is clear that tympanosclerosis of both the tympanic membrane and the contents of the middle ear (including the promontory) can occur in patients who have a history of childhood otitis media even if a VT has not been inserted. We need

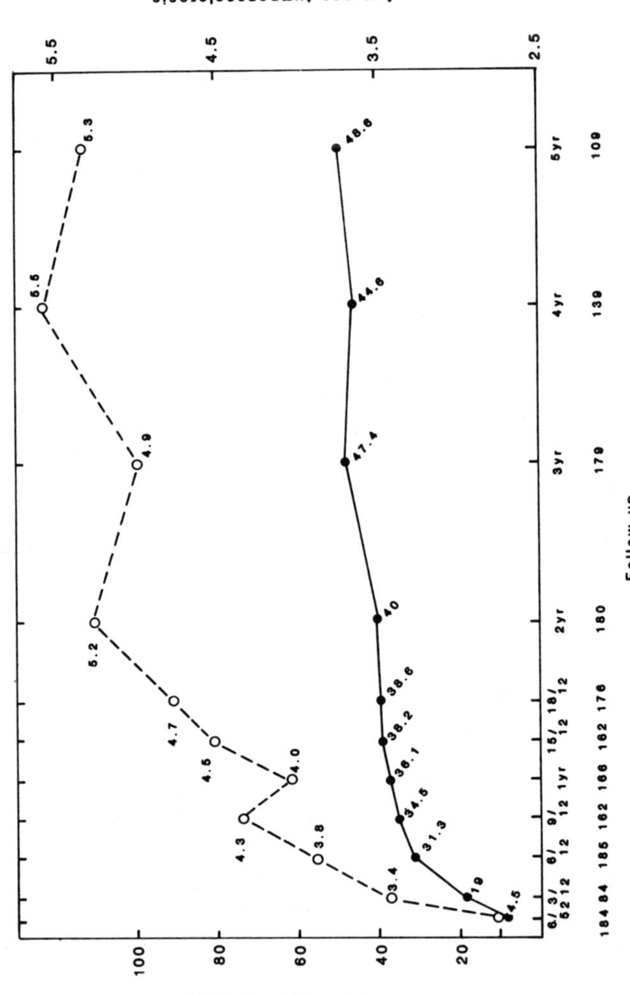

Fig 6–5.—The cumulative incidence for the development of tympanosclerosis in all cases (*solid line*) and the average tympanosclerosis score for those treated by insertion of more than 1 VT (*dashed line*). (Courtesy of Maw AR: *J Laryngol Otol* 105:614–617, 1991.)

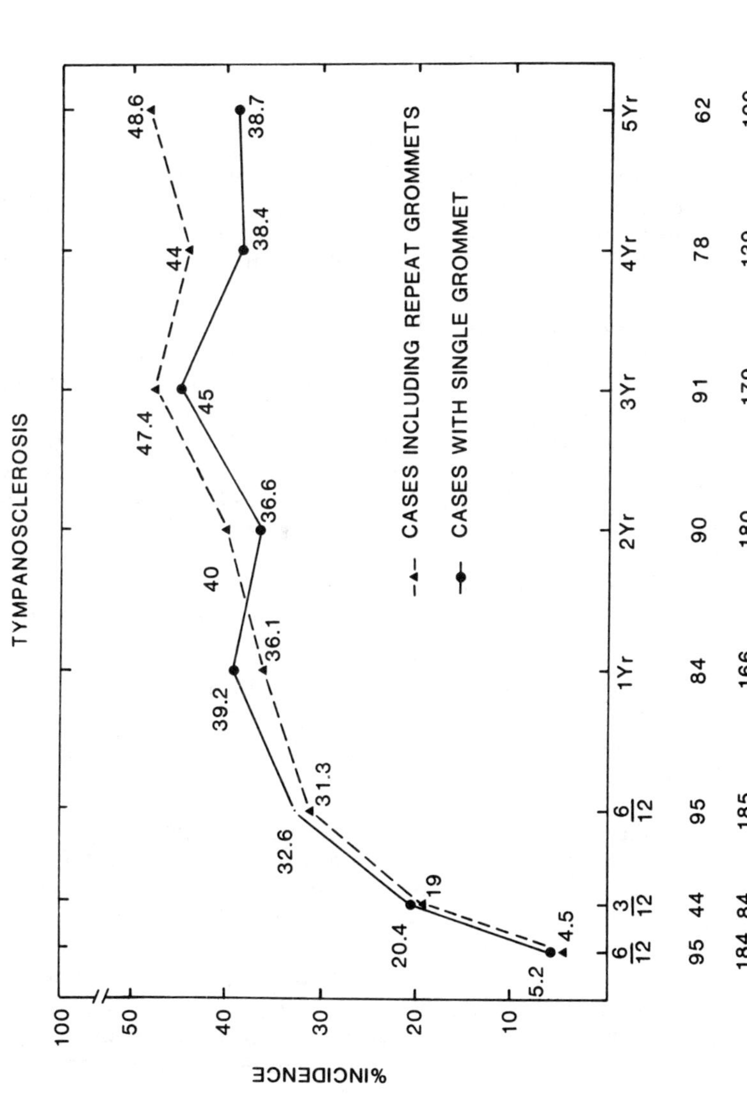

Fig 6–6.—The percentage incidence of tympanosclerosis in all cases (*dashed line*) and in those cases treated with VT insertion on only 1 occasion (*solid line*) during a 5-year postoperative follow-up. (Courtesy of Maw AR: *J Laryngol Otol* 105:614–617, 1991.)

a study to determine the incidence of tympanosclerosis in patients who have not had VTs, as well as in those who have undergone insertion.—M.M. Paparella, M.D.

The Deep Oval Window

Kapur TR (Stoke-on-Trent, England)

J Laryngol Otol 105:721–724, 1991 6–19

Background.—The relationship of the oval window to the promontory appears to vary. Sometimes the oval window appears to be relatively superficial; at other times, it seems deep. One cause of failure of total ossicular chain reconstruction using cortical bone grafts may be "deep oval window". This anatomical variation was better defined, and its approximate incidence was determined.

Methods and Observations.—Fifty temporal bones were studied. The visual impressions of superficial and deep oval windows appears to correspond fairly closely with the depth of the inferior wall of the fossula fenestra vestibuli. The depth of the superior and anterior fossula fenestra vestibuli walls did not seem to have such a dominating relationship when determining the deep oval window. In 86% of the specimens, there was not a well-defined posterior wall. When scar tissue forms between the superior, inferior, and anterior walls, the gap between the postero-superior part of the promontory and posterior tympanic wall could permit aeration of the deep oval window region. Closing this gap by a solid shelf of ponticulus or scar tissue may cause a localized malaeration of the fossula in most cases in which the oval window is deep.

Conclusions.—In these specimens, the visual impressions of the superficial and deep oval windows corresponded fairly well with the depth of the inferior fossular wall, more so than with any other measurement. Little overlap was seen between the groups.

▶ Our studies suggest that obstructive sites are an important part of the pathogenesis in chronic otitis media. Therefore, circumventing those sites is an important part of the management of patients with the disease. This finding of the deep oval window, which would necessarily be accompanied by a high promontory, plus the possibility of the umbo being attached to the promontory could result in an obstructive site being one of the pathogenetic factors of chronic otitis media. As this article suggests, the windows do vary; they can be deep, they can be wide, they can be narrow, there can be a high promontory, a shallow promontory, a protuberant fallopian canal or no fallopian canal. All these anatomical pathologic factors will be important in the pathogenesis of otitis media, as well as in treatment using ossiculoplasty with total or partial ossicular replacement prostheses.—M.M. Paparella, M.D.

Fibroblast Growth Factor Improves Healing of Experimental Tympanic Membrane Perforations

Mondain M, Saffiedine S, Uziel A (INSERM U254; Saint Charles Hosp, Montpellier, France)

Acta Otolaryngol (Stockh) 111:337–341, 1991 6–20

Introduction.—Several treatment methods have been proposed to promote the healing of perforations of the tympanic membrane. Fibroblast growth factor (FGF), a potent mitogen for mesodermal and neuroectodermal cells, was evaluated to determine its influence on the healing of tympanic membrane perforations in rats.

Methods.—Calibrated tympanic membrane perforations were performed in 30 rats. Each rat received 40 μL of a solution containing FGF at different concentrations in the left ear and 40 μL of placebo in the right ear. The quality of healing was observed by otomiscroscopy and by light microscopy of histological sections.

Results.—The mean time of healing was significantly shorter in the eardrums treated with 400 ng or 2,000 ng of FGF, compared with the placebo-treated ears. The higher dose of FGF was associated with a high rate of myringitis; this was not observed when 400 ng of FGF was given. Healing time did not differ significantly between the rats treated with 200 ng of FGF and the nontreated rats. Light microscopic studies revealed that the quality of healing was apparently comparable in both the treated and nontreated tympanic membranes.

Conclusion.—At a dose level of 400 ng, FGF accelerates the healing of traumatic tympanic membrane perforations in rats. Further studies are necessary to define the effect of FGF on nontraumatic tympanic perforations. Fibroblast growth factor may become an alternative to myringoplasty for the treatment of tympanic membrane perforations.

▶ This animal study is fascinating. Fibroblastic growth factor does improve the healing of experimentally induced perforations of the tympanic membrane. We can look forward to clinical studies in which FGF may be studied in patients in lieu of myringoplasty.—M.M.Paparella, M.D.

Anatomy of the Temporalis Fascia

Wormald PJ, Alun-Jones T (Groote Schuur Hosp, Cape Town, South Africa)

J Laryngol Otol 105:522–524, 1991 6–21

Background.—The use of autologous temporalis fascia for tympanoplasty has become commonplace. Because otolaryngologists are sometimes confused about the layers of the temporalis fascia, the anatomy of these different layers was reviewed.

Methods.—Light microscopy was used to study the superficial and deep layers of the temporalis fascia. Any histological difference between

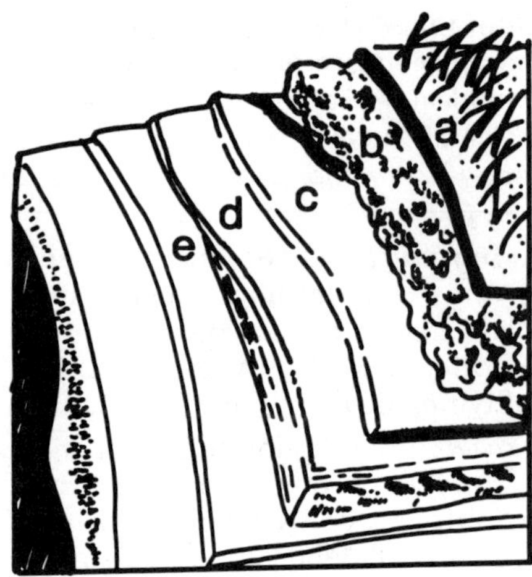

Fig 6–7.—Diagram showing the different layers of the scalp: *a,* skin; *b,* subcutaneous fat; *c,* superficial temporal fascia; *d,* deep temporal fascia; and *e,* periosteum. (Courtesy of Wormald PJ, Alun-Jones T: *J Laryngol Otol* 105:522–524, 1991.)

the 2 was noted. The physical characteristics of the layers were also assessed by measuring their Young's modulus in wet and dry states.

Findings.—Anatomically, the superficial layer is part of the epicranial aponeurosis. It covers the entire lateral aspect of the skull. The deep temporal fascial layers, measuring 10 cm × 12 cm exactly cover the temporalis muscle. The fascial layers have a separate arterial and venous suppy that enables them to be used as a homograft, rotation flap, or free microvascular flap. There were not histological differences between the 2 layers, nor was there any significant difference in elasticity. The fascial state of hydration was the most significant factor affecting elasticity (Figs 6–7 and 6–8).

Conclusions.—Much has been written about the use of temporalis fascia in the tympanoplasty, thereby prompting the need for a published otolaryngology study of the anatomy of the temporal fascial layers.

▶ Because otologists very commonly use temporalis fascia in both tympanoplasty and tympanomastoidectomy, this study of the tissue is long overdue. It has always been my contention that temporalis fascia represents collagen that can be removed in other places around the ear, either postauricularly or

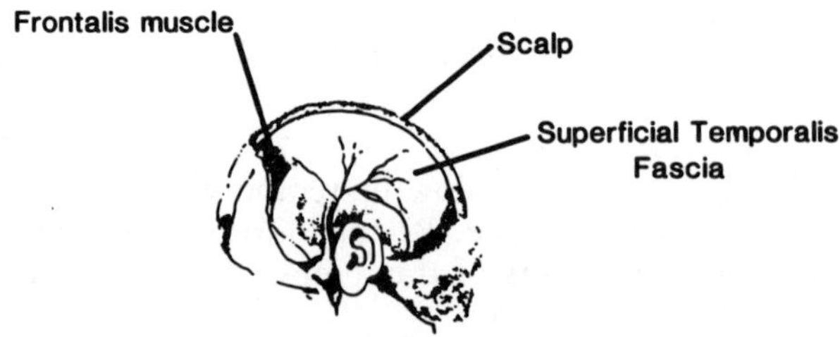

Fig 6–8.—Diagram showing the attachments of the left superficial temporal fascia. (Courtesy of Wormald PJ, Alun-Jones T: *J Laryngol Otol* 105:522–524, 1991.)

endaurally. When temporalis fascia is not available, I use postauricular collagen or collegen from other places. Sometimes I use periosteum and have found the results to be just as good. Temporalis fascia is collagen.—M.M. Paparella, M.D.

New Alloplastic Tympanic Membrane Material

Grote JJ, Bakker D, Hesseling SC, van Blitterswijk CA (Univ Hosp, Leiden, The Netherlands)

Am J Otol 12:329–335, 1991 6–22

Background.—Previous alloplastic devices for tympanic membrane closure have failed clinically or have only been assessed in animal studies. Researchers have developed a total alloplastic middle ear prosthesis for use in patients with an empty middle ear. It consists of a canal-wall segment of macroporous hydroxyapatite, from which an ossicular chain of dense hydroxyapatite is suspended. An alloplastic tympanic membrane of polymer was devised to connect the ossicular chain.

Study.—The biocompatibility of Polyactive, a polyether polyester copolymer, was examined after implantation in the rat middle ear. In addition to light and electron microscopy and morphometric study, autoradiographical studies were performed.

Observations.—Implants were totally covered by tympanic-membrane epidermis and epithelium by 4 weeks after placement. A mild foreign-body reaction was noted. More than half of the material was degraded after 1 year, but there was no resultant toxicity. Fibrous tissue and bone grew into the polymer, indicating mechanical interlocking of the implant. Contact was evident as early as a week after implantation, and it occurred with both submucosal and bone/muscle tissue implants.

Implications.—This degradable material can be effectively used both as temporary support in repairing large perforations and as a tympanic membrane in a total alloplastic middle ear prosthesis. The material is especially useful for fixing the hydroxyapatite ossicular chain to the canal wall of a prosthesis. Degradation products have not proved to be toxic in the first year after placement.

► This study, in which a polyether polyester copolymer was implanted in the middle ear was done in rats. Toxicity was nonexistent, and more than half the material was degraded after 1 year. This material apparently has possible clinical application to support a tympanoplastic graft. When doing tympanoplasty, it is always important to try to maintain an air space, particularly between the eustachian tube and the round window. Therefore, I try not to use Gelfoam or other similar materials to pack into the middle ear. Instead, I use grafting techniques such as overlay techniques, using the adjacent canal so as to avoid using Gelfoam in the middle ear. If I need to support the graft, I will use Gelfilm, again maintaining the middle-ear air space that helps eustachian tubal function and development of a cavum minor, posttympanoplasty.—M.M. Paparella, M.D.

Realities in Ossiculoplasty

Toner JG, Smyth GDL, Kerr AG (Royal Victoria Hosp, Belfast)

J Laryngol Otol 105:529–533, 1991 6–23

Background.—Closure of the air-bone gap is a reliable indicator of technical success in performing ossiculoplasty. This is meaningful in comparing materials or techniques, but it does not evaluate the effect on binaural hearing. It is important to evaluate the contribution of the other ear. A patient-oriented approach to the results of ossiculoplasty was developed.

Methods.—Previous research has indicated that an air conduction level of 30 dB must be attained in the operated ear for the speech frequencies, or be within 15 dB of that of the other ear, to insure a significant benefit. A Glasgow plot to illustrate hearing status was reviewed. The addition of a horizontal and vertical axis at 30 dB identified 3 categories of preoperative auditory status: unilateral, asymmetric bilateral, and symmetric bilateral hearing loss. This allows a graphic method of predicting the benefit of ossiculoplasty. One hundred patients with open mastoidectomy and 100 with staged combined approach tympanoplasty (CAT) were evaluated using this system.

Results.—The total average increase in air conduction for patients with CAT was 7 dB for those with an intact chain and 14.5 dB for those with myringostapediopexy (MSA). For patients with an open cavity, air conduction decreased by 1.7 dB in those with an intact chain and by .7 dB in those with MSA. The results were better when patients with worse postoperative hearing were excluded; however, poor outcomes would not be avoided by prediction. For many patients, the overall auditory status failed to improve.

Conclusions.—The surgeon must determine which conductive hearing losses can be improved surgically and the extent to which a patient's hearing loss can be relieved. Care must be taken to avoid making unduly optimistic statements to the patient. The surgeon must be aware of his or her own success rates in both closure of the air-bone gap and air conduction change.

▶ Ossiculoplasty is an important part of tympanoplasty and reconstruction of the middle ear. Too often in past studies, rosily optimistic results have been reported. I give credit to Toner, Smith, and Kerr because I believe they are trying to provide the real observations as we typically see them in such patients who have ossiculoplasty. Although many patients will have slight improvement, some will have none. We need to be forthright with our patients regarding the possible benefit of ossiculoplasty. As always, the ossiculoplasty cannot be isolated but will be connected to many other factors such as eustachian tubal dysfunction and chronic persistent pathologic conditions, as well as the patient's ability to heal after surgery.—M.M. Paparella, M.D.

Hearing Results With Incus and Incus Stapes Prostheses of Hydroxylapatite

Wehrs RE (St Francis Hosp, Tulsa, Okla)
Laryngoscope 101:555–556, 1991 6–24

Introduction.—Bony prostheses used to be made from the homograft incus to repair defects of the ossicular chain. Although excellent hearing was obtained, the use of human tissue carried disadvantages. Hydroxylapatite replacement prostheses now are available.

Applications.—The incus prosthesis is used to correct a break caused by a defect in the incus (Fig 6–9). The incus-stapes prostheses replaces the stapes superstructure as well, extending from the stapedial footplate to the handle of the malleus (Fig 6–10).

Results.—Between 1987 and 1989, 86 patients underwent middle ear reconstruction in the course of tympanoplasty. An ossicular defect was repaired using a hydroxylapatite incus or incus-stapes prosthesis. Of 60 patients with incus defects, 33 (55%) had an air-bone gap of 10 dB or

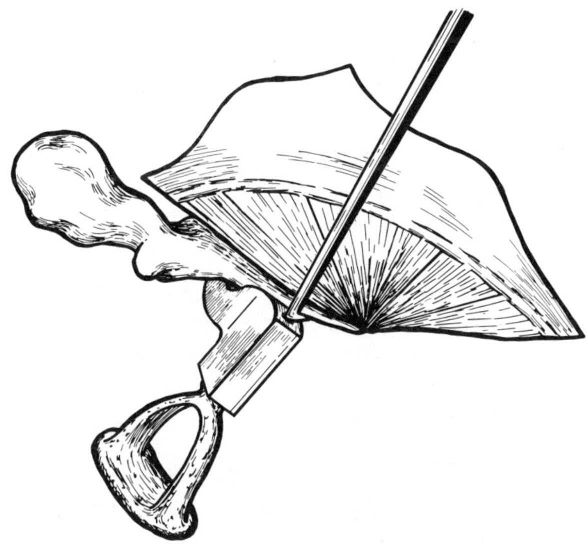

Fig 6–9.—The motion of the incus prosthesis is tested by exerting gentle pressure on the body of the prosthesis and noting the motion of the stapes, stapedial tendon, or round window reflex. (Courtesy of Wehrs RE: *Laryngoscope* 101:555–556, 1991.)

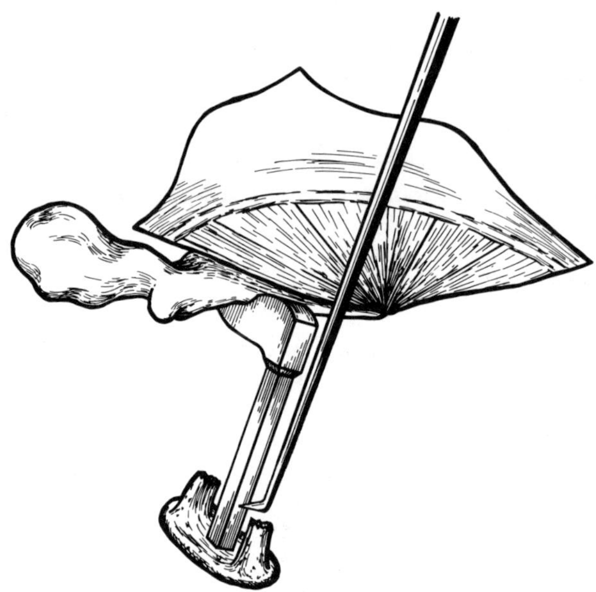

Fig 6–10.—Centering the shaft of the prosthesis on the stapedial footplate and checking its motion. (Courtesy of Wehrs RE: *Laryngoscope* 101:555–556, 1991.)

less and another 30% had a gap of 10–20 dB. In 12% of the cases there was an air-bone gap exceeding 30 dB, indicating failure. Of the 26 patients with a defect of the stapes superstructure as well as of the incus, 46% had an air-bone gap of 10 dB or less and 19% had a gap of 10–20 dB. The remaining patients had a fair outcome with an air-bone gap of 20–30 dB.

Discussion.—Incus and incus-stapes prostheses of hydroxylapatite appear to be satisfactory substitutes for homograft prostheses. The hearing results compare favorably with those obtained using bony prostheses.

▶ Hydroxylapatite has been found to be an apparently innocuous and fairly useful material for ossiculoplasty. Other materials have also been proven safe and useful. The results will depend not only on the substance or material used, but on the skill of the surgeon and on the many variables relating to the disease process itself.—M.M. Paparella, M.D.

Induced Atelectasis of the Middle Ear and Its Clinical Behavior

Luntz M, Eisman S, Sade J (Sackler School of Medicine; Tel-Aviv Univ, Ramat Aviv, Israel)

Eur Arch Otorhinolaryngol 248:286–288, 1991 6–25

Introduction.—Although atelectatic ears are frequently managed by inserting ventilating tubes (VTs), some patients may require repeated tube insertion. Some physicians prefer to use long-standing VTs; however, over time, many of these ears become "self-ventilated". Methods of determining whether a given atelectatic ear fitted with a VT still requires a tube ventilation were explored.

Procedure.—A group of 26 patients had received VTs in 36 ears because of nonadhesive atelectasis or retraction pockets. The average time of VT placement was approximately 7 months before admission to the study. The tympanic membrane had returned to its physiological position shortly after tube insertion. The tube was sealed by adhesive paper placed over its aperture using the operating microscope.

Results.—Four ears remained free of atelectasis after 10 days; their VTs were then removed. In the other ears, atelectasis or a retraction pocket reappeared, and the findings were generally similar to those present before VT insertion. Removal of the seals led to the resolution of atelectasis. Successful tympanometric testing further confirmed the effectiveness of the VT seal.

Implications.—The presence of some air in atelectatic ears rules out significant tubal narrowing and organic obstruction as causes of chronic middle ear underaeration. Reversion of atelectatic ears after sealing of a VT suggests that some controlling mechanism may be operative. Diffusion of gases into and out of the tissues or mucosal vessels is a possible mechanism.

▶ The authors nicely describe some of the problems and implications of the use of VTs in patients who have atelectasis. One of the important facts not emphasized in this study is that a collapse of the middle ear occurs when a patient has atelectasis. Because there is little or no space in which to insert a tube, extrusion is ensured rather rapidly. Clinically, if atelectasis is not accompanied by a hearing loss or other clinical problems (such as an early formation of cholesteatoma), our policy is to leave these atelectatic ears alone. However, when there is a clinical problem, the use of a VT and a carefully done underplant tympanoplasty (a widening of the middle ear both in terms of depth and diameter) accompanied by a VT will help guarantee a long-term successful result. If the ventilation tube extrudes after tympanoplasty, atelectatis will recur and the tube will have to be reinserted.—M.M. Paparella, M.D.

Management of Retraction Pockets of the Pars Tensa

Mills RP (Ninewells Hosp, Dundee, Scotland)

J Laryngol Otol 105:525–528, 1991 6–26

Background.—Retraction pockets of the pars tensa occur fairly commonly in patients with previous ear disease, especially otitis media with effusion (OME). The retraction pockets have been classified into 4 grades (Fig 6–11). The morbidity associated with retraction pockets of the pars tensa and the use of cartilage/perichondrium grafts were assessed.

Methods.—A group of 73 patients with retraction pockets of the pars tensa in 93 ears was studied. Of these, 32% had otalgia and 31% had episodes of aural discharge. Audiometric data was adequate for 75 ears, and the mean air-bone gap calculations were determined by using 500 Hz, 1,000 Hz, 2,000 Hz, and 4,000 Hz.

Results.—A total of 30% of the ears had air-bone gaps of less than 10 dB. In 93%, the air-bone gap was less than 30 dB, whereas 7% had air-bone gaps of more than 40 dB. Of this latter group, 7 patients were selected for surgery. The retraction pockets were elevated and everted in all patients. In 6 patients, a composite graft of cartilage and perichondrium was used to reinforce the thinned tympanic membrane. Four patients underwent ossiculoplasty. The retraction pockets remained completely everted in the early months, but by 12 months some degree of retraction recurred in 4 of the 6 patients who were followed for more than 12 months.

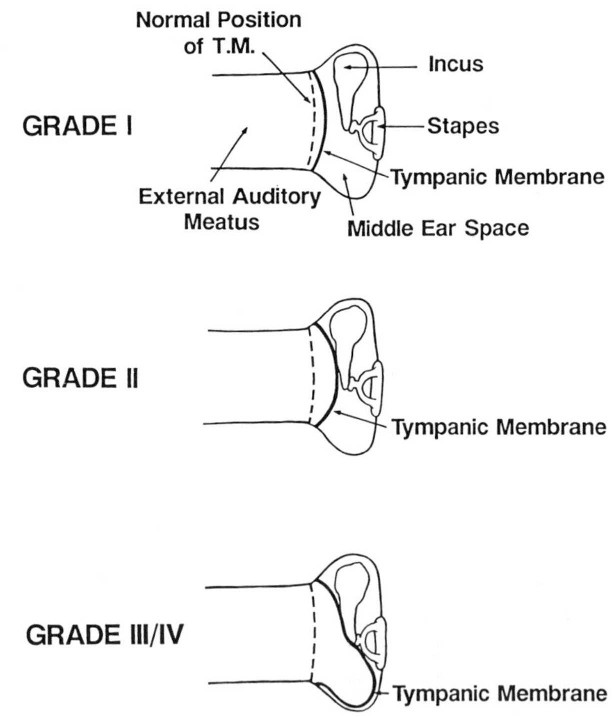

Fig 6–11.—Classification of the retraction pockets of the pars tensa proposed by Sade. (Courtesy of Mills RP: *J Laryngol Otol* 105:525–528, 1991.)

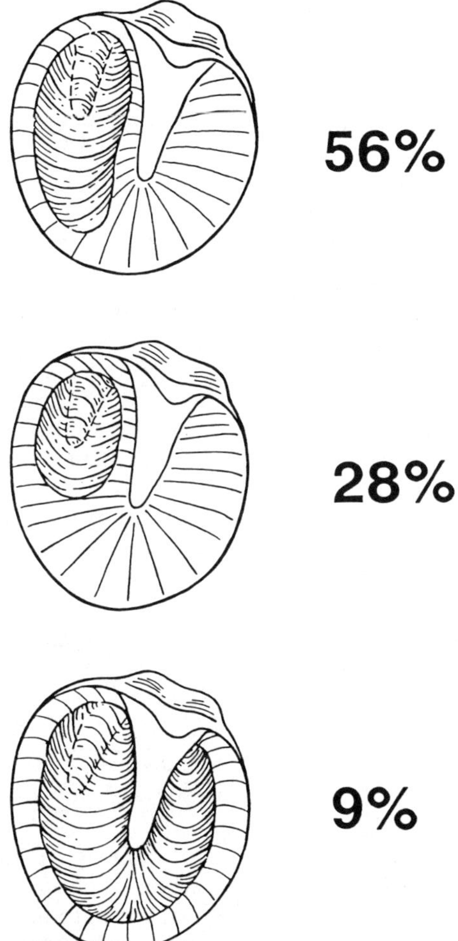

Fig 6–12.—The 3 most common patterns of drum retraction observed in the patient survey. (Courtesy of Mills RP: *J Laryngol Otol* 105:525–528, 1991.)

Conclusions.—The most common drum area to be affected by the retraction was the posterosuperior quadrant (Fig 6–12). The early results of the cartilage/perichondrial graft were promising; however, a progressively increasing recurrence rate for drum retraction was noted as time passed.

► This study describes what most of us see: the common site for a retraction pocket is the posterosuperior quadrant. An even more important site would be a region of the pars flaccida itself. Mills' methods of diagnosis and treatment seem reasonable. If clinical problems exist they should be treated;

they can be treated conservatively or more actively depending on the nature of the clinical problem.—M.M. Paparella, M.D.

The Effect of Mastoid Surgery on Atelectatic Ears and Retraction Pockets

Avraham S, Luntz M, Sadé J (Meir Hosp, Kfar Saba, Israel; Tel-Aviv Univ, Ramat Aviv, Israel)

Eur Arch Otorhinolaryngol 248:335–336, 1991 6–27

Background.—Atelectasis, the displacement of the tympanic membrane (TM) toward the promontory, has been graded. Grade 1 is a slight retraction of the TM, whereas grade 2 involves the drum touching the incus or stapes. In grade 3, the TM is inclined on the promontory; grade 4 changes involve the drum adhering to the promontory; and in grade 5, the TM is adherent and perforated. The management of atelectatic ears and retraction can be expectant, conservative, or surgical. Tympanoplasty limits the surgical treatment to the drum, whereas tympanomastoidectomy involves the mastoid. The benefits of different types of mastoid surgery in preventing the reformation of atelectatic ears were assessed.

Patients.—In 40 children and 53 adults, tympanoplasty was performed on 84 ears; tympanoplasty plus a mastoid operation was performed on 27 ears. Grades 1–3 atelectatic ears were considered reversible, and grades 4–5 were considered irreversible.

Findings.—The ears treated with tympanoplasty alone maintained better aeration of the middle ear than the ears treated with surgery involving the mastoid cell system.

Conclusions.—When conservative treatment of the atelectatic ear fails, a tympanoplasty confined to the TM and ossicular chain is the treatment of choice. If an associated retraction pocket deteriorates into a retraction pocket cholesteatoma, then more extensive surgery is needed.

► My observations have been similar to those described in this study. Surgical treatment of atelectasis in the absence of chronic pathologic conditions in the mastoid does not need be accompanied by a mastoidectomy to provide an increased air reservoir. Tympanoplasty alone works as well as, if not better than, tympanoplasty with mastoidectomy in patients who have atelectasis. I attempt to increase the air reservoir of the middle ear proper by increasing the diameter by extensive removal of attic and posterior bony anulus and also by increasing the depth of the mesotympanum by incising the tensor tympani, lateralizing the malleus, and using grafting techniques that do not compromise the middle ear space.—M.M. Paparella, M.D.

Inflammatory Disease of the Anterior Epitympanum

Collins ME, Coker NJ, Igarashi M (Baylor College of Medicine, Houston)

Am J Otol 12:11–15, 1991 6–28

Background.—Surgery for middle ear disease frequently reveals hidden pathologic conditions in the sinus epitympanic or the anterior epitympanic recess, an anterior extension of the epitympanum. Inflammatory disease can make access to this region difficult.

Anatomy.—In 94 horizontally sectioned human temporal bones, 48 of which had inflammatory disease, the epitympanic sinus was consistently present but quite variable in degree of development. The space first appeared at a level above the ampulla of the superior semicircular canal. Its medial wall was formed by the capsule of the fallopian canal superiorly and by the semicanal of the tensor tympani muscle inferiorly (Fig 6–13). The size of the sinus was similar in normal ears and in those with chronic inflammation.

Inflammation.—The same inflammatory changes involving the middle ear and mastoid were evident in the epitympanic sinus. Effusion and purulent exudate was often noted in the pneumatized areas. Rarefying osteitis occassionally involved the ossicles or attic wall (Fig 6–14). Osteitic changes were seen involving the ossicles or septa in 5 of 26 cases with acute inflammation.

Intervention.—Improved ventilation of the attic and mastoid is the goal of any reconstructive middle ear operation. Fischs' epitympanectomy requires complete exenteration of all air cells in the attic, as well as removal of air cells in the anterior epitympanic space. The tympanic isthmus may be widened either by radical epitympanectomy with opening of the epitympanic sinus or by posterior tympanotomy (Fig 6–15). This ap-

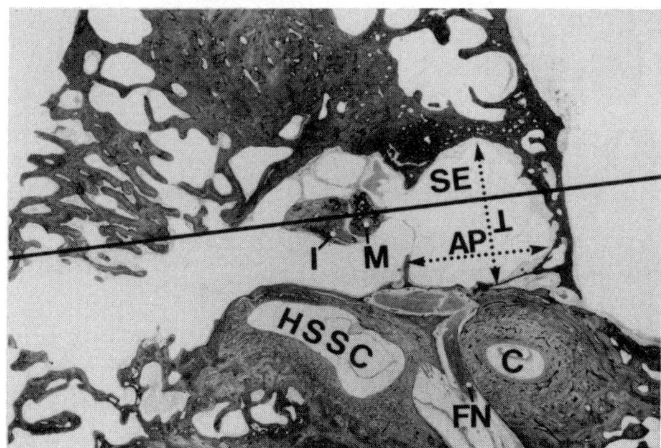

Fig 6–13.—*Abbreviations: M,* head of malleus; *I,* incus; C, cochlea; *HSSC,* horizontal semicircular canal; *FN,* facial nerve. The sinus epitympani (*SE*) and related structures along with the anteroposterior (*AP*) axis and the perpendicular (⊥) used to estimate relative size. (Courtesy of Collins ME, Coker NJ, Igarashi M: *Am J Otol* 12:11–15, 1991.)

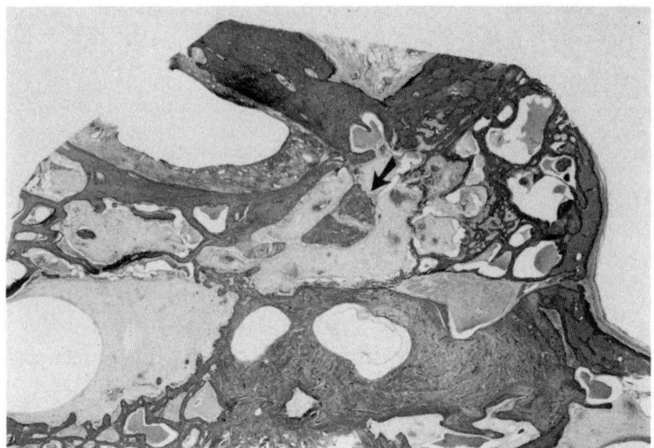

Fig 6–14.—Severe inflammation of the antrum and attic extending into the anterior epitympanic recess. Osteitis of the head of the malleus is present (*arrow*). (Courtesy of Collins ME, Coker NJ, Igarashi M: *Am J Otol* 12:11–15, 1991.)

proach provides good exposure for removing a diseased area and also a means of improving ventilation of the attic and mastoid.

▶ The pathology or nature of the inflammatory disease of the compartments of the middle ear cleft varies in chronic otitis media. In some patients, the disease will be diffuse and uniformly distributed throughout the middle ear cleft; in other patients, the disease may be localized to the attic, localized to the mastoid with exclusion of the mesotympanum, and so forth. Therefore, it

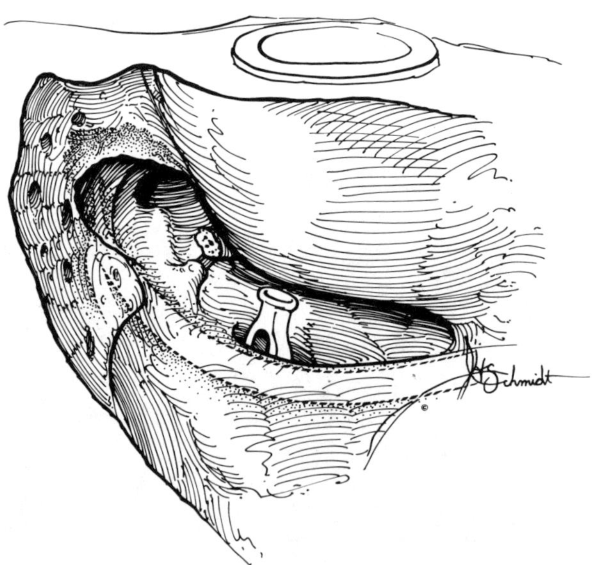

Fig 6–15.—Surgical view of the tympanic isthmus enlarged by posterior tympanotomy and by opening the anterior epitympanic recess. (Courtesy of Collins ME, Coker NJ, Igarashi M: *Am J Otol* 12:11–15, 1991.)

is important to look at the various compartments or sections of the middle ear cleft to see which are most actively involved in the pathogenesis and, therefore, treatment of the disease process. This study seems to substantiate the observation that obstructive sites are a part of this pathogenesis.—M.M. Paparella, M.D.

Surgery vs. Natural Course of Chronic Otitis Media: Long-Term Hearing Evaluation

Colletti V, Fiorino FG, Indelicato T (Univ of Verona, Verona, Italy)
Acta Otolaryngol (Stockh) 111:762–768, 1991 6–29

Background.—Assessments of the efficacy of surgery in chronic otitis media (COM) should not neglect the natural history of the disease. Whether tympanomastoid surgery modifies the natural trend of hearing deterioration in COM was investigated.

Methods.—A group of 41 patients with bilateral COM undergoing unilateral operations was studied. Thirteen had chronic otitis media with cholesteatoma; 24 had chronic otitis media without cholesteatoma; and 4 had tympanosclerosis. All the patients had the same type of disease in both ears and symmetric hearing loss. The contralateral ear was used as a comparison for assessing the natural course of the untreated disease vs. tympanoplasty. Auditory evaluations were done just before surgery and at 1–14 years after surgery.

Findings.—Both nonoperated and operated ears showed a progressive reduction in the hearing theshold as a function of time. Comparison of the threshold shifts between the 2 ears showed that the long-term functional results of tympanoplasty are satisfactory.

Conclusions.—Tympanomastoid surgery, arresting active chronic ear disease, prevents further damage to the middle and inner ear. The procedure should be considered an effective method for improving hearing function in COM.

► Colletti and coworkers accurately conclude that COM is caused by intractably pathologic tissue from granulation tissue or cholesteatoma or both. It is interesting that the ears that underwent mastoid surgery were found to have granulation tissue almost twice as often as cholesteatoma. In our own series, the ratio is closer to 50:50, and this is an observation that I have found in other countries as well. The point is that chronic, intractably pathologic tissue and its sequelae and complications can result from granulation tissue as well as from cholesteatoma. After patients have failed medical therapy, use of the treatment described in this article is the only way to bring the disease process under control and avoid sequelae in the inner ear and elsewhere.—M.M. Paparella, M.D.

Medical Treatment of Chronic Otitis Media: Steroid or Antibiotic With Steroid Ear-Drops?

Crowther JA, Simpson D (Stobhill Gen Hosp, Glasgow, Scotland)

Clin Otolaryngol 16:142–144, 1991 6–30

Background.—Ear drops that contain gentamicin and hydrocortisone have been effective in the treatment of active noncholesteatomatous chronic otitis media. However, whether this efficacy is caused by the contained steroid or by the combination of antibiotic and steroid has not been established.

Study Design.—Sixty-four patients with active noncholesteatomatous chronic otitis media were randomly assigned to receive either gentamicin with hydrocortisone ear drops or betamethasone ear drops for as long as 4 weeks. Activity in the ear, defined as the presence of mucoid or mucopurulent secretions in the middle ear or mastoid, was assessed at 2 weeks and 4 weeks.

Outcome.—Gentamicin with hydrocortisone drops was significantly more effective than betamethasone drops, producing inactivity in 80% of the treated ears. Only 29% of the ears treated with betamethasone were inactive. The same range of organisms were grown in both treatment groups.

Conclusion.—The effectiveness of gentamicin with hydrocortisone ear drops in the treatment of active noncholesteatomatous chronic otitis media may be attributed to the combination of antibiotic and steroid.

► *Pseudomonas* organisms continue to be common causative organisms of chronic otitis media, with chronic mastoiditis resulting from chronic intractable granulation tissue. Therefore, the use of gentamicin accompanied by a steroid seems logical. We need to be concerned about the ototoxic effects of medications at all times; however, I think the medication described in this study is safe as well as effective.—M.M. Paparella, M.D.

The Hypotympanum and Infralabyrinthine Cells in Chronic Otitis Media

Nadol JB Jr, Krouse JH (Mass Eye & Ear Infirmary, Harvard Med School, Boston)

Laryngoscope 101:137–141, 1991 6–31

Background.—Little research has focused on the role of the hypotympanum in chronic active otitis media; instead, emphasis has been placed on the role of recurrent cholesteatoma or unexenterated cells in the mastoid cell system in the etiology of recurrent disease. Seven cases of chronic otitis media in which clinical evidence suggested that the sole location of suppurative disease was the hypotympanum and infralabyrinthine cell tract were evaluated.

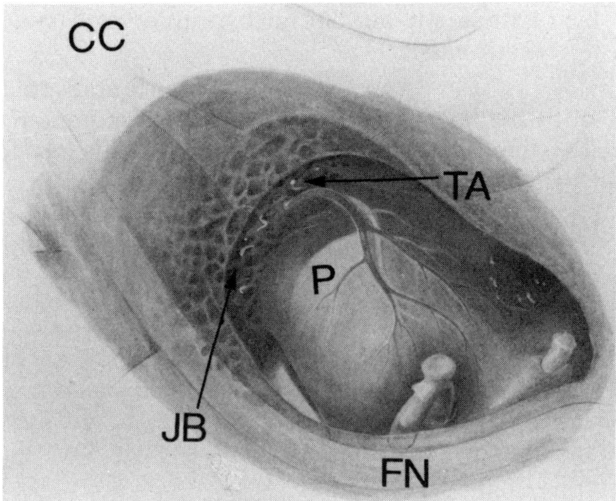

Fig 6–16.—Surgical anatomy of the hypotympanum, which is limited anteriorly by the petrous portion of the carotid canal *(CC)*, inferiorly by the jugular bulb *(JB)*, posteriorly by the facial nerve *(FN)*, superiorly by the promontory *(P)*, and laterally by the bony tympanic annulus *(TA)*. (Courtesy of Nadol JB Jr, Krouse JH: *Laryngoscope* 101:137–141, 1991.)

Patients.—The patients were 4 women and 3 men, aged 19 - 69 years. Follow-up ranged from 5 months to 23 years. Revision procedures were performed in 5 cases. The operative findings were granulation in the hypotympanum in 2 patients; granulation in peritubal and hypotympanum cells in 1; granulation filling hypotympanum cells with a disease-free mastoid bowl in 1; and residual cholesteatoma in hypotympanum and infralabyrinthine cell tracts skeletonizing the carotid artery and jugular vein in 1 patient. In the patients who underwent revision surgery, exentera-

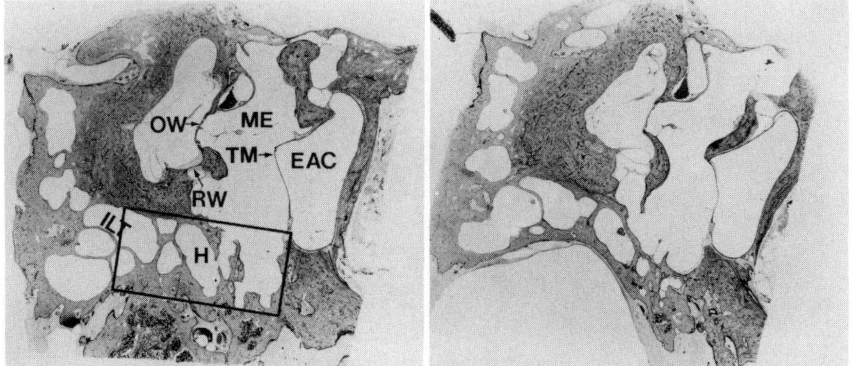

Fig 6–17.—*Abbreviations: EAC,* external auditory canal; *TM,* tympanic membrane; *M,* malleus; *ME,* middle ear; *OW,* oval window; *RW,* round window; *H,* hypotympanum; *ILT,* infralabyrinthine cell tract. **Left,** vertical section through a normal adult human temporal bone. The *H* is indicated by the boxed enclosure. The *ILT* extends from the *H* to the petrous apex. Hematoxylin = eosin; original magnification × 4.7. (Courtesy of Nadol JB Jr, Krouse JH: *Laryngoscope* 101:137–141, 1991.)

tion of the hypotympanum and infralabyrinthine cell system area resulted in asymptomatic ears.

Conclusions.—In these 7 cases, clinical evidence indicated that recurrent chronic otitis media was limited to the hypotympanum and infralabyrinthine cell system. Otolaryngolists should carefully inspect the hypotympanum in primary surgery for chronic ear disease. Exenteration of the hypotympanic and proximal infralabyrinthine cell tract is advocated when these areas contain cholesteatoma or extensive granulomatous disease (Figs 6–16 and 6–17).

► Earlier studies have suggested that the anterior epitympanum can be a focus of infection. This study suggests that the pathologic conditions can be limited to the hypotympanum and infralabyrinthine cellular system. Once again, the location of the pathologic condition may be generalized or more localized, and the otologist needs to consider these variations and treat them accordingly.—M.M. Paparella, M.D.

Tympanic Membrane Microstructure in Experimental Cholesteatoma

Wright CG, Bird LL, Meyerhoff WL (Univ of Texas Southwestern Med Ctr, Dallas)

Acta Otolaryngol (Stockh) 111:101–111, 1991 6–32

Objective.—Introduction of propylene glycol into the middle ear of the chinchilla produces structural changes in the tympanic membrane that are associated with cholesteatoma. This may be a useful model for so-called "papillary" cholesteatoma, which is believed by some to occur in humans when epidermis migrates through the tympanic membrane.

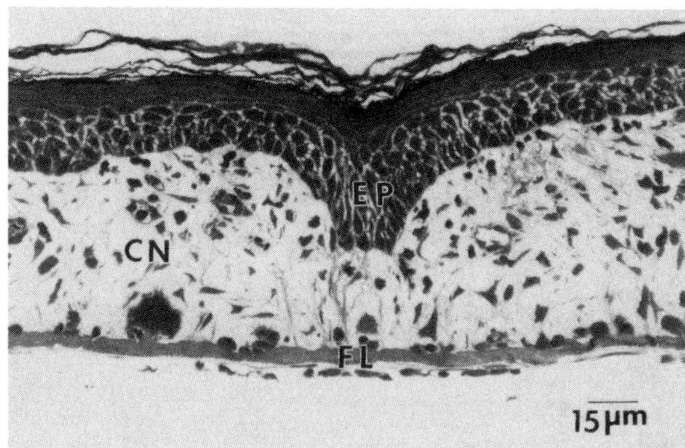

Fig 6–18.—Light micrograph of a tympanic membrane cross section at 2 weeks after propylene glycol administration. A papillary projection of epidermal cells *(EP)* is seen extending into the thickened connective tissue *(CN)* of the lamina propria. In this case, connective tissue hyperplasia is restricted to the portion of the tympanic membrane lateral to the fibrous layer *(FL)*. Some inflammatory cells are seen on the medial side of the fibrous layer near the center of the micrograph; however, the medial

aspect of the tympanic membrane remains denuded of mucosal cells in this area. (Courtesy of Wright CG, Bird LL, Meyerhoff WL: *Acta Otolaryngol (Stockh)* 111:101–111, 1991.)

The microstructural changes that occur when 50% propylene glycol is placed in the chinchilla middle ear were determined.

Observations.—The epidermal and mucosal layers of the tympanic membrane were destroyed 2 days after application of propylene glycol; however, the epidermal basal lamina remained intact over the lateral aspect of the lamina propria. The tympanic membrane became much thicker in the first 2 weeks after treatment, largely because of the growth of connective tissue in the lamina appropria adjacent to the fibrous layer (Figs 6–18 and 6–19). The epidermal basement membrane became fragmented at approximately 2 weeks, allowing the skin cells from the hyperplastic epidermis to migrate through gaps into the thick connective tissue of the lamina propria. Parts of the fibrous layer were often highly distorted at this stage. The mucosal cells appeared after approximately a week; in some areas they proliferated to form hyperplastic foci. Repair of the mucosal basal lamina was quite variable.

Discussion.—These findings support the view that cholesteatomas induced by applying middle ear irritants arise when epidermis penetrates through the structurally altered tympanic membrane. Rapid and uneven growth of connective tissue in the lamina propria distorts the fibrous layer and causes its structure to be severely disrupted in some areas of the tympanic membrane. Similar tympanic membrane changes have been observed in humans.

▶ It is easy to develop animal models to create chronic otitis media with intractable granulation tissue, thus mimicking the clinical situation. Chronic otitis media and chronic mastoiditis in animals occur as a natural continuum of experimentally induced serous otitis media. It is more difficult to create an

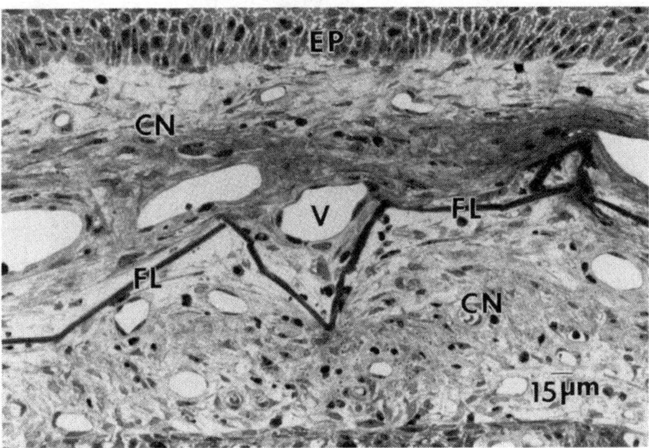

Fig 6–19.—Light micrograph showing marked hyperplasia of connective tissue *(CN)* and wavelike distortion of the fibrous layer *(FL)* of the tympanic membrane 2 weeks after propylene glycol application. Several widely dilated blood vessels (1 of which is marked by V) are seen lateral to the fibrous layer. *EP* = epidermis. (Courtesy of Wright CG, Bird LL, Meyerhoff WL: *Acta Otolaryngol (Stockh)* 111:101–111, 1991).

animal model to study cholesteatoma as it occurs in humans. Therefore, any animal model is very interesting and useful for studying the mechanisms of the formation of cholesteatoma in animals. The use of propylene glycol appears to stimulate epidermal migration through the structurally altered tympanic membrane, thereby resulting in cholesteatoma.—M.M. Paparella, M.D.

Mode of Growth of Acquired Cholesteatoma

Wells MD, Michaels L (Univ College and Middlesex School of Medicine, London)

J Laryngol Otol 105:261–267, 1991 6–33

Introduction.—Cholesteatoma is characterized by squamous epithelium in the middle ear cleft. Some cholesteatomas developing from re-

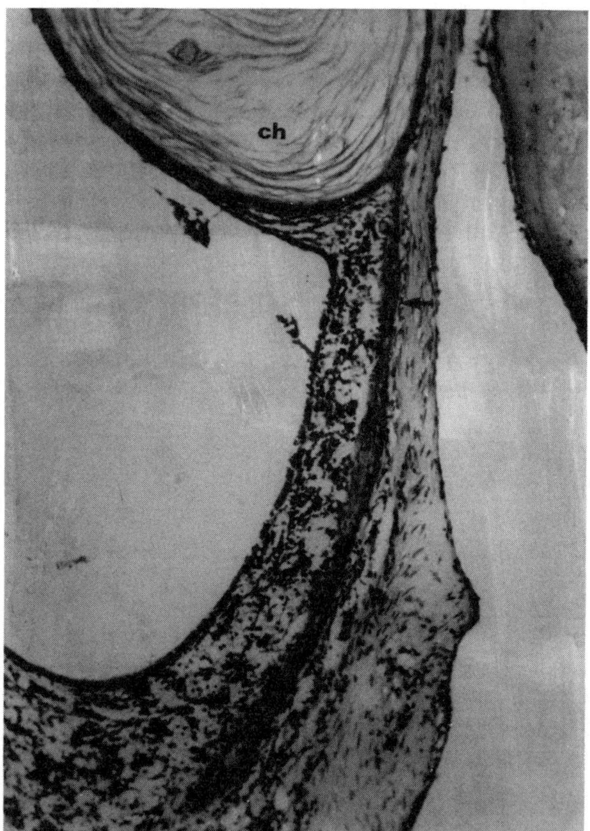

Fig 6–20.—Downgrowth of squamous epithelium *(arrow)* from cholesteatoma sac *(ch)*. (Courtesy of Wells MD, Michaels L; *J Laryngol Otol* 105:261–267, 1991.)

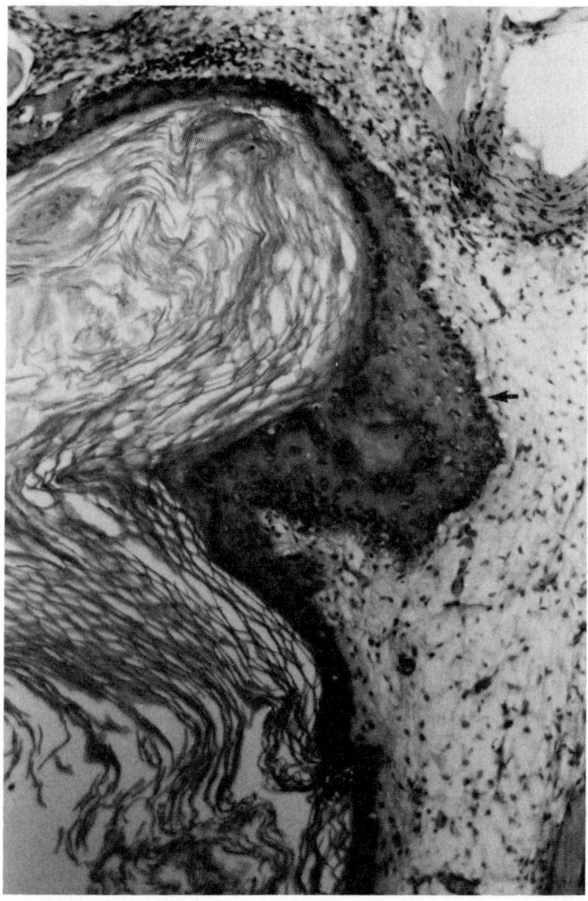

Fig 6–21.—Thickened epithelium shown *(arrow)*. (Courtesy of Wells MD, Michaels L: *J Laryngol Otol* 105:261–267, 1991.)

traction pockets of the tympanic membrane; however, their origin and mode of growth remain unclear. The origin and mode of growth of acquired cholesteatoma were studied.

Study Material.—Four temporal bones were removed at autopsy from 2 adults, aged 60 and 81 years, and 1 child, aged 11 years, with acquired cholesteatomas. The temporal bones were processed and stained by standard histological techniques.

Findings.—Histopathologic examination of the temporal bones confirmed that the origin of acquired cholesteatoma is the squamous epithelium in the retraction pockets of tympanic membrane. Persistent retraction pockets are formed secondary to chronic inflammation and fibrosis in the middle ear that are associated with chronic otitis media resulting in the loss of connective tissue of the tympanic membrane. The growth of cholesteatoma is similar to tongues of squamous epithelium extending from the deeper part of the sac into the middle ear, thereby replacing the mucosal layer of the tympanic membrane (Fig 6–20). The squamous epithelium may be thickened at the site of the growth (Fig 6–21). Keratin pearl formation is also a frequent finding.

Conclusion.—Acquired cholesteatoma originates from retraction pockets. Inflammation is an important factor in the growth of cholesteatoma. Active growth of the squamous epithelium of the retraction pockets may be enhanced in the presence of chronic otitis media.

▶ Cholesteatoma can develop in various ways. Its origin is often the retraction pockets. This study nicely documents histological findings that demonstrate that retraction pockets can and do become cholesteatomas. Therefore, if we can identify a retraction pocket that will become a cholesteatoma, we would be wise to treat it early, before an extensive cholesteatoma develops.—M.M. Paparella, M.D.

Patterns of Epithelial Migration in the Unaffected Ear in Patients With a History of Unilateral Cholesteatoma

Moriarty BG, Johnson AP, Patel P (Queen Elizabeth Hosp, Birmingham, England)

Clin Otolaryngol 16:48–51, 1991 6–34

Introduction.—Squamous epithelium on the normal human tympanic membrane migrates in a spiral centrifugal manner. This migration serves to remove debris from the ear canal and has a role in the healing of tympanic membrane perforations. Whether an inherent abnormality in the tympanic membranes of certain patients causes faulty epithelial migration leading to the development of cholesteatoma was determined.

Patients.—A group of 15 patients who had undergone mastoid exploration in 1 ear for cholesteatoma and who had a normal contralateral ear on otoscopic examination participated in the study. The tympanic membranes in the unaffected ears were marked in a standard pattern using India ink. The progress of the ink dots was recorded by regular photography during a 4-month period until all the ink dots had disappeared from the tympanic membrane.

Results.—All the patients showed the typical spiral centrifugal pattern of epithelial migration on the tympanic membrane of their unaffected ear. The epithelial migration superiorly from the umbo along the malleus handle and into the attic region was continuous and uninterrupted. The speed of epithelial migration superiorly along the malleus handle varied from .04 mm to .11 mm per day.

Conclusion.—Defective epithelial migration is not the initiating factor in the development of acquired cholesteatoma.

▶ This study is interesting. It demonstrates that the migratory pattern of epithelium in a radial fashion on the tympanic membrane is normal in the unaffected ear of patients who have unilateral cholesteatoma. Of course, we don't know if the migratory pattern would have been abnormal or normal before the formation of cholesteatoma in the involved ear requiring surgery. The fact that one ear develops a cholesteatoma need not mean that the opposite ear will do so, and the conditions may be quite different. The study of migratory patterns in both the tympanic membrane the adjacent ear canal is useful in trying to better understand the pathogenesis of the formation of cholesteatoma in patients.—M.M. Paparella, M.D.

Management of Childhood Cholesteatoma

Mills RP, Padgham ND (Ninewells Hosp, Dundee)
J Laryngol Otol 105:343–345, 1991 6–35

Background.—The 2 main types of cholesteatoma are attic cholesteatoma and that arising from retractions of the pars tensa. The latter type

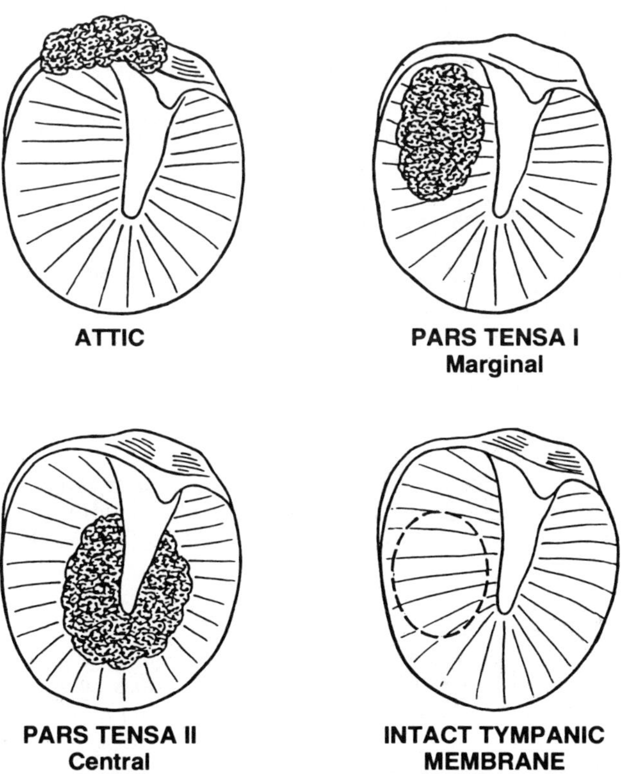

Fig 6–22.—Otoscopic classification of cholesteatoma. (Courtesy of Mills RP, Padgham ND: *J Laryngol Oncol* 105:343–345, 1991.)

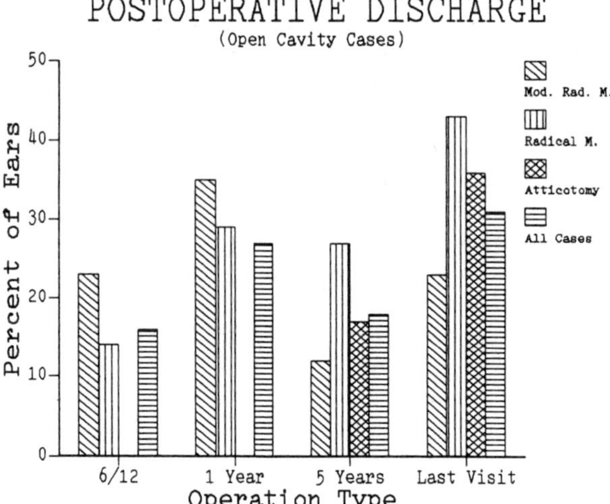

Fig 6–23.—*Abbreviations: Mod. Rad. M.*, modified radical mastoidectomy; *Radical M.*, radical mastoidectomy. Incidence of postoperative discharge in patients undergoing open cavity operations. (Courtesy of Mills RP, Padgham ND: *J Laryngol Oncol* 105:343–345, 1991.)

is subdivided into lesions of the posterosuperior quadrant of the drum and those of the central part. A fourth category in this scheme was proposed so that lesions occurring behind an intact tympanic membrane are also included (Fig 6–22). A series of children with cholesteatoma was reviewed.

Patients and Outcomes.—A total of 54 children with 57 involved ears had surgery for cholesteatoma before their sixteenth birthdays. Most of the children had open cavity operations, including modified radical mastoidectomy, radical mastoidectomy, and atticotomy. The incidence of residual disease was only 6%. Overall, 70% of the ears were free of chronic discharge after surgery (Fig 6–23). The postoperative hearing thresholds were disappointingly low, but they were not generally worse than they were before surgery. The mean postoperative hearing level was 39 dB, and the mean air-bone gap was 29 dB.

Conclusions.—Open cavity surgery offers the most satisfactory results in the treatment of childhood cholesteatoma. Although intact canal wall mastoidectomy can be used in the treatment of patients with limited disease, it should not be the procedure of choice.

▶ I agree with these authors. Open cavity cholesteatoma in children would be preferable to multiple operations that could be avoided if a multistaged closed-cavity approach was used. However, cholesteatomas develop in children in the same manner they develop in adults, in varying locations and to varying degrees. A cholesteatoma can be small and isolated, requiring only an atticotomy or a small antrotomy. Once in a while, congenital cholesteatomas can be treated only with a middle ear approach. Thus, mastoidectomy should be avoided in children if possible, unless the cholesteatoma definitely invades the mastoid per se and requires open cavity tympanomastoidectomy.—M.M. Paparella, M.D.

Otogenic Brain Abscess in Childhood
Murthy PSN, Sukumar R, Hazarika P, Rao AD, Mukulchand, Raja A (Kasturba Med Coll and Hosp, Manipal, India)
Int J Pediatr Otorhinolaryngol 22:9–17, 1991 6–36

Introduction.—Central nervous system complications of middle ear infection are much rarer than in the past; however, they still do occur. Ten patients who were seen before 15 years of age with otogenic brain abscess were reviewed between 1984 and 1990.

Clinical Findings.—Two patients had a temporal-lobe abscess, whereas 8 were seen with cerebellar abscesses. All of the abscesses were ipsilateral to the otitis media. Computed tomography led to a diagnosis in 80% of the cases. Four patients had no neurological abnormalities when admitted to an otolaryngology unit, and they underwent primary mastoid surgery. Headache, vertigo, and vomiting developed within the following week.

Treatment and Outcome.—Half of the patients underwent burrhole aspiration alone or in conjunction with craniotomy for excision of mass lesions. All patients were discharged without neurological deficit. Cholesteatoma and granulations were consistent findings.

Recommendations.—A child suspected of having intracranial extension of middle ear infection must be closely observed. Computed tomography is the single most effective diagnostic measure. The mass effect of an abscess is usually managed by burrhole aspiration if major neurosurgery is not feasible; the abscess may be excised at a later time. Definitive mastoid surgery is indicated after drainage or excision of the brain abscess.

► In the past, some researchers advocated otologic surgery as the first priority in treating the disease and draining the abscess from the intracranial space. In this study, the first priority is intracranial treatment of the abscess via a burrhole aspiration or excision of the abscess, followed by definitive mastoid surgery. I agree with this approach, and I would assume that many otologists would have a similar point of view.—M.M. Paparella, M.D.

Mastoid Misery: Quantifying the Distress in a Radical Cavity
Males AG, Gray RF (Addenbrooke's Hosp, Cambridge, England)
Clin Otolaryngol 16:12–14, 1991 6–37

Introduction.—Symptomatic mastoid cavities are common. Patients who have postoperative symptoms reminiscent of their primary disease may benefit from revision surgery. A method for quantifying the subjective symptoms of radical cavities was evaluated.

Method.—Between 1984 and 1988, 48 patients with troublesome cavities underwent revision procedures. Thirteen patients underwent meatoplasty, 11 had revision mastoidectomy, 11 underwent revision mastoidectomy with meatoplasty, and 4 had mastoid obliteration. All 48 patients were sent a questionnaire compiled by the physicians; 39 replied. The questionnaire asked the patient to rate 5 symptoms, including pain, wax, discharge, smell, and giddiness (defined as dizziness with cold winds or loud sounds) as experienced before and after the revision operation. The scores ranged from 0 points for "never" to 3 points for "always." Thus, the total score for the 5 symptoms could range from 0–15.

Results.—The mean preoperative score was 6.8, and the mean postoperative score was 2.1. The mean improvement was 4.7 points (69%). Dis-

	Never	Some of the time	Most of the time	Always	Total score
Pre-op					
Pain	16	11	6	6	41
Wax	28	7	2	2	17
Discharge	2	6	6	25	93
Smell	2	10	5	22	86
Giddiness	22	10	4	3	27
Post-op					
Pain	25	12	2	0	16
Wax	26	13	0	0	13
Discharge	23	11	2	3	24
Smell	27	9	2	1	16
Giddiness	27	11	0	1	14

Fig 6–24.—All responses superimposed (no. = 39). Total scores were calculated from the responses for each symptom, e.g., total pain score preoperatively is given by: $(16 \times 0) + (11 \times 1) + (6 \times 2) + (6 \times 3) = 41$. (Courtesy of Males AG, Gray RF: *Clin Otolaryngol* 16:12–14, 1991.)

charge and smell were the predominant preoperative symptoms (Fig 6–24). Both symptoms were dramatically reduced after revision.

Conclusion.—This can be used to quantify the subjective symptoms of radical cavities. The preoperative symptom score may be used to predict the likely outcome of revision surgery for symptomatic radical cavities. The questionnaire does not address the problem of hearing loss because the revision procedures performed in this group of patients were not primarily intended to alter the hearing threshold.

▶ The authors' methods of scoring and treating chronic mastoid cavities are of interest. I believe it is difficult, however, to provide a scoring method, because the techniques will vary from surgeon to surgeon. My approach to these patients would be different. Obviously, if there is already a mastoid cavity, then the patient would have a careful mastoidectomy done by circumferential extensive saucerization. This would be followed by removal of normal cortical bone posteriorly, superiorly, and inferiorly, which would reduce the cavity by 50% or more in most patients. This will often be followed by a Thiersch graft several weeks later; the cavity will usually be dry within a matter of a couple of weeks. The matter of scoring is of interest and may be adapted by others; however, it should not be forgotten that the major objective is to achieve a safe, dry ear in all patients.—M.M. Paparella, M.D.

HEAD AND NECK SURGERY

BYRON J. BAILEY, M.D., F.A.C.S.

Introduction

The specialty of otolaryngology–head and neck surgery has had an important year in terms of the exciting advances in both our knowledge of disease processes and our ability to diagnose disease and treat patients more effectively. The new scientific information reported by researchers and clinical observers around the world is quite impressive when one has the opportunity to review the 50 or 60 English language publications in our specialty monitored by the YEAR BOOK staff. We have made an effort to identify and summarize the essence of the best of these articles for you, and we are offering our comments in an attempt to place this information in a useful perspective. Major advances in flap reconstruction of the head and neck using the pectoralis major myocutaneous, the lower trapezius myocutaneous, and the serratus anterior myocutaneous flaps are summarized. Oromandibular reconstruction using vascularized composite free flaps is a hot topic this year. Also, there is considerable interest in the diagnosis and treatment of thyroid cancer, with particular reference to intraoperative diagnosis and surgical strategy (*as well as to*) the changing trends in the surgical management of thyroid malignancy. Carcinoma in situ and early cancer of the larynx continue to be important topics, with particular reference to ultraconservative surgical management. Bilateral true vocal cord paralysis presents a difficult challenge in terms of rehabilitation either by arytenoidectomy or by the use of the new muscle/nerve transfer procedure designed to reinnervate the larynx. New absorbable implants have shown promise in the optimal management of orbital floor blowout fractures. The diagnosis and management of seasonal allergic rhinitis has drawn attention this year as well.

As in previous years, laser surgical procedures, functional endoscopic sinus surgery, and improvements in clinical diagnosis are important areas of interest that physicians are incorporating in their daily clinical activities. As we have sifted through the many publications of the past year, we have been impressed by the volume and quality of subject matter available to include in this volume. This will be my final year as editor of this portion of the YEAR BOOK, and I am continually impressed by the dedication and expertise of the staff of the YEAR BOOK as they boil these articles down to the essence and report them in a precise and readable fashion. I have enjoyed working with this staff to identify the best of what is available in the literature, with particular reference to important information that you might have missed if you read only 2 or 3 specialty journals. We understand the limits of this book, and we hope that we are successful in our effort to bring you a series of capsules that will interest and stimulate you to pursue these subjects in more detail.

Our ultimate goal is to help you identify a few important, new elements that you will be able to integrate into your practice each year. If we have been able to accomplish this with your participation in the learning process, then we believe that our time and effort has been well spent and that your patients will benefit from what we have accomplished.

Byron J. Bailey, M.D., F.A.C.S.

7 Larynx

Arytenoidectomy and Posterior Cordectomy for Bilateral Abductor Paralysis

El Chazly M, Rifai M, El Ezz AA (Cairo, Egypt)

J Laryngol Otol 105:454–455, 1991 7–1

Background.—Arytenoidectomy performed for correcting compromised airways in patients with bilateral adbuctor paralysis has been reported to yield satisfactory results. The treatment of 12 patients with bilateral fixed vocal cords seeking decannulation of their tracheostomies was evaluated.

Technique.—A Kleinsasser's operating laryngoscope with self-retaining chest support was fixed to expose the glottis and supraglottis. Using the microscope, the right arytenoid was infiltrated with adrenaline in the submucosal and muscular planes. An incision was made 10 minutes later to expose the arytenoid, beginning from the posterior half of the vocal ligament and extending over the vocal process, curving parallel to the muscular process (Fig 7–1). A lingual flap of mucosa was then elevated as close as possible to the cartilage. The cartilage was grasped with arytenoid forceps, and as it was rotated in clockwise and counterclockwise directions, the attachments to the surrounding tissues were cut until the cartilage was entirely free. Bleeding was controlled with fine needle point electrocoagulation. The entire periarytenoid pocket was cauterized to promote cicatricial formation to draw the vocal cord laterally. The removal of the posterior third of the vocal ligament completed the posterior cordectomy. The prominent overlapping ventricular bands were then trimmed, and the mucosal flap was put back in place (Fig 7–2).

Conclusions.—Posterior cordectomy appears to be essential to potentiate the outcomes of endoscopic arytenoidectomy. The lingual-shaped

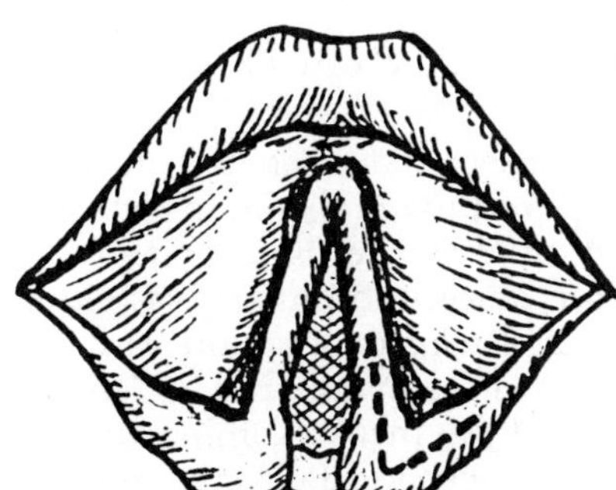

Fig 7–1.—Mucosal incision. (Courtesy of El Chazly M, Rifai M, El Ezz AA: *J Laryngol Otol* 105:454–455, 1991.)

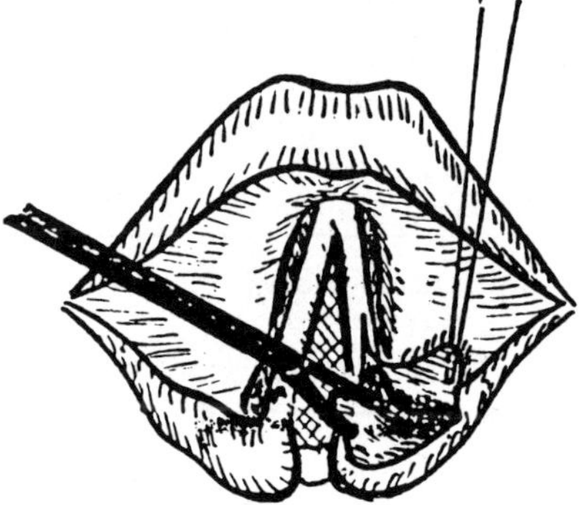

Fig 7–2.—Mucosal flap. Arytenoid cartilage separated and removed. (Courtesy of El Chazly M, Rifai M, El Ezz AA: *J Laryngol Otol* 105:454–455, 1991.)

incision over the arytenoid prevents posterior commissure webbing, and the flap repositioning at the end of the procedure avoids the exposure of raw surfaces with subsequent granulation tissue formation.

▶ Thornell described endoscopic arytenoid excision for bilateral TVC paralysis in 1948; he reported a success rate of 98%. Others have not been able to achieve this level of success, and external arytenoidectomy (as described by Woodman) has generally been more widely used. In recent years, laser arytenoidectomy has been found to be useful in many patients. This study returns to the method of endoscopic surgical excision with 100% decannulation success. Whether the arytenoid is removed surgically with dissection or with the laser, excision of the posterior one third to one half of the cord has been an important step in my experience.—B.J. Bailey, M.D., F.A.C.S.

Muscle Transfer for Laryngeal Paralysis: Restoration of Inspiratory Vocal Cord Abduction by Phrenic-Omohyoid Transfer
Crumley RL (Univ of California at Irvine)
Arch Otolaryngol Head Neck Surg 117:1113–1117, 1991 7–2

Introduction.—Denervation atrophy of the posterior cricoarytenoid (PCA) muscle develops after recurrent laryngneal nerve paralysis and deters the restoration of inspiratory muscle contraction. Cyclical inspiratory drive to the denervated PCA muscle has been restored by transfer of omohyoid muscle.

Technique.—The phrenic nerve was transected low in the neck of adult monkeys. The ansa hypoglossi branch to the omohyoid muscle was transected, and the phrenic nerve was sutured to the distal end of this branch (Fig 7–3). The superior belly of the omohyoid muscle was either detached from the hyoid bone or transected near its junction with the inferior belly; it was left attached superiorly to the hyoid. The cut end of the muscle was then rotated medially behind the thyroid lamina and sutured to the medial edge of the ipsilateral denervated PCA muscle. The

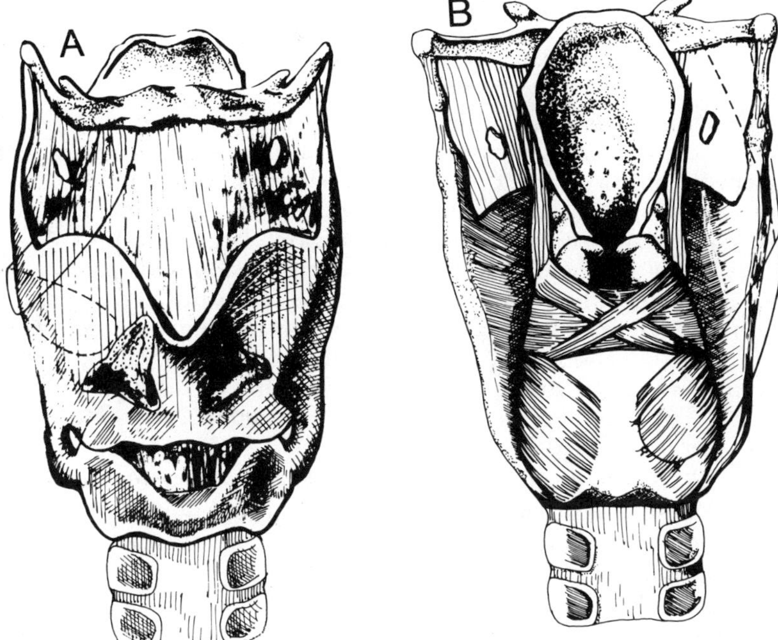

Fig 7–3.—Diagram of phrenic nerve-omohyoid muscle transfer. **A,** anterior view; **B,** posterior view. Superior belly of omohyoid muscle is transected above the tendon. (Phrenic nerve anastomosis to the omohyoid nerve branch is not shown.) The cut end of the omohyoid muscle is trimmed and then sutured to the medial aspect of the ipsilateral posterior cricoarytenoid muscle and the muscular process of the arytenoid. (Courtesy of Crumley RL: *Arch Otolaryngol Head Neck Surg* 117:1113–1117, 1991.)

part of the muscle flap approximating the muscular process of the arytenoid was joined to the process.

Results.—The best results were obtained when the muscle was pedicled on the hyoid bone. Electromyograms confirmed reinnervation of the omohyoid and PCA muscles by the phrenic nerve. Histological study also gave evidence of PCA reinnervation.

Clinical Trial.—The approach was tried in 1 patient who subsequently was able to have tracheotomy decannulation. The procedure has potential for use in long-standing PCA denervation atrophy and also for reinnervating a denervated PCA muscle.

► Crumley has been a major innovator in the quest for laryngeal reinnervation. The technique of using the phrenic nerve to reinnervate the paralyzed PCA muscle has not been successful in humans; however, this may have been the result of either residual innervation by the recurrent laryngeal nerve or PCA muscle atrophy. This abstract provides some grounds for optimism that the procedure may ultimately be useful in a clinical setting.—B.J. Bailey, M.D., F.A.C.S.

Teflonomas of the Larynx and Neck

Wenig BM, Heffner DK, Oertel YC, Johnson FB (George Washington Univ)

Hum Pathol 21:617–623, 1990 7–3

Introduction.—Surgical trauma to the recurrent laryngeal nerve and the presence of tumors in the vocal cord or recurrent laryngeal nerve represent the major causes of vocal cord paralysis. Such paralysis can result in aspiration problems related to open glottic incompetence, ineffective cough, and reduced voice production. Beginning in 1911, patients with vocal paralysis were treated with injections of paraffin into the paralyzed cord; however this procedure was abandoned because extravasation of the paraffin into surrounding tissue frequently produces a "paraffinoma." Teflon paste can be used instead of paraffin; however "Teflonomas" can form, and these are difficult to distinguish from a neoplasm. The complications and results of injecting Teflon into the vocal cord were examined.

Methods.—The records of 7 patients in whom a laryngeal lesion or neck mass developed as a reaction to a Teflon injection were reviewed. An additional case of Teflonoma in a patient treated for vocal cord paralysis at another institution was also studied.

Findings.—The 5 women and 3 men ranged in age from 31 to 72 years. The initial causes of vocal cord paralysis included surgical trauma, postviral neuritis, and primary or metastatic carcinoma. The cause of paralysis remained unknown in 1 patient. Symptoms such as persistent hoarseness or a neck mass were present from 1 month to 15 years after injection of Teflon. The tumors were described as polyploid lesions with the submucosal compartment of the vocal cord. Microscopic analysis of the masses identified a glassy-appearing material that was birefringent under polarized light within the multinucleated giant cells (Fig 7–4). Scanning electron microscopy of the material demonstrated many ovoid-to-spherical shaped particles with a flaky appearance. Of the 8 patients, 5 underwent surgical removal of the Teflon-induced lesion, which improved or eliminated all symptoms. One patient had the material aspirated from the mass.

Conclusions.—Teflon injection still appears to be the treatment of choice for unilateral vocal cord paralysis. Although it seems to be a safe procedure, physicians should be aware of the possible complications that may mimic the presence of a neoplasm.

▶ The results of intracordal Teflon injection for TVC paralysis are generally satisfactory. However, placement of the Teflon bolus a few millimeters from the vocalis muscle may produce a subglottic bulge or a lateral "Teflonoma" that can be seen as a neck mass.—B.J. Bailey, M.D., F.A.C.S.

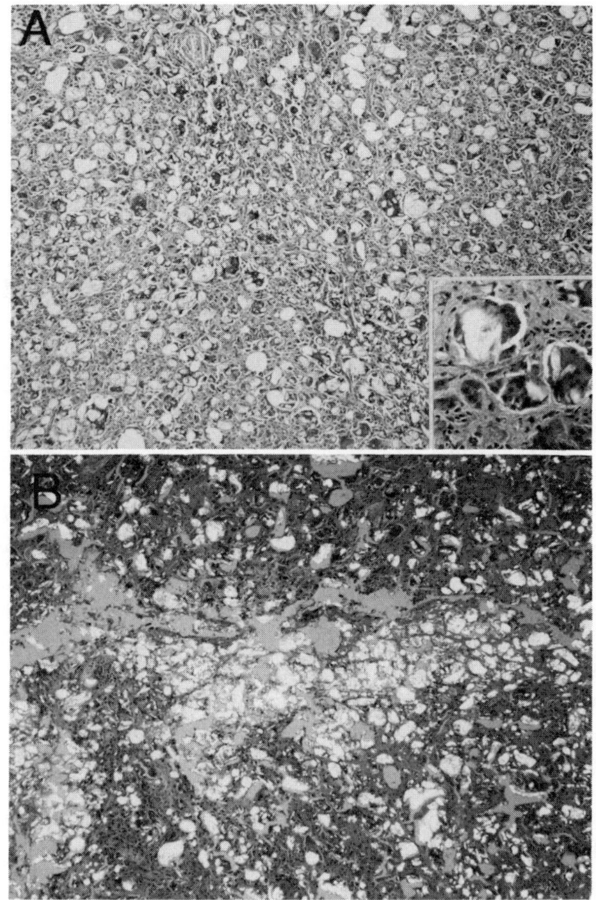

Fig 7–4.—A, neck mass entirely composed of foreign body giant cell reaction. Hematoxylin-eosin; original magnification, × 59. **Inset,** giant cells containing glassy appearing foreign material. Hematoxylin-eosin; original magnification, × 160. **B,** polarization of the foreign material demonstrates its birefringent qualities. Hematoxylin-eosin; original magnification, × 59. (Courtesy of Wenig BM, Heffner DK, Oertel YC, et al: *Hum Pathol* 21: 617–623, 1990.)

Status of the Mucosal Wave Post Vocal Cord Injection Versus Thyroplasty

Gardner GM, Parnes SM (Albany Med College Anbany, NY)
J Voice 5:64–73, 1991 7–4

Background.—Vocal cord injection and thyroplasty are 2 methods that have been used in the treatment of unilateral vocal cord paralysis. The status of the mucosal wave of the vocal folds significantly affects the quality of the voice. Previous studies have shown that vocal cord injection of Teflon (TVCI) often results in a stiff vocal cord with poor voice

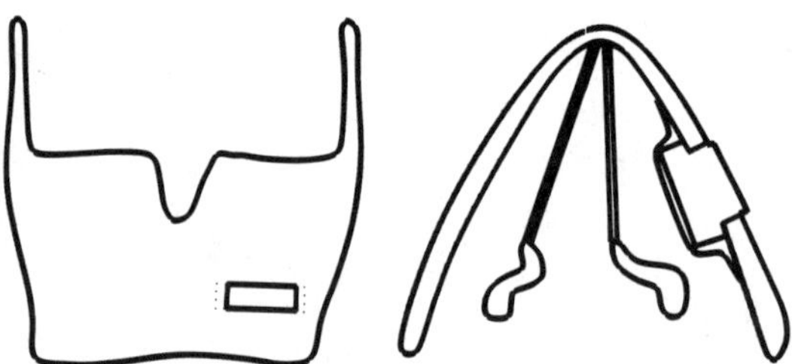

Fig 7–5.—Technique of thyroplasty. The cartilaginous window is created at the level of the vocal cord. The Silastic stent medializes the arytenoid cartilage and vocal cord. The inner perichondrium of the thyroid cartilage is preserved. (Courtesy of Gardner GM, Parnes SM: *J Voice* 5:64–73, 1991.)

quality, whereas thyroplasty may preserve the mucosal wave. The vibratory characteristics and status of the mucosal wave of the vocal cords were assessed in 21 patients who had undergone VCI or thyroplasty.

Methods.—The status of the mucosal wave and the vocal cord vibration evaluated with video stroboscopy in 8 patients who underwent thyroplasty and in 13 patients who underwent vocal cord injection with either Teflon or Gelfoam. Thyroplasty was an Isshiki type I, using Silastic stent (Fig 7–5).

Findings.—Both procedures produced excellent results with regard to mucosal wave and vocal cord vibration, with 50% of the patients undergoing thyroplasty and 45% of patients with TVCI having normal results in 1 or both of those categories. However, only the TVCI group had poor results, and granulomas were present in 3 of 4 patients with poor results. There were no poor results in the thyroplasty group. The results tended to worsen with time in the TVCI group, but this could not be evaluated in the thyroplasty group. Gelfoam vocal cord injection did not adversely affect mucosal wave or vocal cord vibration.

Discussion.—Although both thyroplasty and TVCI are capable of producing excellent results in terms of normalizing mucosal wave and vibratory characteristics of the paralyzed vocal cord, Teflon injection is more likely to decrease the mucosal wave and to stiffen the vocal cord, usually because of granuloma formation. Two basic differences may explain the better results with thyroplasty with regard to mucosal wave and vocal cord vibration. Thyroplasty involves the use of Silastic, which induces little or no foreign body reaction, as opposed to injection of Teflon, which induces granuloma formation. With thyroplasty, the Silastic stent is placed lateral to the inner perichondrium of the thyroid cartilage, where it should not interfere with the motion of the free edge of the vocal cord, as opposed to Teflon injection, which takes place medial to the inner perichondrium.

► A comparative study of vocal cord injection vs. thyroplasty produced results that caused the authors to conclude that thyroplasty is superior. If similar findings are reported in other series, then thyroplasty may emerge as the treatment of choice for most patients with TVC paralysis.—B.J. Bailey, M.D., F.A.C.S.

Laryngeal Dystonia: A Series With Botulinum Toxin Therapy
Blitzer A, Brin MF (Columbia-Presbyterian Med Ctr, New York)
Ann Otol Rhinol Laryngol 100:85–89, 1991 7–5

Background.—Laryngeal dystonia, a neurological disorder of central motor processing, is characterized by action-induced, involuntary spasms of the laryngeal muscles. Most patients with dystonia have adductor laryngeal muscle involvement that produces uncontrolled spasms during phonations, and a "strain-strangle" speech pattern that is commonly called "spastic dysphonia" (SD). In other patients, abductor muscle involvement produces "whispering dysphonia." In rare cases, there is a paradoxical vocal cord motion during respiration with adductor spasms on inspiration. A program of treatment with botulinum toxin (BOTOX) injections was evaluated.

Methods.—More than 200 patients were treated with BOTOX injections during a 5-year period. Some members of this patient group had adductor involvement, whereas others had abductor involvement. The patients with adductor involvement received individualized injections of doses of 1.25 - 3.75 units. The injections were given percutaneously with electromyography (EMG) guidance. In most of the patients with abductor involvement, the larynx was manually rotated away from the side of intended injection, and the hollow EMG needle with syringe was placed posterior to the posterior edge of the thyroid lamina. The needle was then advanced to the cricoid cartilage and moved out under EMG guidance to the best position in the posterior cricoarytenoid (PCA) muscle.

Results.—The treatment benefits appeared within 24 - 72 hours. The improvements were sustained for 2 - 9 months, with an average of 4 months. On average, patients improved to 90% of normal function. However, there were some clinically significant adverse effects, including extended breathy dysphonia and mild choking on fluids.

Conclusions.—Laryngeal BOTOX injection appears to be the treatment of choice for dystonic symptoms of the larynx. Gradual weakening may be achieved by using small dosages and injecting additional toxin as needed.

▶ Blitzer has shown that BOTOX injection into the laryngeal muscles is both safe and effective in the treatment of spasmodic dysphonia. The technique has the following advantages in comparison with surgical procedures: (1) the procedures are performed on ambulatory basis; (2) both TVCs can be treated; (3) EMG control allows injection into the most hyperactive muscles; (4) graded weakening can be achieved; (5) if the muscles are excessively weakened, they will regain strength over time.—B.J. Bailey, M.D., F.A.C.S.

Acoustic Changes in Spasmodic Dysphonia After Botulinum Toxin Injection

Zwirner P, Murry T, Swenson M, Woodson GE (VA Med Ctr, San Diego; Ludwig-Maximilians-Universität, Munich, Germany; Univ of California, San Diego)

J Voice 5:78–84, 1991 7–6

Background.—Recent studies suggest that patients with spasmodic dysphonia (SD) who are treated with botulinum toxin (BOTOX) injected into the thyroarytenoid muscle have dramatic voice improvements. The acoustic changes associated with the phonatory changes after BOTOX injection were characterized.

Methods.—Acoustic recordings were obtained 1 week before and 1 week after injection of BOTOX in the left thyroarytenoid muscle in 19 patients with adductor SD. Acoustic recordings were also obtained in 11 controls during a 2-week interval. Fundamental frequency, standard deviation of fundamental frequency, jitter, shimmer, and signal-to-noise ratio were measured from each subject's longest sustained phonation sample of the vowel quality /a/. The maximum phonation time and the number of phonatory breaks were also measured to define the voice break factor.

Results.—Compared with the controls, patients with SD had significantly higher mean values of standard deviation of fundamental frequency, jitter, shimmer, and voice break factor, and significantly lower mean values of signal-to-noise ratio. After BOTOX injection, there was a significant reduction for standard deviation of fundamental frequency and the voice break factor only.

Conclusion.—The standard deviation of fundamental frequency and voice break factor reflect the vocal fold status of SD change after BOTOX injection. In effect, the "successful" BOTOX injection results in 1 paralytic vocal fold that must still be deemed as a pathologic rather than a "normal" voice condition.

▶ Zwirner et al. studied the acoustical features of speech in patients with SD both pre- and post-BOTOX injection. Their observations caused them to conclude that the improvement in specific vocal features was rather limited. This area of investigation is far from complete, and the number of enthusiasts for BOTOX therapy will not increase rapidly until we have clear answers that will result in more complete, lasting, and predictable results.—B.J. Bailey, M.D.

Management of Vocal Nodules: A Regional Survey of Otolaryngologists and Speech-Language Pathologists

Allen MS, Pettit JM, Sherblom JC (Univ of Maine, Orono)

J Speech Hear Res 34:229–235, 1991 7–7

Purpose.—The role of voice therapy in the management of vocal nodules in children and adults is controversial. The treatment of vocal nodules in children and adults, referral patterns, the effectiveness of therapy, and the adequacy of speech-language pathologists' training in the management of vocal nodules were evaluated.

Study Design.—Questionnaires were sent to all otolaryngologists listed in the *1987 Directory of Medical Specialists* for the state of Maine and to 70 speech-language pathologists (SLPs) who were randomly selected from the *1986 Directory of the Maine Speech-Language-Hearing Association.* Twenty-one (70%) otolaryngologists and 32 (46%) SLPs responded.

Findings.—The type of vocal nodule (recent or established) and the age of the patient (child or adult) significantly affected the preferred treatments and referral patterns of both otolaryngologists and SLPs. For the adult patients, both professional groups agreed on a trial period of voice therapy followed by surgery for recent and established vocal nodules. However, in children, 26% of the SLPs preferred surgery followed by voice therapy for established vocal nodules, compared with only 5% of the otolaryngologists. The physicians preferred voice-therapy–related treatments; however, their treatment selections did not distinguish between recent and established nodules. Although both professional groups believed that voice therapy can be effective, only 5% of the otolaryngologists reported "always" referring patients with vocal nodules to an SLP for voice therapy. Most SLPs indicated that they "always" refer children and adults for medical evaluation. Both otolaryngologists and SLPs indicated that "most" or "some" SLPs were adequately trained to understand the problem presented by vocal nodules, and both chose personal experience as the basis of their opinion regarding the adequacy of training.

Conclusion.—Otolaryngologists and SLPs differ in their treatment of children with established vocal nodules and referral patterns.

▶ Questionnaire surveys are often problematic in the sense that they ask simplistic questions about complex disorders. The clinical appearance of a specific vocal nodule often provides strong clues as to whether or not the lesion will respond to speech therapy. In any event, most agree that referral to SLPs is of great importance in preventing the development of new vocal nodules.—B.J. Bailey, M.D.

Acyclovir in the Treatment of Laryngeal Papillomatosis

Aguado DL, Piñero BP, Betancor L, Mendez A, Bañales EC (Univ Hosp of Canary Islands, Tenerife, Spain)

Int J Pediatr Otorhinolaryngol 21:269–274, 1991 7–8

Background.—Different treatments have been tried to eradicate laryngeal papillomatosis (LP) and prevent recurrence. LP is a pathologic process of viral origin with predominant localization in the larynx and a tendency to recur. Acyclovir has been used successfully against pathologic processes produced by other DNA viruses. Treatment of LP with acyclovir was studied in 3 young patients.

Methods.—A 5-year-old girl and 2 boys, aged 7 and 11 years, were treated. Acyclovir was given after tumor excision using forceps under microlaryngoscopy. The girl was given 300 mg of acyclovir daily for 5 days; the younger boy, 600 mg daily for 5 months; and the older boy, 500 mg daily for 6 months.

Results.—At 18–42 months after therapy, there were no papillomatosis recurrences.

Conclusions.—These children were successfully treated for LP with acyclovir. The number of patients studied was very small, however, and more data are needed to confirm this finding.

▶ Acyclovir has been shown to have therapeutic effectiveness in the management of some patients with recurrent LP. The reported advantages include: (1) ease of administration; (2) few side effects; and (3) direct activity against the etiologic agent.—B.J. Bailey, M.D., F.A.C.S.

Arytenoid Subluxation: Diagnosis and Treatment

Hoffman HT, Brunberg JA, Winter P, Sullivan MJ, Kileny PR (Univ of Calif, San Diego; Univ of Michigan)

Ann Otol Rhinol Laryngol 100:1–9, 1991 7–9

Introduction.—Arytenoid subluxation is the abnormal displacement of arytenoid cartilage that is still partially in contact with the joint space; the condition is difficult to distinguish from recurrent laryngeal nerve paralysis (RLNP). The use of electromyography (EMG) in the diagnosis and treatment of arytenoid subluxation was investigated.

Data Analysis.—In 2 patients with RLNP, CT findings and laryngoscopic photographs were assessed with EMG to assist in distinguishing RLNP from arytenoid subluxation in another patient. Arytenoid subluxation may result from laryngomalacia, acromegaly, prolonged steroid usage, and trauma.

Conclusion.—Arytenoid subluxation has not been consistently associated with any disease process or anatomical abnormality. Definitive diagnosis has been made previously by palpation of the arytenoid at endoscopy; however, CT, MRI, and EMG are equally effective in demonstrating arytenoid subluxation. In this patient, CT was most effective in distinguishing between RLNP and arytenoid subluxation; it appears to be an important factor in prescribing immediate treatment for successful results. The preferred treatment of arytenoid subluxation is medialization laryngoplasty.

► Arytenoid subluxation can be diagnosed by a CT scan. When the diagnosis is made, it is treatable by medialization laryngoplasty. In general, early intervention seems to be associated with a better outcome.—B.J. Bailey, M.D., F.A.C.S.

Rheumatoid Arthritis of the Larynx: The Importance of Early Diagnosis and Corticosteroid Therapy

Dockery KM, Sismanis A, Abedi E (Med College of Virginia)

South Med J 84:95–96, 1991 7–10

Objective.—The larynx is involved in approximately 25% of all patients with rheumatoid arthritis. Five patients with rheumatoid involvement of the larynx were treated successfully with systemic and intraarticular corticosteroids.

Patients.—All 5 patients had a known history of rheumatoid arthritis with laryngeal symptoms of less than 6 months' duration. In addition, all had hoarseness or sore throat, or both; 1 had airway obstruction. Laryngoscopy showed decreased mobility and erythema of the arytenoid.

Treatment-Outcome.—Two patients received oral corticosteroid therapy; both improved within 6 days of treatment. The other 3 patients were treated with an injection of corticosteroid into the cricoarytenoid (C-A) joint under microsuspension laryngoscopy; all showed immediate improvement. The patient with borderline airway obstruction was treated with a prelimnary tracheostomy, followed by corticosteroid injection into the C-A joint.

Conclusion.—The use of systemic and intraarticular corticosteroids in the early diagnosis and treatment of rheumatoid involvement of the larynx is important. Systemic corticosteroid is recommended for patients without airway obstruction, and corticosteroid injection of the C-A joint is recommended when systemic therapy fails or when airway obstruction follows a preliminary tracheostomy. The latter should be considered before an arytenoidectomy is performed, because the immobile joint may represent reversible inflammation rather than complete ankylosis.

► Rheumatoid arthritis involving the larynx is more common than is generally recognized. By increasing our awareness of this disorder, we can make the diagnosis in a more timely manner and begin effective therapy earlier, thereby increasing the likelihood that corticosteroids will be effective.—B.J. Bailey, M.D., F.A.C.S.

Brief Upper Airway (Laryngeal) Dysfunction

Campbell AH, Mestitz H, Pierce R (Repatriation Gen Hosp, Heidelberg, Australia; Repatriation Gen Hosp, Hobart, Tasmania)

Aust NZ J Med 20:663–668, 1990 7–11

Background.—The larynx is designed to prevent aspiration of foreign material into the lungs. Patients who receive light anesthesia experience a more prolonged laryngeal closure (laryngospasm) than usual. The findings and clinical course of 6 patients with recurrent episodes of obstructed breathing caused by a malfunction of the larynx were evaluated.

Patients.—A history and confirmation of attacks of obstructed breathing were obtained from 6 men aged 32–72 years. Spontaneous episodes of obstructed breathing were observed in 2 patients, and stridor could be simulated on endoscopy in the other 4.

Case Report.—Man, 72, a nonsmoking businessman, had soreness and irritability of the throat for 3 weeks before being seen. On several occassions he had coughed violently after ingesting an alcoholic drink; this led to episodes of sudden complete respiratory obstruction followed by difficult respiration. He had had a mild productive cough for many years but had no respiratory problems. During an episode of upper respiratory obstruction, the patient refused laryngoscopy and bronchoscopy. He was treated with amoxicillin and a cough suppressant. He later agreed to bronchoscopy.

Results.—During the fiberoptic bronchoscopy examinations of the 6 patients, the vocal cords appeared normal and moved normally, as did the pharynx and the tracheobronchial tree. During simulated stridor, the vocal cords were severely adducted. Three patients demonstrated some degree of lower airway obstruction, but none of the 3 had a history of asthma. The maximum inspiratory flow appeared reduced and flattened.

Conclusions.—Physicians should recognize that this condition can be confused with other causes of acute dyspnea. Patients who complain of obstructed breathing should be examined and questioned carefully about the characteristic sequence of events that occurs with laryngeal dysfunction. Other causes of laryngeal dysfunction, such as laryngospasm caused by hypocalcemia, vocal cord paresis, and structural abnormalities, should also be excluded before making the final diagnosis.

▶ Brief, frightening episodes of airway obstruction are hard to explain in light of our current knowledge. The authors propose that throat irritation may sensitize laryngeal receptors, thereby causing attacks of laryngeal closure. Fortunately, these episodes do not appear to be life threatening, and they seem to respond to relaxation and gentle breathing.—B.J. Bailey, M.D., F.A.C.S.

Improved Technique for Inserting a T Tube in Patients With Subglottic Stenosis

Kato R, Kobayashi T, Watanabe M, Kawamura M, Kikuchi K, Kobayashi K, Ishihara T (Keio Univ, Tokyo)
Ann Thorac Surg 51:327–329, 1991 7–12

Introduction.—A silicone rubber T tube is usually inserted through the tracheostomy stoma by forcing the vertical portion with a forceps; however, this may be difficult in patients with subglottic stenosis. An improved technique was developed for insertion of a T tube through a tracheostomy stoma in such patients.

Technique.—The patient is placed in a supine position and sedated; the trachea, larynx, and oropharynx are anesthetized. Before the procedure, a dilator cone is made from a Rob-Nel catheter, with the external diameter of the wider end cut to match the external diameter of the T tube. The narrower end is cut. This allows insertion of another catheter through the horizontal limb of the T tube, which is pulled out the proximal end of the vertical limb. The dilator cone is placed on the proximal end. The catheter is then inserted into the stoma and pulled out the mouth. While the patient holds his breath, the narrow end is pulled and the proximal end of the T tube is passed through the subglottic space. If

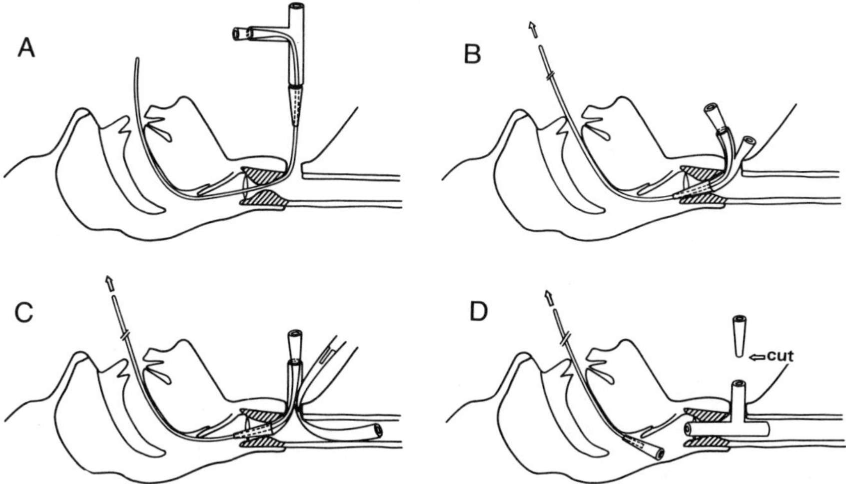

Fig 7–6.—A, the Rob-Nel catheter carrying the T tube and dilator cone is inserted into the tracheostomy stoma and pulled out the mouth. (The vertical limb of the T tube is depicted horizontally and the horizontal limb vertically because of the supine position of the patient. **B,** the tip of the Rob-Nel catheter is pulled vigorously. The cone-shaped dilator facilitates the insertion of the proximal portion of the vertical limb through the stenotic segment. **C,** when the distal portion of the vertical limb is long, it is inserted first. The proximal portion is folded onto the distal portion and inserted with the help of the Rob-Nel catheter. Forceps are used to facilitate insertion of the distal portion. **D,** when the T tube is in the proper position, the Rob-Nel catheter is pulled back a little through the vertical limb of the T tube. The catheter is cut at the tapering portion, and the dilator cone is retrieved by pulling the catheter out the mouth. (Courtesy of Kato R, Kobayashi T, Watanabe M, et al: *Ann Thorac Surg* 51:327–329, 1991.)

it is long, the distal potion of the vertical limb is inserted before the proximal portion. When the tube is appropriately positioned, the catheter is pulled back and cut and the dilator cone is removed (Fig 7–6).

Results.—The procedure was used with good results in 4 patients with subglottic stenosis. In each patient, the usual technique was tried, but it failed because of kinking or folding of the proximal vertical limb of the T tube.

Conclusion.—This procedure is easy and can be performed with local anesthesia. If the T tube cannot be placed by the usual method, this technique should be tried before more complicated techniques are used.

► Although we have no experience with this technique, it appears to be an ingenious method for dealing with a difficult airway problem. In some cases, it may avoid the necessity for an open procedure.—B.J. Bailey, M.D., F.A.C.S.

8 Allergy

Pathophysiology and Treatment of Seasonal Allergic Rhinitis

Bousquet J, Chanez P, Michel FB (Hôpital l'Aiguelongue, Montpellier, France)

Respir Med 84 (Suppl A):11–17, 1990 8–1

Introduction.—The treatment of seasonal allergic rhinitis has improved during the past 2 decades. There is a greater understanding of the mechanisms that are responsible for the condition, and many safe and effective medications have been developed. The various therapeutic approaches to seasonal allergic rhinitis were reviewed.

Background.—Knowledge of the mechanisms of allergic rhinitis has been improved by the technique of nasal challenge. The allergic inflammation results from the coupling of mast-cell-bound-immunoglobulin E (IgE) to a specific allergen, which leads to the release of vasoactive mediators. Patients become symptomatic within minutes of nasal challenge with pollen grains. A late phase reaction occurs in 30% to 40% of patients, starting after 2–5 hours and peaking 6–8 hours after the challenge. In addition to rhinorrhea, obstruction, sneezing, and intermittent pruritus, patients may experience conjunctivitis, asthma, and skin symptoms.

Treatment.—The types of therapy available include allergen eviction, antiallergic treatment, anti-receptor treatment, symptomatic treatment, and allergen-specific immunotherapy. Among the first-line drugs are H_1-receptor antagonists that may be administered orally. The newer preparations do not cause sedation. Corticosteroids are the first-line treatment for nasal symptoms. Disodium cromoglycate appears to be highly effective in allergic conjunctivitis. Topical vasoconstrictors may cause side effects with prolonged use. Anticholinergic drugs are both safe and effective for rhinorrhea. Specific immunotherapy appears to be of value in selected patients with severe rhinitis, in those with asthma, and in patients who are not allergic to many pollen species.

Conclusion.—Both pharmacotherapy and immunotherapy play a role in the treatment of seasonal allergic rhinitis. Either topical corticosteroids or nonsedative antihistamines should be chosen as the initial medication.

▶ Seasonal allergic rhinitis continues to be one of the most common and troubling disorders in medicine. Most patients begin treatment with over-the-counter medications; this may be all that is required for the milder symptoms. We have been pleased by the customary effectiveness of seasonal steroid nasal sprays, antihistamines, and decongestants to control symptoms—even those symptoms that are moderately severe. This study provides a nice review of recent developments in the treatment of allergic rhinitis.—B.J. Bailey, M.D., F.A.C.S.

Changes in Non-Specific Nasal Reactivity and Eosinophil Influx and Activation After Allergen Challenge

Klementsson H, Andersson M, Baumgarten CR, Venge P, Pipkorn U (Univ Hosp, Lund, Sweden; Free Univ of Berlin; Univ Hosp, Uppsala, Sweden)
Clin Exper Allergy 20:539–547, 1990 8–2

Objective.—Several studies have suggested that eosinophils may play a contributory role in the genesis of increased reactivity of the airways. To investigate further the time-course of the allergen-induced changes in nasal nonspecific reactivity was studied in relation to the changes in the local cell populations (particularly the eosinophils) on the nasal mucosal surface.

Methods.—After an initial nasal methacholine challenge, 16 subjects with strictly seasonal allergic rhinitis were challenged with allergen outside the relevant pollen season. For 24 hours they were monitored at intervals for nasal symptoms, changes in nasal reactivity, eosinophil influx and activation, and markers of inflammation. Every second hour after the allergen challenge, the subjects were rechallenged with methacholine. Seven subjects underwent the same challenge procedure without an initial allergen challenge (controls). A nasal lavage was performed before each methacholine challenge to monitor the influx of cells and to determine the changes in the levels of eosinophil cationic protein (ECP) and toluenesulfonylarginine methyl ester (TAME)-esterase activity. A brush specimen was collected from the nasal mucosal surface before nasal challenge and at 24 hours.

Results.—The allergen challenge produced a significant increase in nonspecific nasal reactivity at all observation points for as long as 24 hours. The volume of secretion increased from .051 to .255 mL as early as 2 hours after allergen challenge. During a similar timing, the allergen challenge induced a significant increase in the proportion of eosinophils on the mucosal surface, from an initial .8% to 6.2% of the cells at 2 hours. In contrast, none of these increases were evident in the control group. There was a significant correlation between the levels of ECP and eosinophils in the lavage fluid and between the levels of ECP and TAME-esterase. However, there was no significant correlation between the increases in nonspecific nasal reactivity and the number of eosinophils or levels of ECP at any of the observed time points.

Conclusion.—No clear-cut relationship was demonstrated between the changes in nonspecific reactivity and the influx and activation of eosinophils. It appears that the allergen-induced changes in nonspecific nasal reactivity, although time related, are independent events that represent a complex phenomenon.

► Recently, there has been great interest in several nasal response phenomena. It is hypothesized that nasal inflammation of one type (infection, pollution, irritation) sensitizes the nose to other types of stimuli (allergic stimuli, temperature change, etc). In fact, this has been reported as an explanation for the increased incidence of allergic rhinitis that is ascribed to higher levels of air pollution, smoking, etc. Methacholine provides a specific nasal stimulus that evokes a glandular secretory response without an influx of eosinophils or alterations of mucosal responsiveness. When the subjects were subsequently challenged with allergens, there was no evidence of a synergistic link between the 2 forms of nasal response.—B.J. Bailey, M.D., F.A.C.S.

Masqueraders in Clinical Allergy: Laryngeal Dysfunction Causing Dyspnea

O'Hollaren MT (Oregon Health Sciences Univ)

Ann Allergy 65:351–357, 1990 8–3

Background.—Laryngeal dysfunction is often overlooked as a cause of dyspnea. Failure to reach this diagnosis may lead to inappropriate treatment for "refractory asthma." Function disorders in which abnormal vocal cord movement impedes glottic airflow occur in adults and children. These disorders are treatable once they are diagnosed correctly.

Diagnosis and Management.—Before a diagnosis of laryngeal dysfunction is considered, it is necessary to rule out anaphalaxis, vocal cord tumor, foreign body aspiration and other laryngeal syndromes that may produce symptoms. Dyspnea produced by paradoxical vocal cord motion (PVCM) may be increased by stressful situations precipitated by exercise, and they may produce wheezing. Some patients exhibit PVCM after an influenza-like illness. Treatment of PVCM is usually multidisciplinary. Speech therapy is important for successful management. Laryngeal relaxation techniques and biofeedback are also helpful. The most common dyspnea-producing disorder is bilateral vocal cord paralysis resulting from previous thyroid surgery. Meige syndrome sometimes causes laryngeal muscle spasms. Patients with suspected Meige syndrome should be referred to a neurologist as well as an otolaryngologist and a speech pathologist. Abductor spastic dysphonia may produce dyspnea in patients on exertion. It has been misdiagnosed as vocal cord paralysis. Patients with spastic dysphonia with a psychogenic component often benefit from psychotherapy, biofeedback, and speech therapy. Laryngospasm may occur in response to glottic or supraglottic stimulation. Pediatric patients who undergo general anesthesia experience this reflex laryngeal closure more often than adult patients. Metabolic disorders may also produce laryngospasm. There are numerous therapeutic interventions available; however, if the possibility of laryngeal edema from an allergic cause exists, epinephrine could be used.

Summary.—In some patients, the site of origin of dyspnea is the larynx. Allergists need a complete understanding of the normal function of laryngeal anatomy and physiology to accurately diagnose these cases. Recognition of PCVM, Meige syndrome, abductor spastic dysphonia, laryngospasm, and other disorders will facilitate timely and accurate diagnosis and treatment.

▶ Paradoxical vocal cord motion is an uncommon disorder that may masquerade as laryngeal edema or even asthma. Interestingly, most of these patients are women, and many of them have some link with the health care professions (nurse, therapist, counselor, etc). Speech therapy and psychotherapy are reported to be helpful.—B.J. Bailey, M.D., F.A.C.S.

9 Trauma

Poly(L-Lactide) Implants in Repair of Defects of the Orbital Floor: An Animal Study

Rozema FR, Bos RRM, Pennings AJ, Jansen HWB (Univ of Groningen, The Netherlands)

J Oral Maxillofac Surg 48:1305–1309, 1990 9–1

Introduction.—Surgery for traumatically induced defects of the orbital floor may prevent residual diplopia and enophthalmus. Autografts, xenografts, and allografts have been used. Although nonresorbable alloplastic implants are widely used, there are many potential complications. Resorbable alloplastic material may be preferable. The implant must provide temporary support of the orbital tissues but disappear completely.

Procedure and Findings.—A high-molecular-weight, as-polymerized poly(L-lactide) (PLLA) was used to repair artificial orbital defects in goats (Fig 9–1). At postoperative follow-up, the specially designed .4-mm thick PLLA implant gave sufficient support to the orbital tissue during healing. Based on the animal studies, full resorption of the implant can be estimated at approximately 3.5 years. It would be preferable to shorten this resorption time to avoid the complications that accompany nonresorbable implants.

Conclusions.—The PLLA was well tolerated, with no clinically detectable inflammatory or foreign-body reaction. Positive results may make the high-molecular-weight, as-polymerized PLLA useful in the management of human orbital blowout fracture.

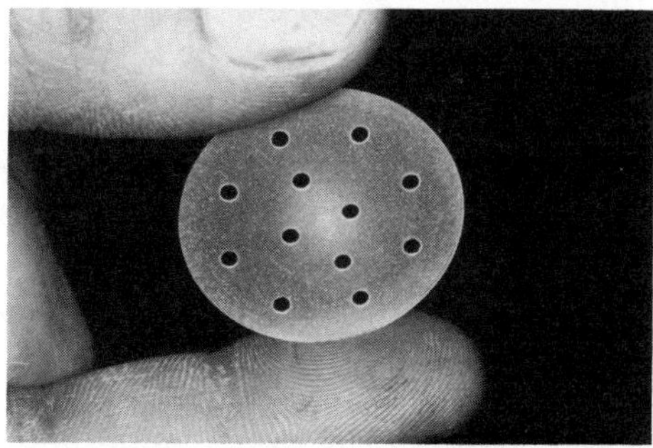

Fig 9–1.—Photograph of the PLLA implant. The implant has a glassy appearance. (Courtesy of Rozema FR, Bos RRM, Pennings AJ, et al: *J Oral Maxillofac Surg* 48:1305–1309, 1990.)

High-Energy Orbital Dislocations: The Possibility of Traumatic Hypertelorbitism

Markowitz BL, Manson PN, Yaremchuk M, Glassman D, Kawamoto H (Maryland Inst of Emergency Med Services Systems, Baltimore; Univ of California, Los Angeles)

Plast Reconstr Surg 88:20–30, 1991 9–2

Background.—Although isolated reports of traumatic hypertelorbitism have appeared, the clinical and radiographic features have not been established. Therefore, a series of patients was reviewed to document traumatic hypertelorbitism and its treatment.

Patients.—From 1983 to 1987, 7,160 patients with blunt injuries were admitted to 1 trauma center. Of these patients, 10% had facial injuries, and approximately 10% of these had high-energy fractures as characterized by CT. Five patients with high-energy orbital dislocations, some of whom had traumatic hypertelorbitism, were also observed. An additional patient from another institution was also seen for late repair of the condition.

Findings.—High-energy trauma to the upper midface produced fractures of both orbits, zygomas, and nasoethmoidal areas that resulted in lateral transposition, enlargement, and divergence of the orbits. The interorbital, intercanthal, and interpupillary distances were increased and used as criteria to confirm the diagnosis of hypertelorbitism. Half of the patients were blind bilaterally, and 1 patient was blind unilaterally (Fig 9–2).

Conclusions.—The reconstruction of these complex injuries involves the most advanced principles of facial fracture management. Definition of the injury by CT permits reconstruction by stabilization in 3 dimensions, stressing control of facial width and cranial base landmarks as anatomical guides to reconstruction. Facial skeletal anatomy is restored through complete exposure, rigid internal fixation, and immediate bone grafting.

The Transconjunctival Approach for Treating Orbital Trauma

Waite PD, Carr DD (Univ of Alabama, Birmingham)

J Oral Maxillofac Surg 49:499–503, 1991 9–3

Background.—Greater emphasis on open reduction of zygomatic fractures has necessitated a search for incisions that allow adequate access and esthetic results. Results of the transconjunctival incision were reviewed in 12 patients with maxillofacial fractures.

Methods.—The patients (mean age, 25 years) had a variety of diagnoses. The results were assessed by examination and radiographs, and either preseptal or postseptal dissection was done. The approach began with a lateral canthotomy, in which the lateral aspect of the lower lid

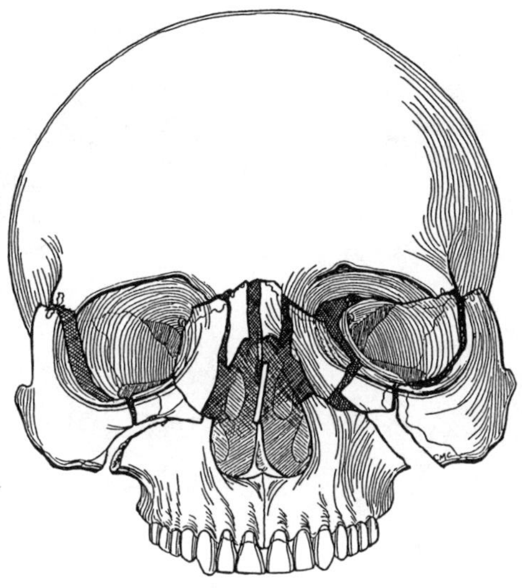

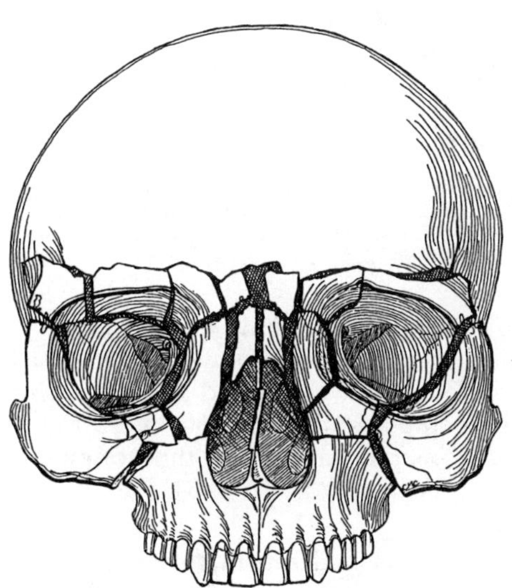

Fig 9–2.—The fractures responsible for traumatic hypertelorism include bilateral zygomatic, naso-ethmoid, and 3- or 4-wall orbital injuries. When the frontal bone is involved, the orbital roof is also displaced. The comminuted fractures are dislocated laterally. **Above,** traumatic hypertelorism without frontal bone involvement (3-wall orbital fractures). **Below,** traumatic hypertelorism with frontal bone involvement (4-wall orbital fractures). (Courtesy of Markowitz BL, Manson PN, Yaremchuk M, et al: *Plast Reconstr Surg* 88:20–30, 1991.)

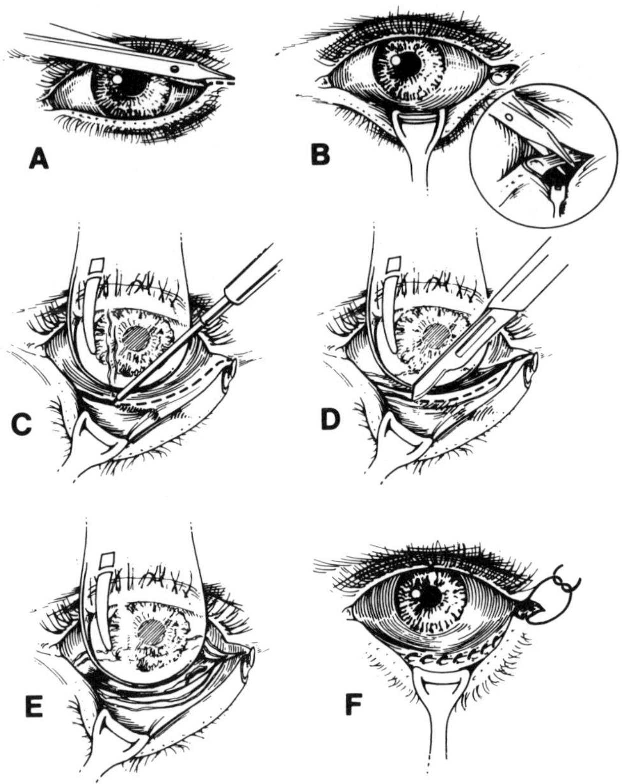

Fig 9–3.—Diagram demonstrating the transconjunctival approach to the orbital rim and floor. **A,** lateral canthotomy; **B,** cantholysis completion; **C,** transconjunctival incision; **D,** periosteal incision; **E,** elevation of periosteum and periorbita; and **F,** conjunctival closure and canthal tendon repair. (Courtesy of Waite PD, Carr DD: *J Oral Maxillofac Surg* 49:499–503, 1991.)

was detached from the inferior limb of the lateral canthal tendon. A conjunctival incision was then made between the tarsal plate and inferior fornix, and the periosteum was incised when the infraorbital rim was identified. The periosteum and periorbita were then elevated, and the orbital floor was reconstructed. Finally, the conjunctiva was closed and the canthal tendon was repaired (Fig 9–3). Patients were followed for a mean of 12 months.

Results.—All 12 patients had satisfactory results. Esthetically, the results were excellent, with the transconjunctival incision and lateral canthotomy being undetectable within 1 to 2 months. When a lateral canthotomy and cantholysis were performed, access was always adequate. Fracture reduction and plate placement were no more difficult than with a subciliary or brow incision. Subconjunctival ecchymosis and periorbital edema often occurred, lasting for 1–2 weeks. There were no immediate or delayed complications.

Conclusions.—The transconjunctival approach is recommended as the primary approach to the orbital floor and the infraorbital and lateral rims. This approach reduces complications and provides the same access as other surgical techniques. The globe must be meticulously protected to avoid corneal abrasions or other damage.

Early Treatment of Orbital Floor Fractures With Catheter Balloon in Children

Gatot A, Tovi F (Ben-Gurion Univ of the Negev, Beer-Sheva, Israel)

Int J Pediatr Otorhinolaryngol 21:97–101, 1991 9–4

Background.—The incidence of orbital floor fractures in children, either isolated or associated with other local fractures, is higher than is recognized. Early diagnosis and treatment are important. The transantral restoration of the injured orbital floor with catheter balloon was evaluated.

Methods.—A group of 15 children with orbital floor fractures was treated. The catheter balloon was introduced transantrally; it stabilized and supported the torn but still vascularized periosteum at the edges of the fracture. The catheter balloon also served as a guide for further proliferation and new bone formation (Fig 9–4).

Results.—The technique was used to repair pure blowout fractures in 4 cases. Orbital floor fractures associated with disruption of the orbital ridge, zygomatic bone, and/or maxillary sinus were repaired in the other 11 cases. All children had satisfactory outcomes. Transient anesthesia in the dermatome of the infraorbital nerve was the only complication noted in 11 patients.

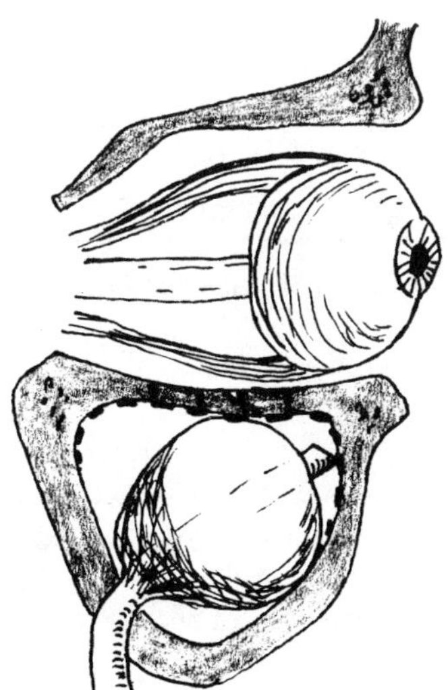

Fig 9–4.—After the reduction of the herniated soft tissues, the catheter balloon supports the periosteum of the orbital floor. (Courtesy of Gatot A, Tovi F: *Int J Pediatr Otorhinolaryngol* 21:97–101, 1991.)

Conclusions.—Early repair using the catheter-balloon technique appears to be a viable alternative in the repair of orbital flood fracture in children.

▶ Rozema et al. (Abstract 9–1) report excellent preliminary results with long-lasting, but ultimately resorbable orbital floor implants. The tissue reaction is much greater on the orbital side of the implant because of the weight and movement of the orbital contents. Because the implant is smooth and has no sharp, angular features, there is a minimal giant cell response. The eventual extrusion of nonresorbable orbital floor implants is probably related to a combination of the local foreign-body reaction, the frequent eye movements, and the tendency for alloplastic materials to become infected. There is great promise for an implant that will have clinical utility with few complications.

Markowitz (Abstract 9–2) emphasizes the severity and complexity of high energy nasofrontal injuries, as well as the importance of the following in their management: (1) precise preoperative evaluation using CT scan; (2) adequate exposure through *large* incisions; (3) immediate bone grafting from missing osseous elements; (4) exact fixation of fractures using mini/microplating; and (5) thorough initial repair to limit the need for delayed reconstruction.

Subciliary and infraciliary incisions to approach the orbital floor carry a low, but significant risk of displacement of the lower lid or ectropion. Abstract 9–3 makes a good case for the transconjunctival approach, which we have used much more often in recent years. Its authors indicate that this approach may be either preseptal or retroseptal; the preseptal approach is advantageous because it avoids the orbital fat. However, the preseptal approach is sometimes followed by fibrosis that distorts the position of the orbital septum and tarsal plate.

Gatot (Abstract 9–4) describes the successful use of a catheter balloon in the maxillary antrum to stabilize orbital floor fractures in children. Surgeons who use this technique must be knowledgeable regarding the small size of the antrum in patients younger than 10 years of age, the presence of unerupted teeth in the anterior wall of the maxilla, and the effects of nasal and sinus surgery on subsequent facial growth.—B.J. Bailey, M.D., F.A.C.S.

Comparison of Functional Recovery After Nonsurgical and Surgical Treatment of Condylar Fractures

Takenoshita Y, Ishibashi H, Oka M (Kyushu Univ, Fukuoka, Japan)

J Oral Maxillofac Surg 48:1191–1195, 1990 9–5

Purpose.—Condylar fractures require the restoration of proper occlusion, function, and normal facial contour. Although most condylar fractures are treated nonsurgically, open reduction of condylar fractures is often reported. The outcome after surgical and nonsurgical reduction of condylar fractures was compared.

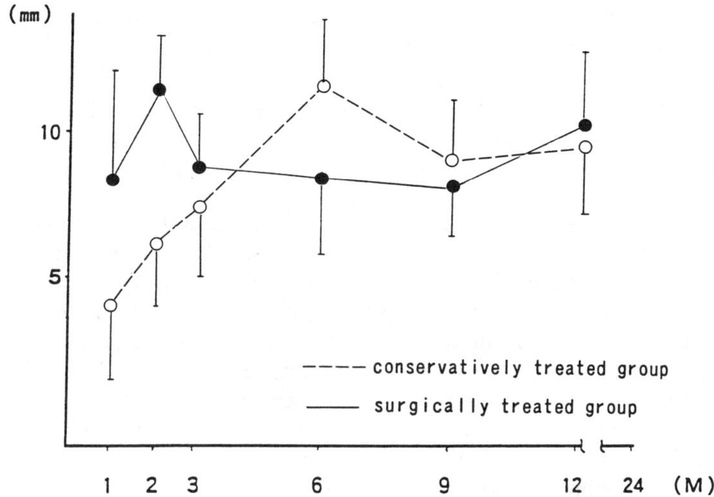

Fig 9–5.—A graph showing the changes (mean ± SD) in laterotrusive excursion of the mandible. (Courtesy of Takenoshita Y, Ishibashi H, Oka M: *J Oral Maxillofac Surg* 48:1191–1195, 1990.)

Patients.—Of 36 patients with condylar process fractures, 20 were treated by closed reduction and 16 were treated surgically. The average follow-up was 11.6 months. Patients with dislocated or severely displaced fractured condylar processes were recommended for surgery; however, some refused to be operated on and were therefore treated nonsurgically. Maxillomandibular fixation (MMF) was applied before operation to correct disturbed occlusion and was then routinely discontinued approximately 3 weeks after application. Active jaw movement with physiotherapy followed.

Results.—There were no postoperative infections or other complications. All the patients regained acceptable joint function (Fig 9–5). During the first year of follow-up, all patients maintained an adequate interocclusal relation with good occlusal contacts. None of the patients complained of pain at follow-up visits.

Open Reduction and Internal Rigid Fixation of Subcondylar Fractures Via an Intraoral Approach

Lachner J, Clanton JT, Waite PD (Univ of Alabama, Birmingham)
Oral Surg Oral Med Oral Pathol 71:257–261, 1991 9–6

Introduction.—The treatment of facial fractures attempts to achieve anatomical reduction and restore function while alleviating patient discomfort and promoting postsurgical care. The results of a specific technique using miniplates for intraoral open reduction and internal fixation of subcondylar fractures were reviewed. This method was found to be easier than a preauricular or submandibular incision; and it posed less risk to the patient's facial nerve.

Methods.—Fourteen patients, 3 women and 11 men (average age, 24 years) underwent intraoral open reduction of subcondylar fractures. The reduction surgeries were assessed by radiographs immediately after surgery, and all patients were followed for 12 months after the operation.

Technique.—The patient received general anesthesia and the subcondylar fracture was reduced. This was followed by the repair of any other fractures. The condylar neck was reached via an incision over the anterior border of the ascending ramus. After later reflection of the periosteum and masseter muscle to the posterior edge, the mandibular notch was located and the periosteum of the proximal segment was raised only the amount necessary for placement of the plate. A 4-hole Würzburg miniplate was first attached to the proximal segment with 1 or 2 screws; the patient was then placed in maxillomandibular fixation and the fracture was reduced. The plate was connected to the distal segment (Fig 9–6) and the incision was closed. The patient wore training elastics for 2–10 days after the surgery.

Results.—In these 14 patients, 80% of the fractures showed good reduction (<2 mm) radiographically. All patients had a normal range of

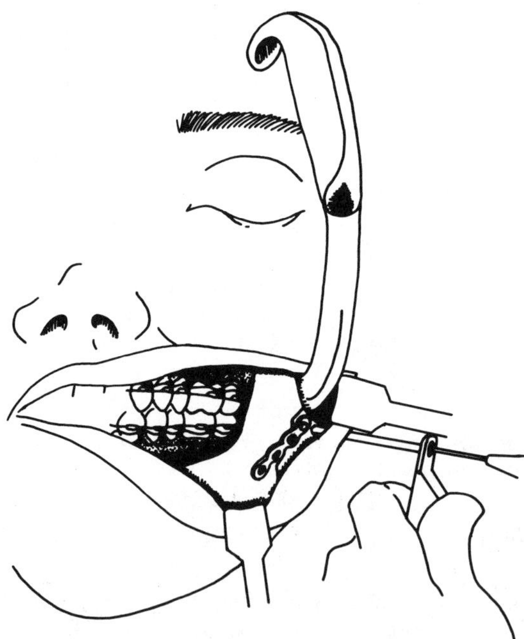

Fig 9–6.—Bauer retractor is positioned in the sigmoid notch, and the fracture is reduced while patient is in maxillomandibular fixation. The miniplate is first fixed to the proximal segment. (Courtesy of Lachner J, Clanton JT, Waite PD: *Oral Surg Oral Med Oral Pathol* 71:257–261, 1991.)

motion (37–43 mm) within 8 weeks of the operation. Four patients experienced clicking, but 2 of these had a history of clicking before the fracture. At 6 weeks after surgery, 53% of the patients said they had mild discomfort when chewing heavily; however, they did not require any medication. At 6 months after the operation, no patients complained of discomfort or other problems related to the surgery.

Implications.—Open reduction surgery should be considered for most low subcondylar fractures because this technique aids in the treatment of any accompanying maxillary fractures. However, this procedure should be used with caution in children and young adults because significant remodeling will occur in these patients.

Monocortical Miniplate Fixation of Mandibular Angle Fractures

Levy FE, Smith RW, Odland RM, Marentette LJ (Univ of Minnesota; Loma Linda Univ)

Arch Otolaryngol Head Neck Surg 117:149–154, 1991 9–7

Introduction.—The use of noncompression monocortical miniplate fixation for mandibular fractures provides reliable rigid fixation and eliminates the need for intermaxillary fixation (IMF). Studies using a variety of internal fixation techniques have shown high rates of complications at the mandibular angle. The use of 1 vs. 2 miniplates in the treatment of mandibular angle fractures was compared in 61 patients with 63 mandibular angle fractures who were treated during a 4-year period.

Methods.—Fracture and treatment characteristics and the occurrence of complications were recorded. Follow-up examinations were usually performed at 1, 2, 4, 6, and 12 weeks. The follow-up was less than 6 weeks in 12 patients; therefore, they were excluded from the analysis.

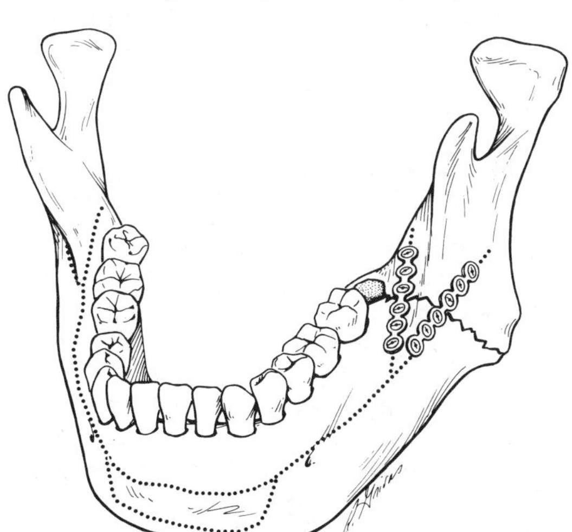

Fig 9–7.—The location of the miniplates used in the treatment of mandibular angle fractures, superimposed on Champy's ideal line of osteosynthesis. (Courtesy of Levy FE, Smith RW, Odland RM, et al: *Arch Otolaryngol Head Neck Surg* 117:149–154, 1991.)

Results.—Associated mandible fractures were present in 31 patients; 51% of these were in the contralateral parasympheal area. Of the patients, 10 were treated with 1 miniplate and no IMF, whereas 9 were treated with 1 miniplate and IMF. The average duration of IMF in this group was 23 days. Two miniplates with no IMF were used in 18 patients, and 2 miniplates with IMF were used in 14 (Fig 9–7); the average duration of IMF in this group was 23.5 days. The 5 (26.3%) complications in the 1 miniplate group included 3 infections, 1 delayed union, and 1 anterior open-bite malocclusion. There was 1 infection in a patient treated with 2 miniplates and IMF, for a significantly lower complication rate of 3.1%.

Conclusion.—For stabilization of mandible angle fractures, the use of 2 miniplates is more effective than the use of 1 miniplate. The complication rate with this procedure is the lowest reported with any plating technique.

Early Immobilization of Mandibular Fractures: A Retrospective Study

Maloney PL, Welch TB, Doku HC (Tufts Univ)

J Oral Maxillofac Surg 49:698–702, 1991 9–8

Background.—Oral and maxillofacial surgeons often treat patients with mandibular fractures. Treatment in a consistent proportion of patients is complicated by bone infection at the fracture site. Early immobilization of mandibular fractures was studied retrospectively.

Methods.—A total of 204 fractures was treated in 131 patients during a 34-month period. Fractures were divided into 5 groups based on time to immobilization, type of reduction, and patient compliance.

Results.—The overall infection rate was 4.4%, which is comparable to previously reported rates. In patients immobilized within 72 hours of injury, there were no bone infections in 111 fractures treated by closed reduction, and there was a 2% incidence of bone infection in 50 fractures treated by open reduction. Of the 161 fractures that were immobilized early in compliant patients, the incidence of bone infection after treatment was .6%. The removal of teeth in the line of fracture was not a significant factor.

Conclusions.—When immobilization is done and antibiotics are given within 72 hours, healing will be timely with closed or open reduction. If the fracture is simple, then delays in treatment will not result in a bone infection. When a compound fracture is not immobilized within 48–72 hours, the patient should be presumed to have an acute infection of bone at the fracture site. When initial immobilization is delayed past 72 hours but less than 10 days and open reduction is necessary, the fracture may be initially stabilized by closed reduction, antibiotics may be given for 10–21 days, and an open reduction may be done with intraosseous fixation. When a compound fracture is older than 7–10 days at first immobilization and an open reduction is done, the patient is at significant risk for postoperative chronic suppurative osteomyelitis. All patients with compound mandibular fractures should receive antibiotics.

▶ It is still an accepted practice to manage almost all condylar fractures conservatively (without open reduction and fixation of the fragments). As far as the reader can tell from the study outlined in Abstract 9–5, conservative management is supported; however, one can't be entirely sure. Open reduction was used in some patients with more severe injuries, but several of the patients with severe fractures refused surgery (and apparently did well). Although we are not told enough about these subgroups to draw firm conclusions, the study does not seem to provide support for open surgical techniques.

Lachner et al. (Abstract 9–6) recommend open management of *low* subcondylar fractures to prevent deviation of the jaw on opening. When there are bilateral subcondylar fractures, the authors believe that plating the side with the lowest fracture is important to restore mandibular height. They also believe that the intraoral approach is useful in preventing complications (scarring, facial nerve injury, etc.). Unfortunately, there is no control group to provide support for their claims of superior results. Until such information is available, we are left with opinions rather than conclusions.

Our local experience with miniplates leads us to agree with Levy et al. (Abstract 9–7) in recommending the use of 2 miniplates in the management of displaced fractures of the mandibular angle—especially in the case of unstable or unfavorable fractures.

Although several large series have failed to show an outcome advantage with early treatment vs. delayed management of mandibular fractures, we agree with Maloney et al. (Abstract 9–8) and others who have shown better results with early treatment. Their approach has suggested a rationale that deserves further confirmatory investigation.—B.J. Bailey, M.D., F.A.C.S.

The Treatment of Acute External Laryngeal Injuries: "State of the Art"

Schaefer SD (Univ of Texas Southwestern Med Ctr, Dallas)

Arch Otolaryngol Head Neck Surg 117:35–39, 1991 9–9

Background.—Although external laryngeal trauma occurs infrequently, a standard treatment of blunt and penetrating laryngeal trauma can be defined from available data. No documented reports support the concept that women or older individuals are at higher risk for laryngeal injuries.

Methods.—A protocol for the general management of laryngeal injury is presented in Fig 9–8. If the airway is not significantly injured, the patient's history should be taken and a physical examination should be accompanied by flexible nasolaryngoscopy. This technique offers better

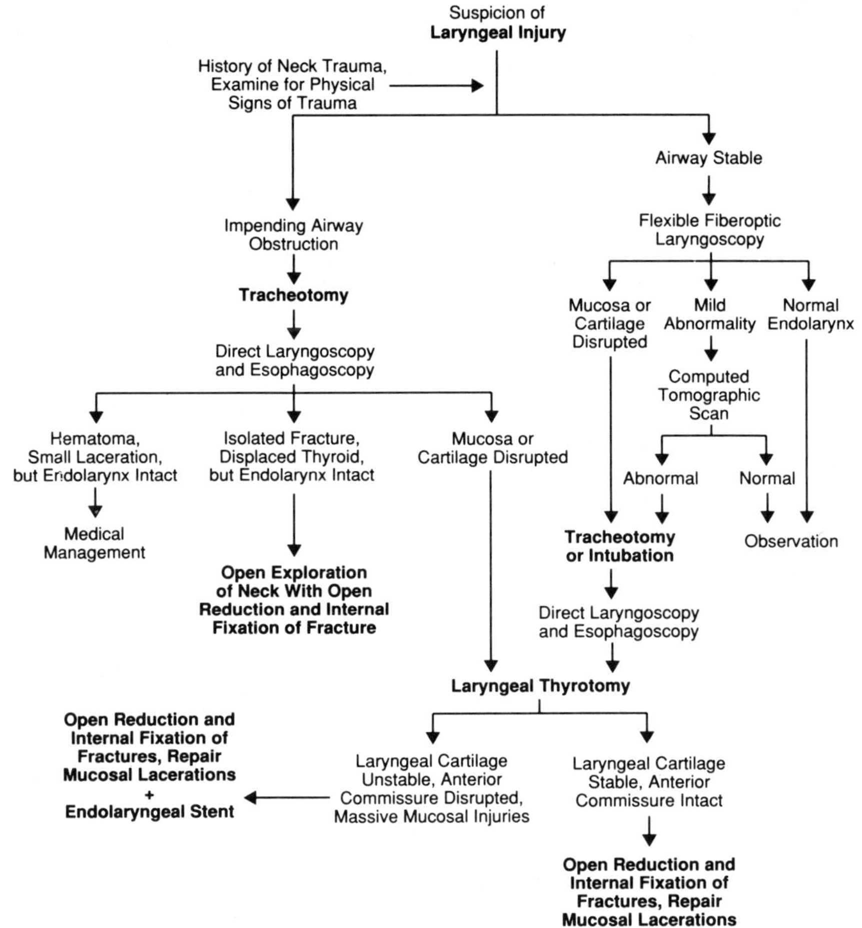

Fig 9–8.—A management protocol for the acutely injured larynx. (Courtesy of Schaefer SD: *Arch Otolaryngol Head Neck Surg* 117:35–39, 1991.)

patient compliance and visualization capabilities than indirect laryngoscopy. If the airway is compromised, then the least traumatic procedure possible, such as tracheotomy under local anesthesia, should be used to establish the airway. Rigid esophagoscopy should be performed to check for esophageal or pharyngeal lacerations. Laryngeal tomography or laryngography should follow. A laryngeal injury should be managed medically if surgery appears unnecessary.

Surgical Management Decisions.—The indications for surgical management include the need to establish an airway and the necessity to internally fix multiple laryngoskeletal fractures. Certain patients can be managed by airway maintenance for several days and decannulized after their injuries have resolved spontaneously. Patients with large mucosal

Moving?

I'd like to receive my ***Year Book of Otolaryngology–Head and Neck Surgery*** without interruption.

Please note the following change of address, effective: ______

Name: ______

New Address: ______

______

City: ______ State: ______ Zip: ______

Old Address: ______

______

City: ______ State: ______ Zip: ______

Reservation Card

Yes, I would like my own copy of the ***Year Book of Otolaryngology–Head and Neck Surgery***. Please begin my subscription with the current edition according to the terms described below.* I understand that I will have 30 days to examine each annual edition. If satisfied, I will pay just $59.95 plus sales tax, postage and handling (price subject to change without notice).

Name: ______

Address: ______

City: ______ State: ______ Zip: ______

Method of Payment

❑ Visa ❑ Mastercard ❑ AmEx ❑ Bill me ❑ Check (in US dollars, payable to Mosby-Year Book, Inc.)

Card number ______ Exp date ______

Signature ______

LS-0907

*Your *Year Book* Service Guarantee:

When you subscribe to the ***Year Book***, we'll send you an advance notice of future volumes about two months before they publish. This automatic notice system is designed to take up as little of your time as possible. If you do not want the ***Year Book***, the advance notice makes it quick and easy for you to let us know your decision; and you will always have at least 20 days to decide. If we don't hear from you, we'll send you the new volume as soon as it's available. And, of course, the ***Year Book*** is yours to examine free of charge for 30 days (postage, handling and applicable sales tax are added to each shipment).

NO POSTAGE
NECESSARY
IF MAILED
IN THE
UNITED STATES

BUSINESS REPLY MAIL
FIRST CLASS MAIL PERMIT No. 762 CHICAGO, IL

POSTAGE WILL BE PAID BY ADDRESSEE

Chris Hughes
Mosby-Year Book, Inc.
200 N. LaSalle Street
Suite 2600
Chicago, IL 60601-9981

NO POSTAGE
NECESSARY
IF MAILED
IN THE
UNITED STATES

BUSINESS REPLY MAIL
FIRST CLASS MAIL PERMIT No. 762 CHICAGO, IL

POSTAGE WILL BE PAID BY ADDRESSEE

Chris Hughes
Mosby-Year Book, Inc.
200 N. LaSalle Street
Suite 2600
Chicago, IL 60601-9981

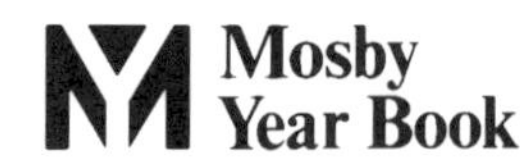

Dedicated to publishing excellence.

lacerations, displaced fractures, exposed cartilage, or vocal fold immobility should undergo laryngeal exploration after tracheotomy and endoscopy and within 24 hours of injury. Minor lacerations should also be examined because they can alter the voice. Endolaryngeal stenting should be reserved for wounds that disrupt the anterior commissure, for comminuted laryngeal skeletal fractures, and for massive mucosal injuries.

Conclusions.—Knowledge gained in the past 3 decades has allowed early treatment of laryngeal trauma to improve patient outcome, voice quality, and airway health.

▶ Schaefer has had a long-term interest in the management of laryngeal trauma, and his latest study emphasizes the following important treatment guidelines: (1) careful evaluation with CT scan and fiberoptic endoscopy; (2) immediate airway management; (3) standardization of reconstructive techniques; and (4) proper use of stents.—B.J. Bailey, M.D., F.A.C.S.

Pediatric Penetrating Head and Neck Trauma

Martin WS, Gussack GS (Emory Univ)

Laryngoscope 100:1288–1291, 1990 9–10

Introduction.—Children who have penetrating trauma to the head and neck are at high risk for vascular, ocular, neurological, and aerodigestive damage. The charts of 21 children who sustained penetrating injuries to the face or upper neck in 1986 through 1989 were reviewed.

Patients.—The study group included 17 boys and 4 girls with a mean age of 10.2 years. Sixteen had been shot and 5 had been stabbed. All injuries were categorized according to the location of the entry wound. Three patients received wounds in area 1, the forehead and ears; 13 patients sustained injuries in area 2, the midportion of the face; and 6 patients had entrance wounds in area 3, extending from the lower lip to the hyoid bone. In 1 patient, a shotgun wound included both areas 2 and 3.

Results.—Three patients died, but most of the remaining children survived with minimal permanent disability. Significant problems included 7 vascular injuries, 5 ocular injuries, 6 CNS injuries, 2 cases of pneumothorax, and 1 cervical esophageal penetration. Stab wounds were just as likely to cause severe injury as were gunshot wounds. The outward appearance of the injury may appear relatively minor in children because of the elasticity and recoil of their soft tissue.

Conclusion.—Penetrating injuries of the head and neck require prompt attention in children. An organized diagnostic and treatment algorithm based upon the classification system of Gant and Epstein for penetrating maxillofacial trauma was reviewed. Once a safe and effective airway is instituted and cardiopulmonary resuscitation is performed, a complete physical examination is in order. Additional examinations and

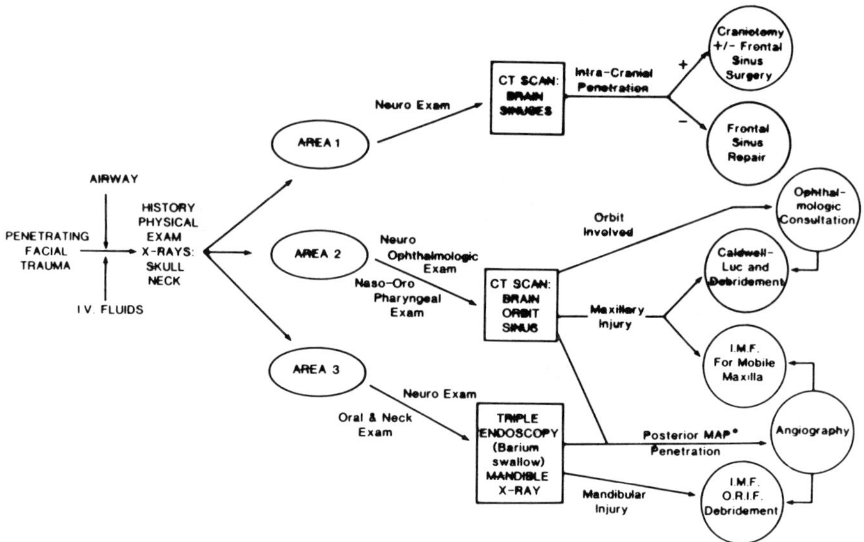

Fig 9–9.—A treatment algorithm for penetrating facial trauma based on 3 anatomical areas of the face. (Courtesy of Martin WS, Gussack GS: *Laryngoscope* 100:1288–1291, 1990.)

procedures are then planned (Fig 9–9), depending on the area of the injury.

▶ Most of the penetrating head and neck trauma that we encounter involves adults, and it is uncommon to be confronted with children with gunshot wounds and stabbing injuries in most communities. Unfortunately, the incidence is increasing in our society, and we must be prepared to deal with such cases in a methodical, rational sequence of steps. Children have a much less substantial "protective reserve" than adults, and any unnecessary delays can be disastrous.—B.J. Bailey, M.D., F.A.C.S.

Head and Neck Burns: Evaluation and Current Management
Osguthorpe JD (Med Univ of South Carolina)
Arch Otolaryngol Head Neck Surg 117:969–974, 1991 9–11

Introduction.—More than half of the 150,000 patients who are hospitalized each year in the United States with burn injury have involvement of the head and neck region. As many as 7% have inhalation injury as well. Advanced fluid replacement and care in specialized burn units have markedly lowered mortality in patients incurring injuries to 75% to 90% of the body surface. Death is most often the result of respiratory complications or sepsis.

Management.—When inhalation injury is diagnosed laryngoscopically, airway compromise is managed by intubation; tracheotomy is used for

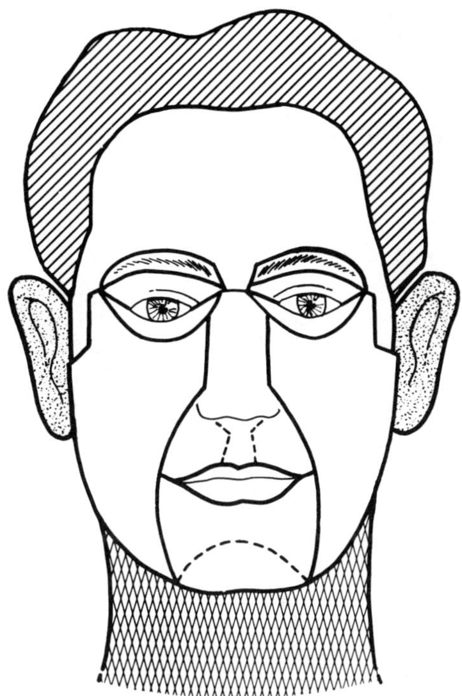

Fig 9–10.—The esthetic units for graft reconstruction of the face are outlined. Hypertrophic scarring at the junctions of these units (and grafts) is common and requires dermabrasion. The 10-degree–20-degree upward angulation of the graft junctions at the corners of the mouth and eyelids minimizes ptosis. (Courtesy of Osguthorpe JD: *Arch Otolaryngol Head Neck Surg* 117:969–974, 1991.)

long-term care. Sloughing mucosa and mucus are removed by repeated bronchoscopy. Sepsis can be minimized by early removal of the burn eschar and autografting. Patients with extensive injuries may receive temporary coverage with cadaver allograft skin, porcine xenograft, or a skin substitute until autograft becomes available. Reconstructive measures are best taken using the concept of esthetic units (Fig 9–10).

Long-Term Care.—Thicker skin grafts generally provide the best color match and texture. Hypertrophic scarring and contracture are minimized by early pressure on the grafts and by stretching exercises. Masks are worn during the day for as long as a year after injury. Even the best care may not prevent suboptimal cosmetic results in the most severely burned patients, and the patients must be prepared for this. Revision is delayed for at least 6 months and often for a year.

▶ The otolaryngologist/head and neck surgeon can be particularly helpful in the care of patients with severe head and neck burns. Evaluation of the airway and assessment of inhalation injury are vital steps in many instances. This study provides an excellent review of the management options from the perspective of facial aesthetic units. This is an excellent update.—B.J. Bailey, M.D., F.A.C.S.

Parotid Duct Injury: Is Immediate Surgical Repair Necessary?

Lewis G, Knottenbelt JD (Groote Schuur Hosp, Cape Town, South Africa)
Injury 22:407–409, 1991 9–12

Objective.—The infrequency of parotid duct injuries means that few prospective treatment studies are available. Nevertheless, the need to repair acute injuries so that salivary fistulas and sepsis will not occur is generally accepted. The outcome of nonoperative management was examined prospectively in 19 patients with duct injuries confirmed by the methylene blue dye method (Fig 9–11).

Observations.—Nearly half of the patients had healing without complications. In 7 patients, a short-term salivary fistula developed, whereas sialocele developed in 4. None of the complications required surgical treatment. All patients were asymptomatic after a mean follow-up of 1 month.

Conclusions.—Conservative management of parotid duct injuries is effective and safe, and acute repair can no longer be recommended. There is no evidence that parotid atrophy is likelier in patients managed nonoperatively.

▶ Immediate repair with stenting of the parotid duct has become standard practice in the event of laceration. The authors point out that this may be problematic in practice because of the difficulty in differentiating duct laceration from general glandular laceration. Cannulation, sialography, and exploration of the wound are important adjuncts that may have to be used to obtain a definitive assessment of the injury. In any event, the goal is to restore the integrity of the duct and to avoid stenosis by using a stent.—B.J. Bailey, M.D., F.A.C.S.

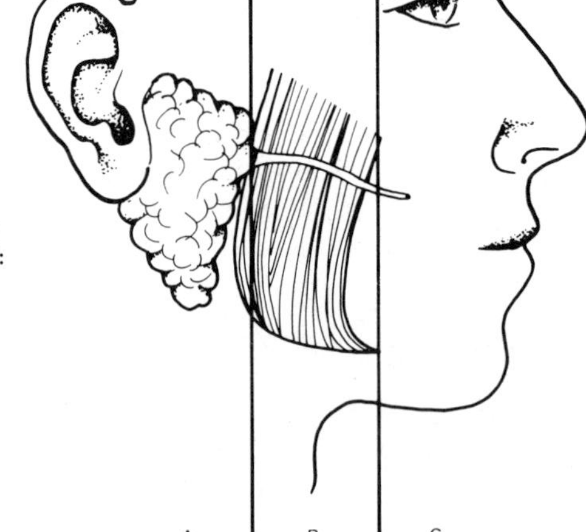

Fig 9–11.—Classification of site of ductal injury. (Courtesy of Lewis G, Knottenbelt JD: *Injury* 22:407–409, 1991.)

10 Head and Neck Oncology

Median Mandibulotomy: A Critical Assessment

Dubner S, Spiro RH (Mem Sloan-Kettering Cancer Ctr, New York)

Head & Neck 13:389–393, 1991 10–1

Introduction.—A reconstructed mandible rarely will function as well as one that is divided and repaired. Mandibulotomy can provide excellent access to selected oral and oropharyngeal tumors, and it produces minimal functional disability and a relatively good cosmetic outcome.

Patients.—Mandibulotomy was performed in 313 patients from 1959 through 1988, most often for tumor removal. The median patient age was 58 years. The oropharynx and oral cavity were the most common sites of tumor. In 60 cases, mandibulotomy was part of a salvage procedure after radiotherapy failed. Another 175 patients received planned postoperative radiotherapy.

Technique.—A notched osteotomy is favored for enhancing vertical stability (Fig 10–1). A paramedian rather than a midline osteotomy is made through the symphysis, allowing division between the lateral incisor and canine teeth where the tooth roots diverge. Although the manidibulotomy is repaired with wire, in-

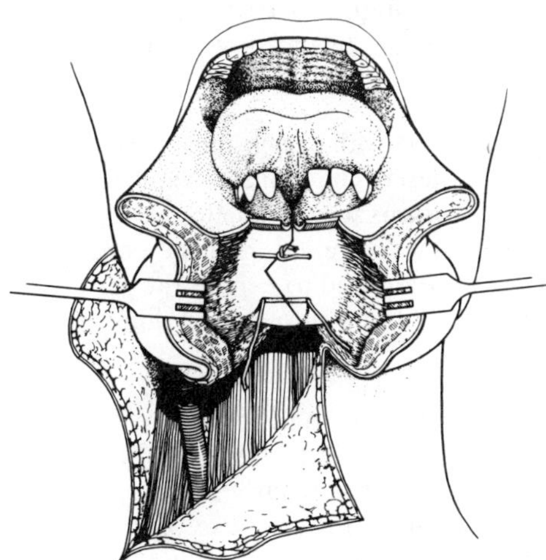

Fig 10–1.—Median mandibulotomy with wire repair. (Courtesy of Dubner S, Spiro RH: *Head & Neck* 13:389–393, 1991.)

terest now centers on titanium miniplates to achieve bony fixation. Interdental wiring or splints are used for stabilization.

Outcome.—Complications occurred in 44% of the patients, and there were 2 postoperative deaths. Most problems were related to wound sepsis, pneumonia, or tracheitis. Patients with squamous cancer had a 5-year disease-free survival of 53%. Local recurrences were noted in 20% of the patients.

Conclusions.—Mandibulotomy offers a worthwhile alternative to jaw reconstruction for selected patients who require tumor removal. It does not provide adequate access to massive tumors. Radiotherapy is a reasonable alternative for patients with small or inaccessible tumors.

▶ The "take-home" message of this study is that it is not necessary to perform segmental resection as frequently as we once believed. Only when the tumor is known to invade or envelop the bone is it mandatory that a section be removed. In most instances, mandibulotomy and a "mandibular swing" approach can provide excellent access to the tumor. Marginal resection in the region of tumor encroachment is usually sufficient to excise the primary tumor.—B.J. Bailey, M.D., F.A.C.S.

Transoral Approach to the Upper Cervical Spine

Merwin GE, Post JC, Sypert GW (Univ of Florida College of Medicine)

Laryngoscope 101:780–784, 1991 10–2

Introduction.—Although its use is logical, the transoral approach to the upper cervical spine is seldom used because of fear of exposure and infection. The approach was utilized in 16 consecutively treated patients who required exposure from the clivus through C3 to treat cord compression caused by rheumatoid disease, tumor, or craniovertebral anomalies.

Technique.—A Dingman mouth gag was used with cheek retractors to gain exposure after the induction of general anesthesia. The limits of exposure were mapped under fluoroscopic guidance, and incisions were made in the form of a horizontal "H" (Fig 10–2). The mucosal flaps were raised, and the constrictor muscles and anterior longitudinal ligament were divided to expose the vertebrae. After the pathologic lesion was removed, a 37-layer closure was done, taking care to make the mucosal closure watertight.

Results.—There were no deaths and no patient had leakage of CSF or meningitis. All the pharyngeal wall incisions healed normally. Nasopharyngeal incompetence was not seen. The patients resumed eating 9 days postoperatively on average. Gross tumor removal was consistently achieved, and pain and weakness were relieved in all patients who had

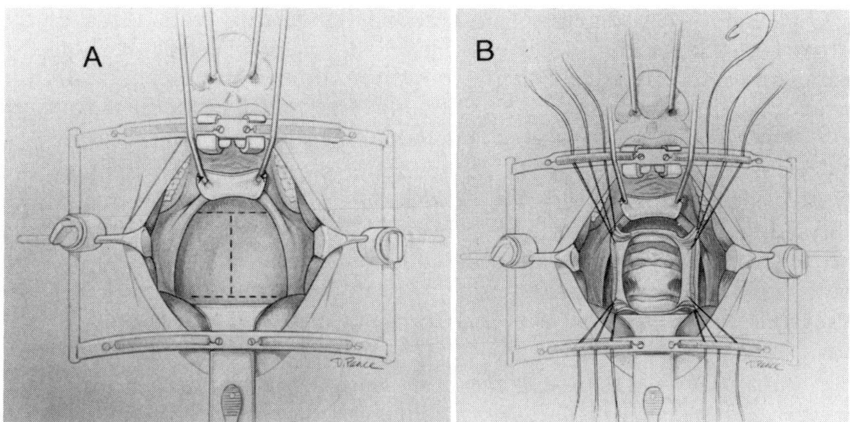

Fig 10–2.—A, surgical exposure using a Dingman mouth gag with custom-fitted silicone rubber sheeting used to retract soft palate and uvula posterosuperiorly. The *dotted lines* indicate a horizontal "H" incision of the pharyngeal mucosa. **B,** elevation and retraction of 3 tissue layers with exposure of cervical spine. The tissue is retracted using 4-0 absorbable sutures, which are also used in the closure. (Courtesy of Merwin GE, Post JC, Sypert GW: *Laryngoscope* 101:780–784, 1991.)

surgery for those reasons. The mean blood loss was 690 cc. One patient became dysphagic for reasons that were not clear.

Conclusion.—Excellent functional results are achieved using a combined otolaryngological/neurosurgical transoral approach to the upper cervical spine. Major complications are few.

► Several authors have observed that the transoral approach to the upper cervical spine is safe and effective. Use of the operating microscope and high speed drill allows rapid and safe removal of bone. Preoperative planning relies on MRI or CT scanning, and intraoperative fluoroscopy adds another margin of safety. Use of a tracheotomy provides the important element of airway protection. The authors emphasize that although the transoral approach is suitable for benign disease, it may not be appropriate for the management of malignant disease.—B.J. Bailey, M.D., F.A.C.S.

Diagnosis of Medullary Carcinoma of the Thyroid (MCT) by Calcitonin Assay Using Monoclonal Antibodies: Criteria for the Pentagastrin Stimulation Test in Hereditary MCT

Guilloteau D, Perdrisot R, Calmettes C, Baulieu JL, Lecomte P, Kaphan G, Milhaud G, Besnard JC, Jallet P, Bigorgne JC (Centre Hospitalier Universitaire, Tours, France; Centre Hospitalier Universitaire, Angers, France; Centre Hospitalier Universitaire, Paris; Centre Hospitalier Universitaire, Marseille, France)

J Clin Endocrinol Metab 71:1064–1067, 1990 10–3

Objective.—The diagnosis of hereditary medullary carcinoma of the thyroid (MCT) is dependent on a calcitonin assay after pentagastrin stimulation. A new calcitonin immunoradiometric assay (IRMA) in which anti-11-7 and anti-24-32 calcitonin fragment monoclonal antibodies are used was compared with classic radioimmunoassays (RIAs).

Method.—The basal levels of calcitonin were measured by RIA and IRMA in 83 controls, 20 chronic hemodialysis patients without known thryoid disease, 7 patients with proven MCT, and 21 patients with recurrent MCT. The pentagastrin stimulation test was performed in 18 normal subjects and in 8 patients from 4 families with confirmed MCT at subsequent surgery. The lowest detectable calcitonin concentration with the IRMA was 2.5 ng/L.

Results.—With the IRMA, the basal level of calcitonin in normal subjects was less than 10 ng/L. After pentagrastrin stimulation, half the normal subjects showed no response in the levels of calcitonin, whereas the other half had levels of calcitonin between 10–30 ng/L. In patients with renal failure, levels of calcitonin were increased between 10 and 52 ng/L. In general, the levels of calcitonin were higher with RIA than with IRMA. In patients with original or recurrent MCT, basal levels of calcitonin ranged from 189 to 28,900 ng/L with the IRMA, and the values showed no overlap with those of normal subjects. After pentagastrin stimulation in family studies, the CT peak was equal to or greater than 38 ng/L. On the basis of the RIA, the diagnosis would have been missed in 4 cases of MCT. However, MCT was correctly identified with the IRMA.

Conclusion.—There are large differences between levels of calcitonin as measured by RIA and IRMA. The IRMA test provides a greater sensitivity to the pentagastrin test and allows better identification of microcarcinoma in hereditary cases of MCT.

Intraoperative Pathologic Diagnosis of Thyroid Neoplasms: Report on Experience With 504 Specimens

Rosen Y, Rosenblatt P, Saltzman E (Brookdale Hosp Med Ctr, Brooklyn)
Cancer 66:2001–2006, 1990 10–4

Objective.—The accuracy of intraoperative frozen section diagnosis was examined in a series of 457 patients who provided 504 specimens of thyroid tissue during a 9-year period. Examination of the permanent sections revealed a malignancy in 57 (11.3%) of the specimens; 50 of these patients had primary thyroid carcinoma, 4 had metastatic cancer, and 3 had malignant lymphoma.

Correlation.—The frozen section diagnosis was malignant in 5.9% of the cases and "deferred" in 5.2% of the cases. The sensitivity of the frozen section diagnosis of malignancy was 53%, whereas the specificity was 100%. The technique had an overall accuracy of approximately 98%.

Malignancy was diagnosed in 62% of the patients with a deferred frozen-section diagnosis. None of the 10 cases of follicular carcinomas was diagnosed as malignant on frozen section study. All of these tumors were well differentiated, and 8 of the 10 were minimally invasive.

Conclusions.—The intraoperative frozen section diagnosis of malignancy in thyroid nodules does not appear to be very sensitive, particularly for follicular carcinoma. The preoperative needle biopsy and intraoperative frozen section study should be considered complementary procedures.

Changing Trends in Thyroid Surgery: 38 Years' Experience

Galloway JW, Sardi A, DeConti RW, Mitchell WT Jr, Bolton JS (Ochsner Clinic and Alton Ochsner Med Found, New Orleans)

Am Surg 57:18–20, 1991 10–5

Background.—Fine-needle aspiration (FNA) of thyroid masses before surgery has been used to prepare and evaluate patients with thyroid disease since the 1950s. The trends in thyroid surgery were determined, and FNA's impact on the treatment of thyroid nodules was evaluated.

Methods.—Between January 1950 and December 1988, 3,035 thyroidectomies were performed. The first 2 years of each decade and the last 2 years of the study period (1988 and 1989) were chosen for retrospective review. During these 10 years, 509 thyroid surgeries were performed.

Findings.—The total number of thyroid operations decreased significantly in the late 1980s, from an average of 112 per year from 1950 to 1981 to 60 procedures during 1987–1988. More than 80% of the patients who underwent thyroid procedures were euthyroid. The use of FNA increased sixfold in the late 1980s when compared with the early 1980s. Total thyroidectomies increased from 7.2% in 1950–1951 to 35%

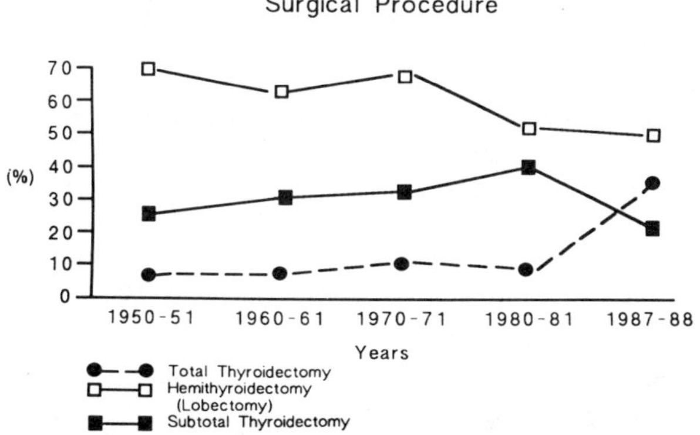

Fig 10–3.—Surgical procedures performed in each study period. (Courtesy of Galloway JW, Sardi A, DeConti RW, et al: *Am Surg* 57:18–20, 1991.)

in 1987–1988 (Fig 10–3). The incidence of papillary carcinoma increased from 29% in 1950–1951 to 79% in 1987–1988, and the incidence of follicular and mixed cell types of carcinoma decreased. Operative cases for carcinoma increased statistically from 6.3% in 1950–1951 to 46.7% in 1987–1988. Although the incidence of total thyroidectomies increased, the complication rate decreased from 4.5% and 6% in 1950–1951 and 1970–1971, respectively, to 1.6% during 1987–1988.

Conclusions.—These findings indicate that the use of FNA has decreased the number of patients undergoing surgery, increased the percentage of cancer as a reason for surgery, and increased the percentage of preoperative pathologic diagnoses. Fine-needle aspiration offers a reliable method for preoperative evaluation of patients with thyroid nodules.

▶ Frozen-section diagnosis during surgery is often the key to selecting an optimal treatment plan from the variety of options that were anticipated preoperatively. In some patients, new intraoperative findings will mandate a strategy different from that which would be clear on the basis of preoperative FNA biopsy. Teamwork among surgeons, pathologists, and radiologists has increased the level of surgical decision-making to an all-time high. Abstracts 10–3 and 10–4 provide specific details about important areas that are seeing rapid advances.

Abstract 10–5 highlights the impact of the refinements in cytopathology that have raised the accuracy of FNA. Patients are the ultimate beneficiaries of our heightened diagnostic accuracy, and the tangible results have reduced both the number of unnecessary primary surgical procedures and the need for reoperations.—B.J. Bailey, M.D., F.A.C.S.

Surgical Strategy in Thyroid Disease

Lando MJ, Hoover LA, Zuckerbraun L (Univ of Kansas, Kansas City; Olive View Med Ctr, Sylmar, Calif)

Arch Otolaryngol Head Neck Surg 116:1378–1383, 1990 10–6

Introduction.—To provide important thyroid surgery experience for residents, the preoperative evaluation and surgical strategy have been standardized for safety and consistency. The specifics of surgical procedures were reviewed, with emphasis on the specific problems of preservation of the recurrent nerve; the parathyroid glands; the management of larger, substernal thyroid glands; and the techniques for partial thyroid surgery. Both cancerous and benign conditions were seen in 260 evaluated patients.

Technique.—Inferior identification of the recurrent laryngeal nerve is performed, and the blood supply to the parathyroid glands is preserved when possible. A modified neck dissection is performed for metastatic disease (Fig 10–4). Completion thyroidectomies are preferred to initial total thyroidectomy.

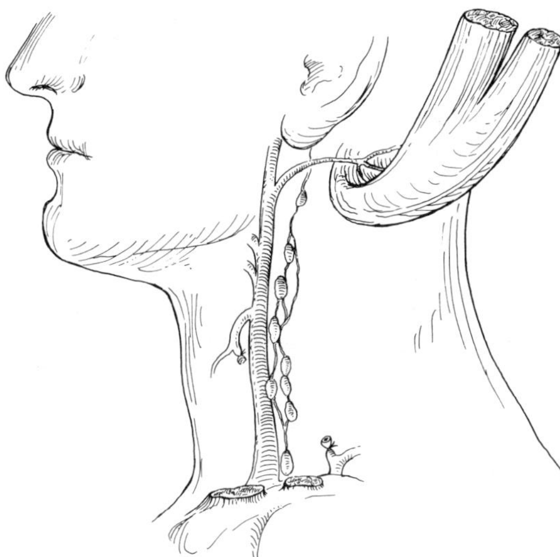

Fig 10–4.—A diagrammatic representation of a modified neck dissection with sternocleidomastoid muscle elevation, which is later reapproximated to allow complete lymph node dissection. (Courtesy of Lando MJ, Hoover LA, Zuckerbraun L: *Arch Otolaryngol Head Neck Surg* 166:1378–1383, 1990.)

Conclusion.—A thorough preoperative workup that utilizes FNA results instead of other imaging techniques assures the development of proper surgical strategy before entering the operating room.

Follicular Thyroid Cancer Treated at the Mayo Clinic, 1946 Through 1970: Initial Manifestations, Pathologic Findings, Therapy, and Outcome

Brennan MD, Bergstralh EJ, van Heerden JA, McConahey WM (Mayo Clinic and Found, Rochester, Minn)

Mayo Clin Proc 66:11–22, 1991 10–7

Introduction.—Follicular thyroid cancer differs histologically and clinically from the papillary variety. Follicular thyroid cancer is less common and is associated with a higher mortality. This reflects its greater tendency to metastasize widely, particularly to the lungs and bones. Several studies of the outcome and survival in patients with follicular thyroid cancer involved only small series of patients. The records of all patients with pure follicular thyroid cancer who were treated at the Mayo Clinic between 1946 and 1970 were reviewed. The diagnosis was confirmed by reexamination of the preserved tissue specimens.

Patients.—Fifty-seven women with a mean age of 50.5 years and 43 men with a mean age of 56.3 years had a confirmed diagnosis of follicular thyroid cancer. A total of 97 patients had palpable nodules, 20% of which were clinically suggestive of a malignant lesion. Seven patients had cervical lymphadenopathy and malignant nodal involvement was confirmed in 6. Twenty patients also had nonthyroidal malignant disease. All patients underwent operation, with total removal of the primary tumor in 97 patients. Of the 88 patients who had no distant metastatic lesions at the time of diagnosis, only 2 of them underwent ablation of the thyroid remnant.

Outcome.—The mean follow-up was 17.4 years. At the end of the study, 19 patients had died of follicular thyroid cancer. The mean follow-up in these patients was 6.4 years (range, 3 months–19 years). Multivariate analysis identified age greater than 50 years, marked vascular invasion, and metastatic involvement at the time of diagnosis to be independent predictors of mortality from follicular thyroid cancer. Of the patients, 34 with 2 or more of these predictors were classified as high risk. The survival rates for these high-risk patients were 47% at 5 years and 8% at 20 years. The survival rates for the 66 low-risk patients were 99% at 5 years and 86% at 20 years. The ratio of papillary cancer to follicular cancer was 8.6:1.

Conclusion.—The identification of high- and low-risk patients may facilitate a more rational approach to the treatment of follicular thyroid cancer.

Lymph Node Metastasis From Papillary-Follicular Thyroid Carcinoma in Young Patients

Frankenthaler RA, Sellin RV, Cangir A, Goepfert H (Univ of Texas MD Anderson Cancer Ctr, Houston)

Am J Surg 160:341–343, 1990 10–8

Background.—Authorities disagree on the pathology, treatment, follow-up, and prognostic factors in pediatric thyroid cancer. A 39-year experience with thyroid carcinoma in young patients was reviewed to better define presentation, characteristics, relative frequency of occurrence by anatomical site, and mortality. Special attention was given to the management of regional lymph node metastasis.

Patients.—A group of 117 patients younger than 20 years of age with papillary or follicular thyroid cancer, or both, was studied. The mean age at presentation was 16 years. The ratio of female to male patients was

Recurrence by ^{131}I Treatment

Site of Recurrence	Iodine 131 (n = 63)	No Iodine 131 (n = 54)	All Patients (n = 117)
Any*	13 (21%)	21 (39%)	34 (29%)
Primary	2 (3%)	3 (6%)	5 (4%)
Neck	9 (14%)	19 (35%)	28 (24%)
Distant	2 (3%)	2 (4%)	4 (3%)

* Some patients had recurrence at multiple sites.

(Courtesy of Frankenthaler RA, Sellin RV, Cangir A, et al: *Am J Surg* 160:341–343, 1990.)

2.9:1. Family history of thyroid cancer was found in 3% of the patients, and 20% had had prior irradiation for chronic adenoiditis (57%), thymic hyperplasia (30%), or acne (13%). There was a mean of 11 years between prior irradiation and the diagnosis of thyroid cancer. A solitary, painless cervical mass was the most common presenting symptom. The mass was in the thyroid in 40% of the patients, and it represented regional lymph node metastasis in 60%. Few patients had either hoarseness or dysphagia, and none had signs of thyroid dysfunction. The duration of symptoms ranged from 1 month to 10 years, with a mean duration of 14.5 months.

Outcome.—During the 39-year study period, the trend in treatment has been toward surgery plus postoperative irradiation with ^{131}I. All patients also received postoperative hormone-suppression therapy. In 79% of the patients, the cancer was papillary-follicular; 12% of these were pure papillary and 9% pure follicular. Soft tissue invasion at the primary site was found in 27%, whereas 6% had strap muscle invasion, and 5% had extracapsular spread from the lymph nodes. Pathologic examination revealed lymph node involvement in 26% of the cases that were clinically N0. Overall, the recurrence rate was 29%. The sites of recurrence, according to whether ^{131}I was received, are shown in the table. The most frequent site of recurrence was the neck. Relapse was rare at both primary and distant sites. All distant metastases were pulmonary. For all sites, the average time to recurrence was 3.5 years. No patients died of thyroid cancer at overall follow-up of 14.5 years.

Discussion.—Surgery and postoperative irradiation with ^{131}I for initial control of local and regional thyroid cancer should lower the rate of neck recurrences and decrease overall morbidity. Near total or total thyroidectomy with modified neck dissection followed by treatment with ^{131}I is recommended. Excellent prognosis is a product of aggressive initial treatment, vigilant surveillance for recurrence, and early treatment when recurrent disease is documented.

Experience in the Surgical Management of Medullary Thyroid Carcinoma

Lannigan FJ, Maisey MN, Watkinson JC, Shaheen OH, Clarke SE (Guy's Hosp, London)

Ann R Coll Surg Engl 73:27–31, 1991 10–9

Purpose.—The results of the surgical management of medullary thyroid carcinoma (MTC) in 12 patients were evaluated. Five patients had tumors that extended beyond the thyroid capsule, 9 had regional lymph node metastasis, and 3 had distant metastasis.

Management.—All patients underwent total thyroidectomy. Eight patients had modified neck dissection for the removal of nodal disease; 4 of these patients required a sternal split to remove mediastinal nodal spread. Another 2 patients underwent partial esophageal resection to obtain macroscopic tumor clearance. Nine patients with nodal disease and/or spread beyond the capsule of the thyroid gland received postoperative radiotherapy.

Results.—There were no perioperative deaths. Serum calcitonin returned to normal levels in 2 patients after radical surgery. Two patients with distant metastases on presentation died of their disease at 3 years and 5 years after surgery. Six patients were alive (with no evidence of disease) between 1 year and 9 years (average, 2.75 years) after surgery. Another patient was still alive at 9 years after surgery despite the presence of liver metastasis.

Conclusion.—An aggressive treatment policy may produce worthwhile survival for patients with advanced MTC. Long-term survival may be achieved even in the presence of distant metastases.

► Thyroid surgery for benign and malignant lesions is a topic of great interest. Standardization of preoperative assessment and surgical management is a desirable, but elusive goal because of the numerous variables of the disease process. Lando et al. (Abstract 10–6) provide a valuable summary of their experience, from which they have distilled a strategy for diagnosis and surgical management. Specific guidelines are presented for dealing with key decision points.

The report from the Mayo Clinic (Abstract 10–7) provides very long-term follow-up (20–45 years) on a series of patients with follicular thyroid cancer. The ominous prognostic features in this group of patients were distant metastases, extra thyroid tumor extension, angioinvasion, increasing tumor size and grade, and age greater than 50 years.

The behavior of papillary and/or follicular carcinoma in patients younger than 20 years of age was studied in the report from the M.D. Anderson Cancer Center (Abstract 10–8). This long-term survey (1949–1987) focused on the pattern of lymph node metastasis and concluded that near-total thyroidectomy, modified neck dissection, and postoperative ^{131}I was the optimal treatment strategy. Because of the need to prevent recurrence, death, and lifelong complications of treatment in young patients, the authors emphasize the need for aggressive initial management.

Medullary thyroid cancer (discussed in Abstract 10–9) accounts for less than 10% of thyroid malignancy. Screening for familial MTC and workup for multiple endocrine neoplasia type II are essential. In the management of these patients, it is important to remember that MTC is associated with a higher rate of recurrence, metastasis, and local invasion of the surrounding tissues.—B.J. Bailey, M.D., F.A.C.S.

Outpatient and Short-Stay Thyroid Surgery

Lo Gerfo P, Gates R, Gazetas P (Columbia Univ; Columbia Presbyterian Med

Ctr, New York; Univ of California, San Francisco)
Head Neck 13:97–101, 1991 10–10

Introduction.—Simple thyroidectomies have an extremely low incidence of complications, and most patients who undergo this procedure are discharged the day after surgery. The results of thyroid surgery performed in an ambulatory surgical setting at the Columbia Presbyterian Medical Center were reviewed.

Patients.—Between 1987 and 1989, a total of 105 women and 29 men (average age, 47 years) underwent 56 total thyroidectomies, 28 subtotal thyroidectomies, and 50 lobectomies in an ambulatory surgery setting. Those patients who had undergone reoperation, neck dissection, sternal splits, or other concomitant procedures were excluded. All patients were believed to be reliable and completely capable of understanding the procedure and complying with postoperative plans.

Procedures.—The surgical technique and recovery room protocol were designed to allow for early identification of life-threatening complications in their anticipated time frame. The recurrent laryngeal nerve was routinely identified and traced, and closure of the wound involved reapproximating the anterior cervical fascia and strap muscles only over the thyroid cartilage and superior portion of the trachea. Local anesthesia was used in 16% of the procedures. Half the procedures were performed for benign disease, but the most common diagnosis was papillary cancer (44%).

Results.—Of the patients, 76 were discharged the day of surgery (including 21 who had total thyroidectomy, 13 who had subtotal thyroidectomy, and 42 who had simple lobectomies). Fifty-three of the 58 patients admitted were discharged the day after surgery. The average postoperative stay was .49 days. Postoperative complications included transient hypocalcemia in 8 patients (6%) and permanent unilateral recurrent laryngeal nerve paralysis in 1 (.75%). All complications occurred in patients who had total thyroidectomies. None of the patients had postoperative complications that required reoperation or readmission. There was no operative mortality.

Conclusion.—By using specific selection criteria, thyroid lobectomy and subtotal thyroidectomy can be performed safely in an ambulatory surgical setting without an increase in morbidity or mortality. It appears that total thyroidectomies may be managed in a similar fashion.

▶ This report, like several others, describes a positive experience with planned same-day thyroid surgery in selected patients. Nearly all of the patients who were admitted were discharged the next day. The 2 keys to success are careful observation in the immediate postoperative period and clear, forceful patient education regarding the early signs and symptoms of complications. Airway obstruction, bleeding, and hypocalcemia are the major concerns after thyroidectomy. Surgeons must act cautiously when shifting some postoperative responsibilities to patients and their families.—B.J. Bailey, M.D., F.A.C.S.

Current Trends in the Surgical Treatment of Solitary Parathyroid Adenoma: A Questionnaire Study from 53 Surgical Departments in 14 Countries

Tibblin S, Bondesson A-G, Udén P (Univ of Kuwait; Lund Univ, Sweden)
Eur J Surg 157:103–107, 1991 10–11

Background.—Parathyroid surgery has become common in surgical practice. There have been many recent modifications of the classic procedure, including the biopsy and intraoperative histological study techniques. The acceptance and influence of these newer measures were examined with special regard to the surgical management of primary hyperparathyroidism caused by solitary parathyroid adenoma.

Methods.—Questionnaires were distributed to 57 departments that were active in this field. Responses were received from 53 departments in 14 countries. The questionnaire determined the frequency with which parathyroid surgery was performed, the principles for treatment of primary hyperparathyroidism, the use of intraoperative histopathologic studies and fat stainings, the number of operations for primary hyperparathyroidism, and which of 6 surgical options would be closest to the departments' practice if an adenoma was found.

Results.—Of the departments, 70% considered intraoperative histological examination to be essential, particularly in Scandinavia and North America. Fat stains were used in 58% of the Scandinavian centers—more commonly than in other areas. Also, 32% of the departments preferred

Mode of Intraoperatively Identifying a Normal Parathyroid Gland in Relation to the Extent of Exploration (%)

Mode of identification	Exploration: Unilateral	Exploration: Bilateral
Intraoperative histology necessary	89	70
Intraoperative fat staining	56	28
Excisional biopsy (1 whole gland)	67	16
Gross inspection alone	0	26

(Courtesy of Tibblin S, Bondesson A-G, Udén P: *Eur J Surg* 157:103-107, 1991.)

excisional biopsy including 1 whole gland to multiple incisional biopsies. Inspection of 3 normal glands without histological identification was preferred by 21% of the departments, whereas 31% preferred bilateral exploration and incisional biopsy (table). Bilateral exploration with incisional biopsy of all 3 normal glands was advocated by 17% when an adenoma was found on the first side to be explored; a similar percentage preferred unilateral exploration with excisional or incisional biopsy of the ipsilateral normal gland.

Conclusions.—Surgical strategy in dealing with primary hyperparathyroidism appears to be changing. The trend is toward less traumatic modes of identifying normal parathyroid tissue, and the reliability of preoperative histological findings seems to have increased. Excisional biopsy is also gaining popularity because it gives more information on the cause of the hyperparathyroidism.

Locally Recurrent Parathyroid Neoplasms as a Cause for Recurrent and Persistent Primary Hyperparathyroidism

Fraker DL, Travis WD, Merendino JJ Jr, Zimering MB, Streeten EA, Weinstein LS, Marx SJ, Spiegel AM, Aurbach GD, Doppman JL, Norton JA (Natl Cancer Inst; Natl Inst of Diabetes Digestive and Kidney Diseases, Bethesda, Md)

Ann Surg 213:58–65, 1991 10–12

Introduction.—Unsuccessful surgery for hyperparathyroidism (HPT) is usually the result of multiglandular disease or parathyroid hyperplasia. The clinical histories, reoperative findings, and results from 145 patients with recurrent or persistent HPT were reviewed.

Methods.—The diagnosis was made by serially increased serum calcium and parathyroid hormone levels. Noninvasive imaging was performed to identify abnormal parathyroid glands.

Results.—Recurrent parathyroid tumors were found in 15 patients who had undergone 28 previous operations for HPT. Of the tumors, 4 were parathyroid carcinomas, and 11 were locally recurrent or atypical adenomas. Patients with carcinoma were more symptomatic and had greater levels of serum calcium and parathyroid hormone. After reoperation for excision of recurrent parathyroid tumors, the patients remained biochemically cured for a median follow-up of 21 months.

Conclusion.—Whether the persistent primary HPT is caused by parathyroid carcinoma or adenoma, aggressive reoperation can successfully result in prolonged cure.

► Tibblin et al. (Abstract 10–11) provide an interesting global perspective on the use of intraoperative histopathologic studies during surgery for parathyroid adenoma. There is a lack of uniformity among surgeons concerning whether both sides of the neck should be explored and how many glands should be biopsied. Although surveying leading surgeons to ascertain preferences is valuable, prospective studies that can compare the safety and effectiveness of various strategies are the greatest need in this field.

The article by Fraker et al. (Abstract 10–12) analyzes the role of local recurrence in patients with persistent HPT after surgery. In most instances, unsuccessful operations result from a failure to identify and remove an adenoma. Inexperience of the surgeon, unusual adenoma location, and multiglandular disease are the most common causes. Special problems and a higher incidence of recurrence are associated with parathyroid carcinoma; however, patients with this carcinoma are a relatively small subgroup within the HPT population.—B.J. Bailey, M.D., F.A.C.S.

Management Decisions in Laryngeal Carcinoma In Situ

McGuirt WF, Browne JD (Wake Forest Univ Med Ctr)

Laryngoscope 101:125–129, 1991 10–13

Introduction.—Carcinoma in situ and carcinoma in situ with microinvasion are neoplastic diseases that are usually difficult to treat. A group of 21 patients with laryngeal carcinoma in situ were treated with transoral endoscopic laser surgery.

Methods.—Diagnostic criteria included loss of differentiation, hypercellularity, atypical appearance of cells, changed polarity of cell orientation, macronucleosis and anisonucleosis, altered cell staining, and atypical mitotic characteristics. Of the 21 patients, 12 had carcinoma in situ and 9 had carcinoma in situ with microinvasion. All patients underwent

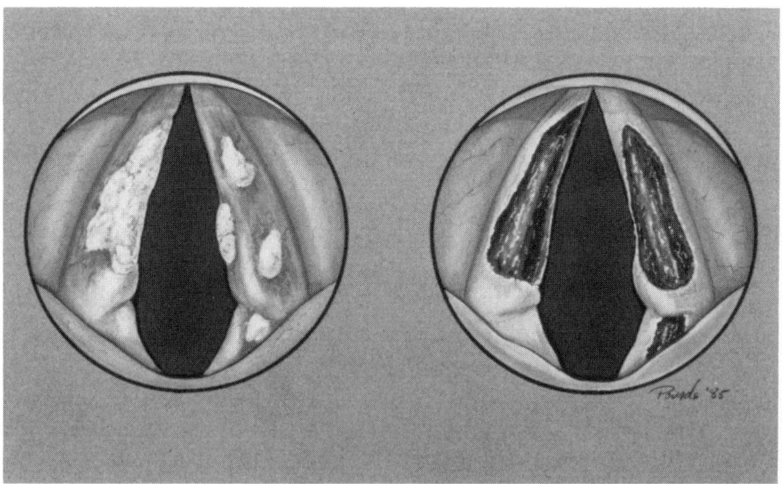

Fig 10–5.—A schematic drawing of laryngeal carcinoma in situ before (**left**) and after (**right**) laser mucosal resection. Note the sparing of the underlying, noninvolved tissue. (Courtesy of McGuirt WF, Browne JD: *Laryngoscope* 101:125–129, 1991.)

laser mucosal dissection of the vocal cord and vaporization of the adjacent and deeper tissues that appeared abnormal on viewing with the operating microscope. The patients had monthly follow-up studies using direct microscopic laryngoscopy, indirect laryngoscopy, or flexible office laryngoscopy.

Treatment technique.—The laryngeal lesions that were diagnosed (according to the criteria) as carcinoma in situ with or without microinvasion were treated by laser mucosal resection of the diseased mucosal and submucosal tissue. Underlying tumor-free tissue was left in place (Fig 10–5). The lesion was initially outlined by laser spot vaporization. The mucosa was tensed and undercut just above the membranous true cord for the superficial lesion. Toluidine blue staining was sometimes used to delineate the abnormal tissue in the first patients treated; however, it is no longer necessary because of experience and the capabilities of the operating microscope.

Results.—Most of the 21 patients have normal larynges after a single operative procedure. Of these patients, 5 have had recurrent or persistent abnormal-looking tissue, and 1 of the 5 required another single laser procedure. All patients are now free of any laryngeal abnormality after a maximal follow-up time of 4 years.

Implications.—These findings indicate that the laser mucosal dissection procedure successfully treats carcinoma in situ with or without microinvasion. Transoral endoscopic laser mucosal resection of this condition is recommended for most patients.

Hemilaryngectomy for Salvage of Radiation Therapy Failures

Rothfield RE, Johnson JT, Myers EN, Wagner RL (Univ of Pittsburgh; Eye and Ear Hosp of Pittsburgh)

Otolaryngol Head Neck Surg 103:792–794, 1990 10–14

Background.—Radiation therapy is the most common treatment for stage I vocal cord cancer. Surgery is usually reserved for patients in whom cancer recurs after radiation therapy. Unfortunately, total laryngectomy is often needed in such cases. An experience with frontolateral hemilaryngectomy was reviewed in patients with recurrence after radiation therapy.

Results.—Between 1977 and 1986, a total of 14 patients was treated with hemilaryngectomy for salvage of stage I vocal cord squamous cell carcinoma after unsuccessful full-course radiation therapy. During this same period, 77 patients had total laryngectomy for salvage after failure of radiation therapy. Hemilaryngectomy failed in 3 patients, and 2 were ultimately salvaged with total laryngectomy. Therefore, the salvage rate with hemilaryngectomy was 79%. The average follow-up was 90 months. The overall cure rate was 93%, with voice preservation in 86%. Age did not affect decannulation, postoperative infection, or initiation of oral intake. Such problems were more common in patients who had radiation therapy, compared with those who had hemilaryngectomy without prior radiation therapy.

Conclusions.—Hemilaryngectomy is an effective salvage technique in selected patients with stage I vocal cord cancer in whom radiation therapy has failed. Hemilaryngectomy offers voice preservation and good cure rates. Although the healing and complication rates are slightly higher than in patients who have hemilaryngectomy with no previous irradiation, they are not unacceptable.

Recurrence After Radiotherapy for Glottic Carcinoma

Viani L, Stell PM, Dalby JE (Univ of Liverpool, England; Clatterbridge Hosp, Wirral, England)

Cancer 67:577–584, 1991 10–15

Objective.—A series of 478 patients with $T_{1-3}N_0$ glottic carcinoma was treated by irradiation. Of these, 320 had not been previously treated; 158 with recurrent disease had undergone radiation therapy elsewhere. Radiation therapy was directed only at the primary site plus a reasonable margin of normal tissue, excluding the lymph node drainage area.

Data Analysis.—For previously untreated patients, the recurrence rate at 5 years was 10%. The recurrence rate was higher in T_2 and T_3 tumors, poorly differentiated tumors, and in patients in poor general condition. Of the recurrent tumors, 82% were pT_3 or pT_4, but 12% of the total laryngectomy specimens had no evidence of tumor. The necrosis rate was 1.4% for T_1 tumors, 4.2% for T_2 tumors, and 2.9% for T_3 tumors. Of the tumors, 60% were transglottic when they recurred, and only 29% were confined to the glottis. Preoperative histological diagnosis was 89% accurate, with a 97% sensitivity and a 91% predictive value for positive results; however, it was only 50% predictive of negative results and 25% specific, indicating that a negative histological report was unreliable.

Survival.—The 5-year survival rate after treatment of the primary recurrence was 39%. Sex, the clinical T stage of the tumor at recurrence, and the length of time to recurrence were significant predictors of survival. A total of 13% of the patients with primary recurrence was untreatable. Hospital mortality after laryngectomy was 3%, and a fistula developed in 32% of patients. Among the evaluable patients at 5 years, 49% were alive with a larynx, 5% were alive without a larynx, 13% were dead of the original cancer, and 33% had died of unrelated causes. The most common cause of death was subsequent lymph node metastases, followed by stomal recurrence and recurrence in the pharyngeal remnant. The 5-year recurrence rate at lymph nodes was 14%. General condition and T stage were significant predictors of node recurrence. Only 17% of the patients had small (N_1) nodes at recurrence, and 27% were unsuitable for treatment. The 5-year survival rate after treatment of node recurrence was 16%. Host and tumor factors and time to recurrence were not significant predictors of survival after node recurrence. The hospital mortality rate after salvage neck dissection was 4.7%. The most common cause of death was uncontrolled recurrence in the neck.

Discussion.—A total of 10% of the glottic carcinomas treated by irradiation recur at the primary site, and most tumors have advanced disease at recurrence. Tumor factors are important predictors of survival after treatment of a primary recurrence. A large proportion of patients survive with a functioning larynx, even after treatment of a T_3 tumor. The causes of failure include stomal recurrence and uncontrolled neck disease. Survival after a nodal recurrence is poor.

Vertical Partial Laryngectomy on Demand

Krajina Z (Zagreb, Yugoslavia)

J Laryngol Otol 104:879–882, 1990 10–16

Introduction.—Cancer of the larynx has a good prognosis after treatment. The value of horizontal partial laryngectomies is well established. However, the value of partial vertical laryngectomies remains controversial. The term "vertical partial laryngectomy on demand" should be applied to all modifications of vertical laryngectomies. Data were reviewed on 120 vertical and frontolateral partial laryngectomies performed at 1 center from 1970 to 1979.

Patients.—Most of the patients were classified preoperatively as $T_2N_0M_0$ and $T_3N_0M_0$. Of the 22 patients with positive lymph nodes, 8 (36%) survived 5 years. Positive cervical nodes were the biggest problem after partial procedures in patient survival. Those patients without cervical metastases had an 84% survival rate. Overall, 90 of the 120 patients were alive 5–10 years after surgery.

Results.—Early postoperative complications included edema of the arytenoid, pneumonia, hemorrhage, swallowing difficulties after 15 days, postoperative wound infection, and histologically positive marginal excision. Most of the patients were decannulated in the first month after surgery. Decannulation was performed much later in patients undergoing postoperative irradiation.

Conclusion.—Vertical partial laryngectomy on demand significantly contributes to the preservation of laryngeal function in patients with unilateral tumor localization. Immediate reconstruction with fascia was very effective, even when longer defects were covered.

► We have had an interest in the conservative management of carcinoma in situ and microinvasive carcinoma for 2 decades (see Abstract 10–13). Although laser excision is a reasonable option for glottic lesions, it is unclear whether it offers any advantage over microsurgical excision. We must remember that this disease process is often quite treacherous when located in the supraglottic region. Even on the true cords, multiple sites are common. Because the epithelium has been changed, surgeons should expect that other lesions will occur sometime in the future. Periodic follow-up for a very prolonged time is appropriate.

We have also employed partial laryngectomy for the salvage of radiation therapy failures (see Abstract 10–14). Vertical partial laryngectomy is a good choice if the patient was initially a suitable candidate for conservation surgery and if the recurrence is diagnosed before extralaryngeal spread has occurred. Surgical excision should be extensive enough to deal with the original tumor presentation—even if the recurrence appears to be small.

The article by Krajina (Abstract 10–16) proposes the use of a new term, "on demand", to describe modifications of vertical laryngectomy. Experienced surgeons frequently choose from a variety of options when dealing with individual patients, and these options may be necessary for either the excision of the tumor or the reconstruction afterward. The term "modified vertical partial laryngectomy" would probably be more appropriate, if it is indeed necessary.—B.J. Bailey, M.D., F.A.C.S.

Surgical Management of Supraglottic Cancer and Its Lymph Node Metastases in a Conservative Perspective

Bocca E (Univ of Milan, Italy)

Ann Otol Rhinol Laryngol 100:261–266, 1991 10–17

Background.—Combined with functional elective or curative neck dissection, supraglottic neck dissection has made an invaluable contribution to the treatment of supraglottic cancer and its lymph node metastases. The history and background of this approach were reviewed.

Discussion.—The concept of supraglottic laryngectomy was slow to be accepted because it upset the traditional principles of cancer surgery. Even in the 1970s it was still not popular in many countries, and some resistance may still be encountered. The supraglottis must be resected in

Recurrence Rate of Functional vs. Classic Neck Dissection

	No. of Cases	*Recurrences No.*	*Recurrences %*
Elective neck dissection			
Functional	672	16	2.38
Classic	226	15	6.63
Curative neck dissection			
Functional	171	52	30.4
Classic	188	90	47.9

Data from reference 39.

(Courtesy of Bocca E: *Ann Otol Rhinol Laryngol* 100:261-266, 1991.)

its entirety whenever the cancer originates within its boundaries. Functional neck dissection completes the conservative perspective of surgical management of the supraglottic cancer and its lymph node metastases. Distinct improvements in the number of recurrences are seen when functional, as opposed to radical, neck dissection is used (table). Because of the high incidence of useless elective neck dissections, a wait-and-see attitude is often preferred. If elective functional neck dissection is considered in continuity with supraglottic laryngectomy, it does not add to the morbidity and operative risks. In stage II to IV disease, results show a progressive discrepancy in favor of surgery over radiation. The factors that play a decisive role in the choice of treatment include the patient's will and condition, the tumor site and stage, the risks of second tumors, radiation tissue damage, salvage surgery, the difficulty in detecting early recurrences, the greater frequency of late recurrences with radiotherapy, and the expertise of the surgeon and radiation oncologist. When the choice is made, it is an all-or-nothing matter; there are few indications for combined therapy.

Conclusions.—The techniques of surgical management of supraglottic cancer have changed, although the principle has not. Compared with radiotherapy, surgery's advantages include respect for function and body image, more effective regional control, and deeper insight into the physiopathologic behavior of cancer. Surgeons must remember that their enemy is cancer of the larynx and lymph nodes, not the larynx and neck themselves.

▶ Bocca has made a major contribution to conservation surgery of the head and neck. As a pioneer with a new concept, his ideas were challenged and his critics were far more vocal (and more numerous) than his supporters. Modified neck dissection is not always the exact procedure that he described; however, the concept is valid in selected situations. As our understanding of cancer behavior expands, the surgical techniques we use will continue to evolve.—B.J. Bailey, M.D., F.A.C.S.

Incisional or Excisional Neck-Node Biopsy Before Definitive Radiotherapy, Alone or Followed by Neck Dissection

Ellis ER, Mendenhall WM, Rao PV, McCarthy PJ, Parsons JT, Stringer SP, Cassisi NJ, Million RR (Univ of Florida)

Head Neck 13:177–183, 1991 10–18

Introduction.—Open diagnostic cervical node biopsy before definitive resection of squamous cell carcinoma of the head and neck is controversial because surgical violation of diseased nodes may enhance tumor dissemination. However, no adverse effect of open neck-node biopsy has been reported for patients who undergo radiation therapy, either alone or combined with resection. Whether surgical violation of the neck compromises the results of subsequent definitive radiation therapy, either alone or followed by resection, was determined.

Patients.—During a 21-year period, 508 patients were treated for head and neck squamous cell carcinoma and clinically positive neck nodes in 660 heminecks; 457 were treated with radiation therapy alone and 203 received radiation therapy followed by neck dissection. A total of 66 patients had incisional or excisional biopsy of a positive neck node before the start of radiation therapy. All patients were observed for at least 2 years or until death. The prognostic factors that were analyzed included biopsy status of the neck, node stage, treatment, node mobility and location, tumor stage, primary site, and control of disease above the clavicles.

Findings.—Overall comparison of the Kaplan-Meier hemineck control curves for the biopsy and no-biopsy groups did not show a statistically significant difference between the groups for any of the 4 neck stages. In 3 of the 4 node stages, the results actually favored those who underwent neck biopsy before treatment.

Conclusion.—The data do not support a potential adverse effect of violating the neck before definitive treatment in patients with head and neck squamous cell carcinoma and positive neck nodes who undergo radiation therapy as the next step of treatment.

▶ Although the authors found no adverse effect of an open biopsy in their analysis, they do not recommend it as a diagnostic step. In fact, they feel that radiation therapy should precede any required surgical procedure. This seems to be a more reasonable strategy when combined therapy is indicated.

In an accompanying commentary, Robbins emphasizes that, although this study is counter to traditional teaching about the violation of surgical planes, it is significant because it provides support for modified neck dissection procedures.—B.J. Bailey, M.D., F.A.C.S.

Standardizing Neck Dissection Terminology: Official Report of the Academy's Committee for Head and Neck Surgery and Oncology

Robbins KT, Medina JE, Wolfe GT, Levine PA, Sessions RB, Pruet CW (Univ of California, San Diego Cancer Ctr)

Arch Otolaryngol Head Neck Surg 117:601–605, 1991 10–19

Background.—The multitude of modified methods for neck dissection has resulted in a nonuniform nomenclature system. The Academy's Committee for Head and Neck Surgery and Oncology, with input from the Education Committee of the American Society of Head and Neck Surgery, has developed a classification system for these procedures.

Classification.—The classification is based on several concepts. First, radical neck dissection is the fundamental procedure with which all other neck dissections are compared. Modified radical neck dissection

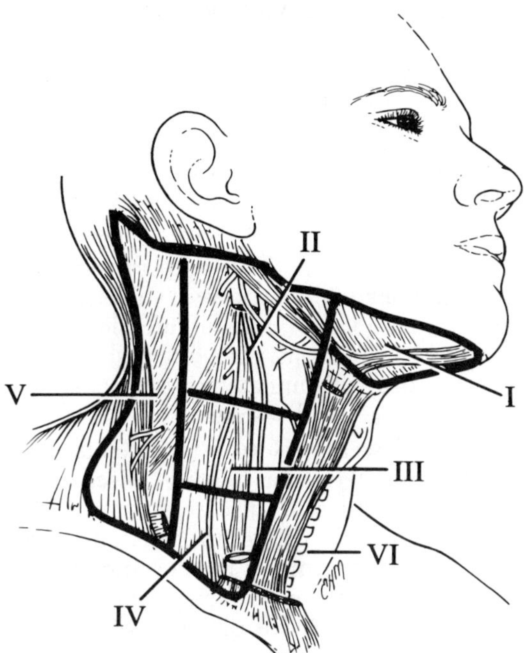

Fig 10–6.—The level system for describing the location of the lymph nodes in the neck. Level *I* indicates the submental and submandibular group; level *II*, the upper jugular group; level *III*, the middle jugular group; level *IV*, the lower jugular group; level V, the posterior triangle group; and level *VI*, the anterior-compartment group. (Courtesy of Robbins KT, Medina JE, Wolfe GT, et al: *Arch Otolaryngol Head Neck Surg* 117:601–605, 1991.)

means preservation of 1 or more nonlymphatic structures. Selective neck dissection indicates preservation of 1 or more groups of lymph nodes. Finally, extended radical neck dissection is the removal of 1 or more additional lymphatic and/or nonlymphatic structures. Selective neck dissection includes supraomohyoid, posterolateral, lateral, and anterior-compartment neck dissection. In radical neck dissection, definitions were recommended for the boundaries of the lymph node groups removed (Fig 10–6). Level I denotes the submental and submandibular group; level II, upper jugular; level III, middle jugular; level IV, lower jugular; level V, posterior triangle; and level VI, the anterior-compartment group.

Conclusions.—Communication among researchers and clinicians should be improved by adherence to the principles of this classification system to describe neck dissection techniques. This system also provides a rational framework to which new terminology can be added.

Is Laterality Important in Neck Node Metastases in Head and Neck Cancer?

Jones AS, Stell PM (Univ of Liverpool, Liverpool, England)
Clin Otolaryngol 16:261–265, 1991 10–20

Background.—Neck node metastasis is the most important prognostic factor in head and neck cancer; however, whether laterality of neck node metastasis affects prognosis is not clear.

Objective.—Data from 2,219 patients with previously untreated squamous carcinomas of the head and neck were studied to identify prognostic factors and to define the importance of laterality in neck node metastases. The survival rates in patients with bilateral neck node metastases were compared with those with unilateral disease matched for age, performance status, tumor stage, and T stage.

Data Analysis.—There were 141 (6.5%) patients with bilateral neck node metastases. The incidence of bilateral disease decreased significantly with increasing age. Bilateral disease was strongly associated with nasopharyngeal tumors, poorly differentiated tumors, and tumor stage T_3 or T_4 at presentation. Furthermore, the combination of these 3 tumor factors significantly increased the incidence still further, i.e., the incidence of bilateral nodes was 25% for patients with all 3 factors. A group

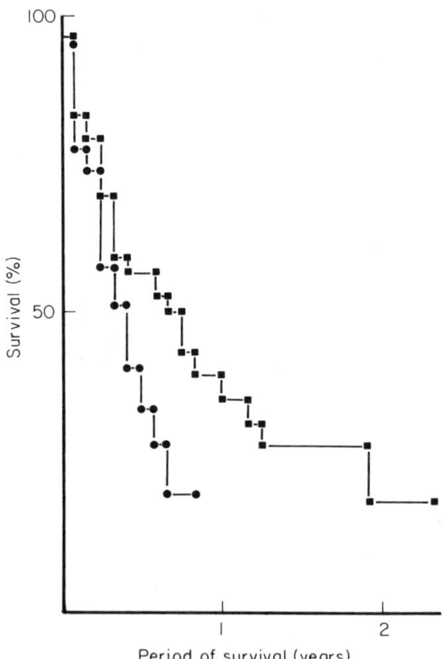

Fig 10–7.—Survival of patients with nodes greater than 6 cm. *Squares* indicate unilateral nodes; *circles,* bilateral nodes. (Courtesy of Jones AS, Stell PM: *Clin Otolaryngol* 16:261-265, 1991.)

of 126 patients with bilateral disease was matched for these main prognostic factors with 126 patients with unilateral disease. Survival was 9% better for patients with unilateral disease, compared with those with bilateral disease; however, the difference was not significant. When the subgroups were analyzed based on the size of the nodes, survival was not affected by laterality among those with nodes smaller than 6 cm; laterality significantly affected survival in patients with massive nodes (>6 cm) (Fig 10–7).

Conclusion.—Bilateral neck node metastases are not associated with a worse prognosis; the survival rates are similar to those of unilateral disease. Treating patients with bilateral disease is worthwhile.

▶ Standardization of neck dissection terminology (see Abstract 10–19) has been accomplished by a committee of the American Academy of Otolaryngology—Head and Neck Surgery. Their monograph has been well received by surgeons who were frustrated by the variety of terms, descriptions, and techniques that have been proposed by a variety of sources.

Jones and Stell (Abstract 10–20) reviewed a very large series and determined the factors of prognostic importance. The bottom line in their study is that bilateral neck dissections are solidly supported by their observations of survival.—B.J. Bailey, M.D., F.A.C.S.

Sequential Immunopathologic Study of Oral Lichen Planus Treated With Tretinoin and Etretinate

Baudet-Pommel M, Janin-Mercier A, Souteyrand P (School of Dentristry, Clermont-Ferrand; Hôpital Calmette, Lille; Hôtel-Dieu, Clermont-Ferrand, France)
Oral Surg Oral Med Oral Pathol 71:197–202, 1991 10–21

Objective.—The distribution and phenotype of inflammatory cells in biopsy specimens from patients with oral lichen planus (OLP) were compared before and after treatment with topical tretinoin and systemic etretinate.

Method.—Immunopathologic studies were performed using monoclonal antibodies before and after a 3-month course of treatment in 25 patients with histologically proved OLP. Ten patients with reticular and hyperkeratotic OLP received topical tretinoin, whereas 10 patients with erosive and reticular OLP associated with cutaneous and/or genital lichen planus received systemic etretinate. A group of 5 patients with reticular OLP received no treatment and served as controls.

Observations.—Before treatment, the biopsy specimens showed an abundance of T lymphocytes with a predominance of helper cells, few B lymphocytes, and a relatively large number of macrophages. After treatment, there was an overall decrease in the density of the infiltrate, without any significant difference in the pattern of distribution between the 2 treatment groups. The percentage of T lymphocytes decreased, and that

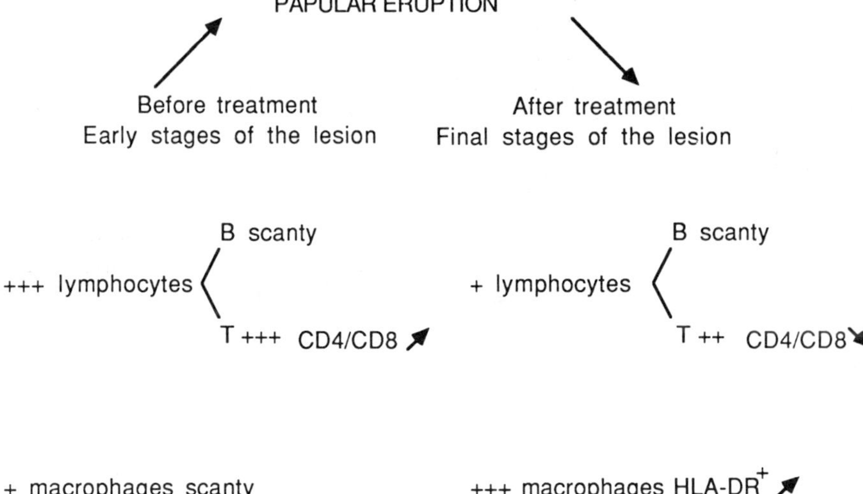

Fig 10–8.—Evolution of infiltrate with retinoid treatment. (Courtesy of Baudet-Pommel M, Janin-Mercier A, Souteyrand P: *Oral Surg Oral Med Oral Pathol* 71:197–202, 1991.)

of macrophages increased. There were 20% fewer CD-3-positive cells. Although the number of CD-4-positive lymphocytes decreased, the number of CD-8-positive lymphocytes remained stable, resulting in a decrease in the CD-4/CD-8 ratio (Fig 10–8). The distribution was unchanged in the untreated patients.

Conclusions.—In the treatment of OLP, both topical tretinoin and systemic etretinate induce resolution similar to a spontaneous evolution, with a few differences in the lymphocyte/macrophage ratio. With retinoid treatment, there appears to be an acceleration of the healing process accompanied by faster renewal of the cellular population and greater deterrence of the lesion.

Response of Oral Leukoplakia to Beta-Carotene

Garewal HS, Meyskens FL Jr, Killen D, Reeves D, Kiersch TA, Elletson H, Strosberg A, King D, Seinbronn K (Univ of Arizona; VA Med Ctrs of Tucson and Phoenix; Good Samaritan Hosp, Phoenix, Ariz)

J Clin Oncol 8:1715–1720, 1990 10–22

Introduction.—Leukoplakia is considered a premalignant lesion. Retinoids, particularly 13-cis retinoic acid, are often able to reverse leukoplakia. Because of the toxicity of these agents, they are often unsuitable for treatment. Beta-carotene, a naturally occurring nontoxic carotenoid that has inhibited oral carcinogenesis in animal studies, was assessed in adults with measurable oral leukoplakia. Beta-carotene was given to patients in a daily dose of 30 mg for 3 months, and responders continued to take it for an additional 3 months.

Findings.—A group of 25 patients, 11 of whom had dysplasia, was evaluated. Of the 24 evaluable patients, 71% had an objective response. Both dysplastic and nondysplastic lesions responded to β-carotene administration. No significant toxicity occurred.

Discussion.—Beta-carotene is active against oral leukoplakia, and its lack of significant toxicity makes it an excellent prospect for the chemoprevention of oral cancer. There also appears to be considerable epidemiological evidence supporting a role for carotenoids in preventing cancer.

Retinoic Acid Suppression of Squamous Differentiation in Human Head-and-Neck Squamous Carcinoma Cells

Poddar S, Hong WK, Thacher SM, Lotan R (Univ of Texas MD Anderson Cancer Ctr, Houston; Texas A&M College of Medicine)

Int J Cancer 48:239–247, 1991 10–23

Background.—Retinoids are vitamin A analogues that inhibit the squamous differentiation of normal and malignant epithelial cells. The ability of the head-and-neck squamous cell carcinoma (HNSCC) cell line 1483 to undergo squamous differentiation was investigated in the presence and absence of β-all-trans retinoic acid (RA).

Methods.—The 1483 HNSCC cell line was established from a biopsy specimen of a tumor in the retromolar trigone of 1 patient. The cell growth in culture was accompanied by an increase in keratinocyte transglutaminase, involucrin, and keratin KI (3 markers of squamous cell differentiation). Greater levels of these markers were found in cells cultured in delipidized serum (DLS), from which endogenous retinoids have been extracted, than were found in cells cultured in fetal bovine serum (FBS), which contains retinoids.

Results.—Treatment with RA reduced the levels of the various differentiation markers in cells cultured in FBS or DLS. This was shown by immunofluorescent labeling of permeabilized cells and immunoblotting of cell extracts using specific monoclonal or polyclonal antibodies. Calcium ionophore stimulated the ability of the cells to crosslink proteins to form envelopes under the plasma membrane, whereas RA inhibited it (Fig 10–9).

Conclusions.—The malignant 1483 HNSCC cells recapitulate the main features of normal squamous cell differentiation in culture, and RA suppresses this differentiation as it does in normal keratinizing epithelial cells.

▶ The pearl of great price in the management of head and neck cancer is prevention. Some of the most exciting opportunities for cancer prevention

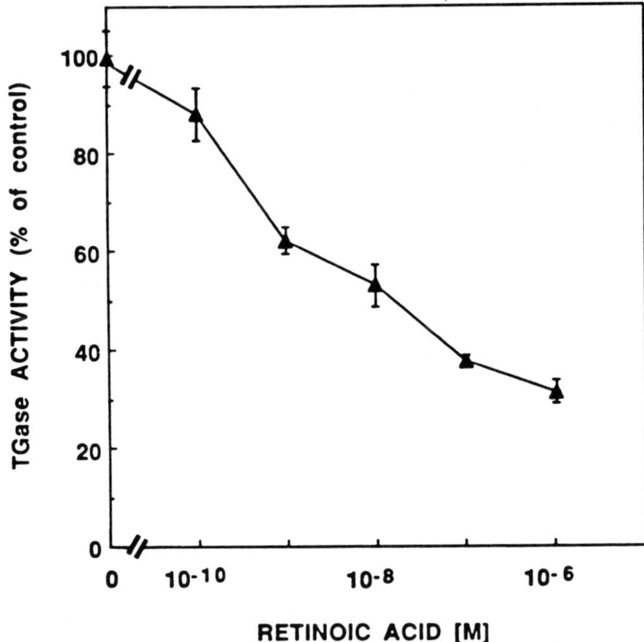

Fig 10–9.—Retinoic acid dose-dependent suppression of keratinocyte TGase activity in 1483 HNSCC cells. The cells were grown in FBS supplemented with RA concentrations in the range between 10^{-10} M and 10^{-16} M. After 7 days, the cells were harvested and the activity of keratinocyte TGase was analyzed. The activity in the control cultures (grown in the presence of .1% DMSO) was 870 ± 35 pmol/min/mg protein. The activity in the treated cells was expressed as a percentage of this control value, which was taken as 100%. (Courtesy of Poddar S, Hong WK, Thacher SM, et al: *Int J Cancer* 48:239-247, 1991.)

involve the ability of vitamin A and certain synthetic vitamin A analogs (known as retinoids) to *inhibit* cell proliferation/growth and *promote* cellular differentiation. The study discussed in Abstract 10–23 joins others in providing guarded optimism that these substances may be useful to: (1) arrest the conversion of premalignant lesions to cancer; (2) prevent primary malignancy development; and (3) reduce the incidence of tumor recurrence and second primaries.

Oral lichen planus is described as a T-lymphocytic inflammatory response to an antigen localized in the basal keratinocytes (see Abstract 10–21). Some experts list OLP as a premalignant lesion, whereas others state that the evidence for this is not conclusive. In any event, retinoids (vitamin A analogs) given for 3 months shortened the clinical course of the disorder.

Retinoids and β-carotene demonstrated a favorable response in oral leukoplakia (Abstract 10–22). They also demonstrated the ability to inhibit squamous differentiation in normal and malignant epithelial cells. The expansion of clinical trials to larger patient populations is the next step. If side effects and cost can be minimized and statistically significant decreases in morbidity and mortality from cancer can be documented, then we are truly on the threshold of a major advance in head and neck oncology.—B.J. Bailey, M.D., F.A.C.S.

Altered Antigen Expression Predicts Outcome in Squamous Cell Carcinoma of the Head and Neck

Wolf GT, Carey TE, Schmaltz SP, McClatchey KD, Poore J, Glaser L, Hayashida DJS, Hsu S (Univ of Michigan Med Ctr and VA Med Research Service; Ann Arbor)

J Natl Cancer Inst 82:1566–1572, 1990 10–24

Background.—The monoclonal antibody UM-A9 identifies an antigen on the basal surface of the epithelial cells that is consistently expressed on all squamous cell carcinomas (SCC). A previous study revealed that cell lines from metastatic or recurrent SCC express the A9 antigen more strongly than the cell lines from the primary tumor of the same donor.

Study.—The prognostic significance of antigen markers was examined in a prospective series of 82 consecutive patients with SCC of the head and neck. All patients were previously untreated, and the resected tumor specimens were studied immunohistologically.

Findings.—The rate of relapse was 58% in patients whose tumors expressed high levels of A9 antigen and 34% in those patients whose tumors expressed low levels of A9 antigen. The disease-free interval was

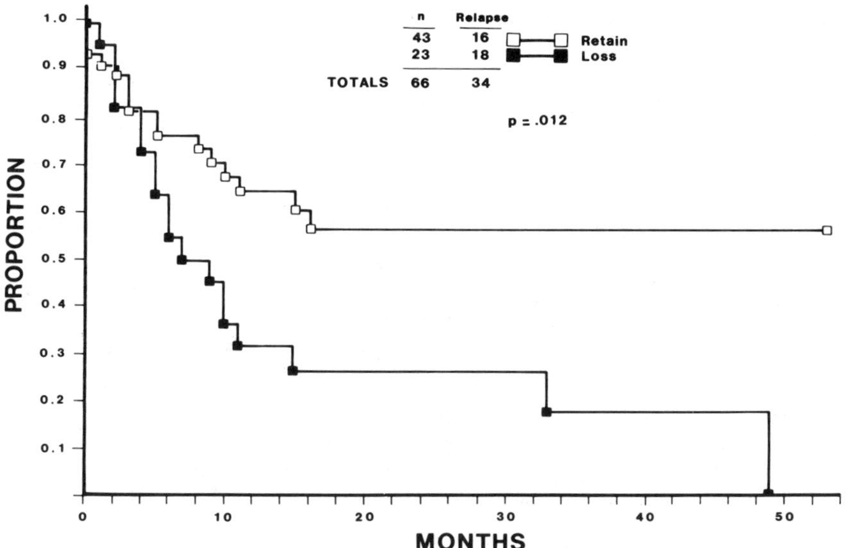

Fig 10–10.—Disease-free interval according to whether blood group antigen expression was retained or lost in the patient's cancer. Disease-free interval was significantly shorter in patients whose tumor did not express normal blood group antigens. ($P = .012$). (Courtesy of Wolf GT, Carey TE, Schmaltz SP, et al: *J Natl Cancer Inst* 82:1566–1572, 1990.)

significantly shorter in the first group of patients. The loss of blood group antigen expression correlated significantly with the high rate of tumor recurrence and decreased disease-free survival (Fig 10–10). Only 5 of the 21 patients with low tumor A9 expression but retention of blood group expression had recurrent tumors, compared with 34 of the other 59 patients.

Discussion.—Studies of A9 and blood group antigen expression may help determine whether patients with SCC should receive more aggressive treatment.

▶ This study concludes that A9 (a monoclonal antibody) is a marker for SCC. When A9 expression was combined with loss of tumor tissue expression of normal A, B, H blood group antigens, tumor behavior was usually found to be quite aggressive. This finding suggests that we may soon be able to use these tools in a clinical setting to plan treatment strategies that are based on what is appropriate for a specific patient rather than being based on "pooled" statistical observations.—B.J. Bailey, M.D., F.A.C.S.

Time to Recurrence of Squamous Cell Carcinoma of the Head and Neck

Stell PM (Univ of Liverpool, England)

Head & Neck 13:277–281, 1991 10–25

Background.—Although the time to malignant recurrence is easy to measure and presumably reflects growth rate, it does not appear to have been studied. The time to recurrence of squamous cell carcinoma (SCC) of the head and neck was investigated in relation to the response to treatment, host, and tumor factors and to prognosis.

Patients.—From 1963 to 1990, 3,215 patients with SCC of the head and neck were seen at 1 center. Of these patients, 515 had a primary tumor recurrence after radiotherapy. Only 1 patient was lost to follow-up. The median potential follow-up was 11 years.

Findings.—The interval from the end of radiotherapy to the diagnosis of a primary recurrence was unrelated to any known host factors and tumor factors except site. However, this interval was the most significant predictor of survival, both from initial presentation and the date of recurrence. The time to recurrence was not related to tumor size at recurrence, which suggests that large recurrences are multicentric. In 67 patients with end-stage disease who were treated by chemotherapy, the time to recurrence predicted response and survival. Response and survival were better among patients with tumors that had a time to recurrence that was longer than the median. Although their increased survival was not significant, their increased response was. The overall survival for patients with a time to primary recurrence above the median was ap-

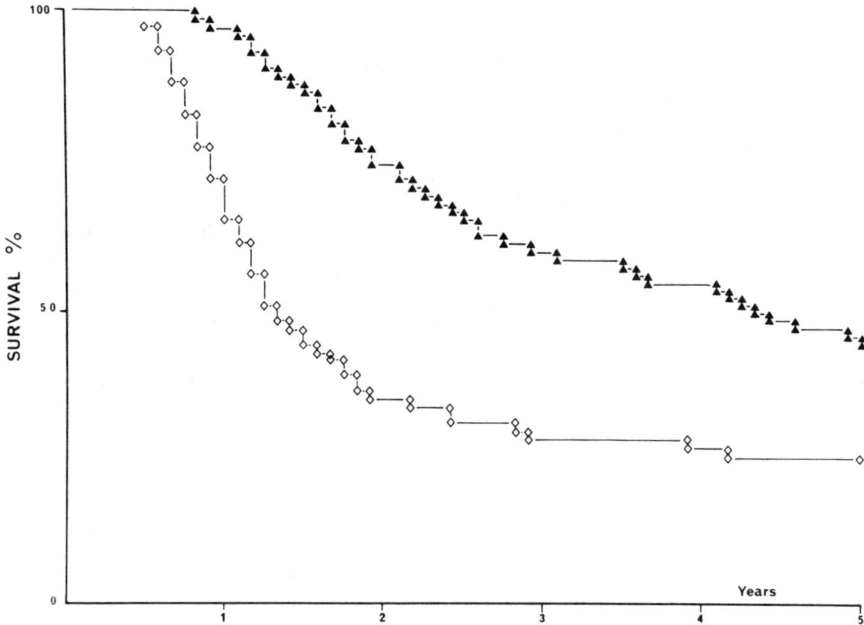

Fig 10–11.—Survival related to time of recurrence: (*solid triangles*) patients with time to recurrence greater than the median; (*open diamonds*) patients with time to occurrence less than the median. (Courtesy of Stell PM: *Head & Neck* 13:277–281, 1991.)

proximately 20% better at 5-year follow-up than for patients with recurrence below the median (Fig 10–11).

Conclusions.—If the time to recurrence reflects tumor growth rate, then the latter is an independent variable that predicts survival. Multivariate analysis confirms that time to recurrence is the most powerful predictor of survival in these patients.

▶ According to Stell, the time to recurrence after radiation therapy predicts both survival and response to treatment. It is interesting that the time to recurrence does not correlate with tumor size. This raises questions concerning the usefulness of tumor size in regard to treatment aggressiveness and patient counseling. Caution should be used in drawing inferences suggesting that radical surgical intervention should be used in patients in whom recurrence develops quickly, because this study does not provide evidence that such a strategy would result in increased patient survival.—B.J. Bailey, M.D., F.A.C.S.

Esthesioneuroblastoma With Intracranial Extension

Meneses MS, Thurel C, Mikol J, Ramina R, Maniglia JJ, Arruda WO, Cophignon J (Lariboisière Hosp, Paris; Hospital das Nações, Curitiba, Brazil)
Neurosurgery 27:813–820, 1990 10–26

Introduction.—Esthesioneuroblastoma is a rare neoplasm of the nasal cavities that can extend to the paranasal sinuses. Intracranial extension usually occurs in the late phase of the illness and significantly worsens the prognosis. Primary intracranial esthesioneuroblastomas are rarely found. These tumors grow relatively slowly and are considered to be radiosensitive. Total resection with radiation therapy is the preferred treatment.

Patients.—Four females and 1 male (aged 15 to 59 years) received a diagnosis of esthesioneuroblastomas with intracranial extension. All 5 patients underwent craniofacial neurosurgery in collaboration with otorhinolaryngologists. The postoperative course was uneventful in all 5 cases. One patient had a recurrence 10 months after operation and died. The other 4 have remained free of recurrence at follow-up. Electron microscopic study confirmed the histological diagnosis. However, the histogenesis of this tumor remains a subject of debate.

▶ Esthesioneuroblastoma presents a treatment challenge when there is intracranial extension; this occurs in more than 10% of patients. When other factors are favorable, a combined approach to the anterior skull base by neurosurgeons and otolaryngologists provides the best solution according to current knowledge. The best estimates for a cure are in the range of 40% to 60% when the disease is confined to the nose and sinuses. The presence of intracranial extension or distant metastasis may reduce this by about one half. Some authors have suggested that stereotactic radiation therapy (radiosurgery) may provide an alternative to surgery.—B.J. Bailey, M.D., F.A.C.S.

Cryosurgery in 50 Cases of Tongue Carcinoma

Li Z (Xinqiao Hosp, Congqing, People's Republic of China)
J Oral Maxillofac Surg 49:504–506, 1991 10–27

Background.—Cryosurgery is a useful therapeutic measure in many fields. Its use in the treatment of tongue carcinoma was evaluated in 50 patients.

Methods.—A group of 34 men and 16 women (average age, 52 years) was treated during a 10½-year period. Of the lesions, 47 were SCC, and 32 were located in the middle third of the tongue. There were 12 T1, 35 T2, and 3 T3 lesions. All patients received first-time treatment with cryosurgery in the outpatient clinic under local anesthesia. Radical neck dissection was done in 48 patients 3 weeks after cryosurgical control of the primary tumor. The patients were followed for 3–10 years.

Results.—Of the primary lesions, 90% were controlled by cryosurgery, with similar control rates for the T1 and T2 lesions. The recurrence rate was 10%. There was a total of 14 deaths (9 from cancer) in the series of 50 patients. The 3-year survival rate was 71.9%, and 5-year survival was 72.2%. Complications of respiratory distress in 3 patients and sloughing of necrotic tissue in 3 patients each were easily controlled.

Conclusions.—Cryosurgery is an effective and safe technique for carcinoma of the tongue. This method can provide only local treatment and control only the primary lesion. Treatment of the regional lymphatics must be planned by some other method.

▶ Reports don't get much more controversial than this one from China. Primary tongue cancer was treated with cryosurgery, and radical neck dissection (RND) was performed 3 weeks later in less than one half of the patients. Of the group, 38 had T2 or T3 lesions; our department would recommend RND or modified RND for these patients. Radiation therapy would also be recommended for most of the T2 and T3 lesions. The results are surprising to me. I would have expected them to be worse than reported. Looking on the bright side, the message may be that there is a place for cryosurgery in the management of small tongue carcinomas. The difficult work of identifying exactly which group is ideal for cryosurgery remains to be done.—B.J. Bailey, M.D., F.A.C.S.

Hematoporphyrin Photodynamic Therapy: Is There Truly a Future in Head and Neck Oncology? Reflections on a 5-Year Experience

Gluckman JL (Univ of Cincinnati Med Ctr)

Laryngoscope 101:36–42, 1991 — 10–28

Background.—Photodynamic therapy appears to be successful in the treatment of superficial cancers; poorer results are achieved in the treatment of more advanced tumors, regardless of site. However, there has been no vast experience in any organ system or at any center. To evaluate the current status and future possibilities of this therapy in managing patients with head and neck cancer, a 5-year experience in 41 patients was reviewed.

Methods.—The patients were divided into 3 groups: 8 had advanced cancers treated with purely palliative intent, 25 had clinically focal superficial early cancers, and 8 had field cancerization of the mucosa—or "condemned mucosa". A photosensitizer was administered 72 hours before therapy; hematoporphyrin derivative was used initially, and dihematoporphyrin ether was used subsequently. The lesions were treated with surface illumination or tumor implantation with an argon pumped-dye laser in 36 cases or a gold vapor laser in 5 cases. The light dose was 50–100 J/cm^2. Tumor response was determined at 1 month, and the patients were followed for 6–60 months.

Results of Patients With "Condemned Mucosa" Treated With Photodynamic Therapy

Site	Previous Treatment	Response	Duration (Months)	Comments
Oral cavity	—	CR	11	
Oral cavity	—	CR	6	
Oral cavity	—	CR	12	Recurrence
Oral cavity	Surgery	CR	53	
Palate	Surgery	CR	8	Died of cirrhosis
Oral cavity	—	CR	6	
Buccal mucosa	Surg + RT	CR	10	
Oral cavity	Surgery	PR	5	Recurrence, surg

(Courtesy of Gluckman JL: *Laryngoscope* 101:36–42, 1991.)

Results.—In the advanced cases, all of which were treated early in the series, palliation was no more effective or longer lasting than with standard therapies. Skin photosensitivity actually worsened the quality of life in some patients. Of the superficial early cancers, 11 of the 13 oral and oropharyngeal lesions had complete responses; however, 4 recurred between 8 and 12 months. Of the 6 laryngeal cancers, there was only 1 satisfactory result; this patient was lost to follow-up at 36 months. Of the 6 miscellaneous superficial cancers, there was only 1 complete response, which recurred at 12 months. Of the patients with condemned mucosa, all but 1 achieved a complete response (table) and did very well in the short term.

Conclusions.—Hematoporphyrin photodynamic therapy appears to have no role in palliation of the advanced cancers of the upper aerodigestive tract; however, it is excellent treatment for condemned mucosa. The technology is insufficiently advanced for routine use in the treatment of early focal cancers. Additional fundamental basic science study is needed before a formal multi-institutional study can be done.

▶ Photodynamic therapy appeared on the scene rather dramatically about 5 years ago. Early reports were quite enthusiastic, and it seemed that an important new tool had been developed to use against head and neck malignancies. There have been problems in obtaining an even distribution of the injected hematoporphyrius throughout the tumor and in gaining access to all of the tumor. The depth to which laser energy could be projected was a problem in many patients. This study finds photodynamic therapy to be very useful in the management of extensive "condemned mucosa", and until better photodynamic therapy technology is available, even that limited usefulness will be of sufficient value to continue its clinical use.—B.J. Bailey, M.D., F.A.C.S.

Preliminary Trial of Nonrecombinant Interferon Alpha in Recurrent Squamous Cell Carcinoma of the Head and Neck

Vlock DR, Johnson J, Myers E, Day R, Gooding WE, Whiteside T, Pelch K, Sigler B, Wagner R, Colao D, Rust D (Univ of Pittsburgh School of Medicine; VA Med Ctr, Pittsburgh)

Head & Neck 13:15–21, 1991 10–29

Objective.—The responses of squamous cell cancer of the head and neck region (SCCHN) to chemotherapy are usually brief and incomplete. The efficacy of nonrecombinant interferon alpha (IFN) was examined in 14 patients with recurrent or metastatic SCCHN whose tumors were no longer amenable to surgery or radiotherapy. Surgery, radiotherapy, and chemotherapy had all been utilized in 7 patients.

Management.—The patients received 10×10^6 units of IFN intramuscularly per day for 3 days every 4 weeks. Treatment was given for at least 3 months unless toxicity required withdrawal from the trial.

Results.—The treatment was generally well tolerated. One patient had atrial fibrillation; another patient had cardiac arrest after aspiration pneumonia and later died. Only 1 patient had a complete response to IFN therapy (table). In 2 other patients the disease stabilized. Low pretreatment natural killer (NK) cell activity was found in thc 1 patient who had a complete response; activity increased sharply after treatment.

Discussion.—Low-dose cyclical IFN therapy appears to be well tolerated by patients with recurrent SCCHN. It may also have an antitumor effect.

▶ The authors describe the use of IFN in 14 patients who had no other treatment options available. There was 1 complete response, and 2 patients stabilized for 8 and 12 months. The best response was obtained in a patient with initial low NK activity. This would seem to be a logical path for further investigation. It would also be interesting to explore the role of IFN as adju-

Response to Therapy

Response	Number	Median time to progression (months)
Complete response	1	30
Partial response	0	—
Mixed response	1	4
Stable disease	2	10
Progressive disease	10	3

(Courtesy of Vlock DR, Johnson J, Myers E, et al: *Head & Neck* 13:15–21, 1991.)

vant therapy for patients who are in less extreme clinical circumstances than those in this study group.—B.J. Bailey, M.D., F.A.C.S.

Control of Upper Jugular Haemorrhage
Reilly PG, Narula AA, Bradley PJ (St Bartholomew's Hosp, London)
Laryngol Otol 104:976, 1990 10–30

Introduction.—Dissection of squamous carcinoma of the neck often requires removal of the complete jugular vein, because any damage to this vessel can often cause profuse bleeding. An alternative procedure was assessed for control of hemorrhage of the upper jugular vein in the area of the jugular bulb.

Technique.—Locate the lumen of the bleeding internal jugular vein near the base of the skull, and then insert a size 6 Fogarty catheter into the lumen, moving it cephalad until the balloon appears to be into the jugular bulb. Inflate the catheter until the bleeding is under control, and approach the jugular vein and bulb from above through the mastoid to continue. If this procedure does not seem appropriate, one can bring the end of the catheter out of the skin incision upon completion of the surgery. At 48 hours postsurgery, the catheter can be deflated and removed, usually without anesthesia.

Results.—This technique has been used in 3 patients in whom the extent of the tumor was greater than anticipated upon presurgical assessment. When the tumor proves to be unresectable at the time of the operation, the procedure can be stopped—even with profuse per-operative hemorrhage.

Implications.—Although termination of a major tumor resection is not desired, most oncology surgeons will meet with this type of situation during their practice until preoperative imaging techniques improve.

► I have rarely encountered the situation described by the authors; however, I can recall an instance wherein this approach might have been superior to the solution of packing with pressure dressings and hoping that all would turn out well in a few days. Because I have no experience with this technique, I cannot provide any advice; however, the observations in this small group of patients seem favorable.—B.J. Bailey, M.D., F.A.C.S.

A Meta-Analysis of Prophylactic Antibiotics in Head and Neck Surgery
Velanovich V (Letterman Army Med Ctr, San Francisco)
Plast Reconstr Surg 87:429–435, 1991 10–31

Introduction.—Although it is agreed that prophylactic antibiotics are necessary to reduce postoperative infection, the choice of antibiotics and dosing schedule remain controversial. A meta-analysis of published clinical trials of prophylactic antibiotics for head and neck surgery was conducted to determine the most effective regimen.

Methods.—The analysis included 12 randomized, prospective studies with a consistent definition of infection. The pertinent factors were compared to perform sensitivity analysis, including prophylaxis vs. placebo, first-generation cephalosporin vs. multiple agents, and single agent vs. multiple agents or a third-generation cephalosporin.

Results.—Prophylactic antibiotics decreased the incidence of infection by 43.7% compared with placebo. Compared with cefazolin alone, the use of multiple antibiotics decreased the incidence of infection by 14%. There was an improvement of 8.3% with multiple antibiotics vs. a single antibiotic, 13.7% difference in favor of multiple antibiotics vs. cefazolin, and a 4.1% difference in favor of multiple-day vs. single-day prophylaxis (Fig 10–12).

Conclusion.—A 1-day course of clindamycin may be the most effective prophylaxis for patients undergoing head and neck surgery. Clindamycin combined with a third-generation cephalosporin might be effec-

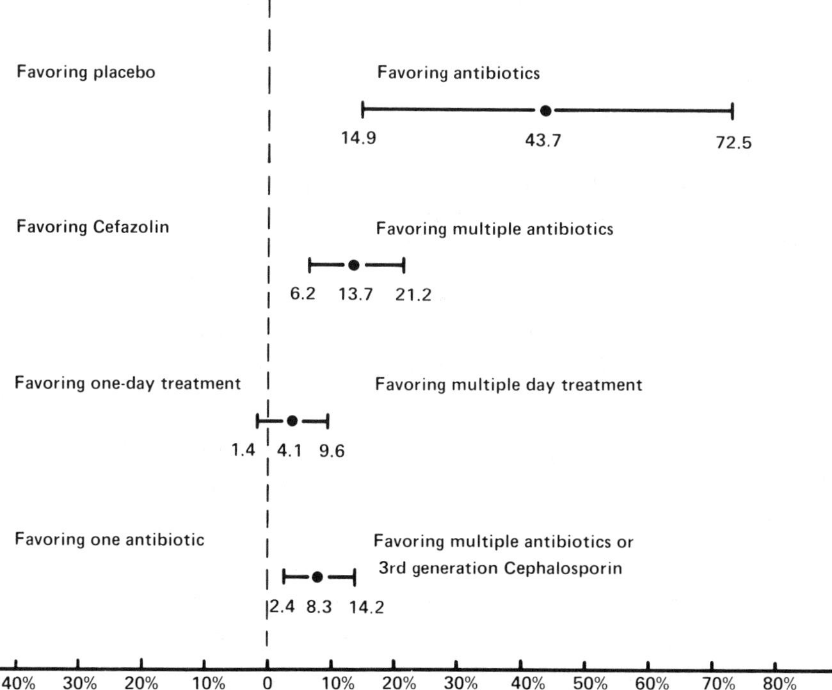

Fig 10–12.—The results of the meta-analysis with the estimates of the overall treatment effect and the 95% confidence intervals for those estimates. (Courtesy of Velanovich V: *Plast Reconstr Surg* 37:429–435, 1991.)

tive against anaerobes, gram-positive bacteria of the oropharynx, and gram-negative bacteria.

▶ There are 2 points of focus in this paper. The first is the process of meta-analysis, which is a sophisticated statistical process that attempts to transform a large number of reported studies into something resembling a large clinical trial. I place more trust in an analysis that clearly reflects the input of biostatistical expertise; this analysis did not do so.

The second focus is the conclusion that a 1-day course of clindamycin is the most effective antibiotic prophylaxis available. My first reaction is that such a strategy will result in a higher late infection rate, particularly in patients who have been irradiated and/or who have undergone more extensive surgical procedures.—B.J. Bailey, M.D., F.A.C.S.

Lymphoproliferative Disorders of the Head and Neck

Green JD Jr, Neel HB III, Witzig TE (Mayo Clinic and Found, Rochester, Minn)

Am J Otolaryngol 12:26–32, 1991 10–32

Hodgkin's Disease.—Patients with Hodgkin's disease most commonly have a painless enlarged cervical node, often low in the neck. Constitutional symptoms are also frequently present. The disease appears to be unifocal in origin, and it often progresses to the contiguous lymph nodes. The stage of disease at the time of diagnosis is the single most significant prognostic factor.

Non-Hodgkin's Lymphoma.—Patients with this disorder pursue a highly variable clinical course. Tumors usually appear as painless node enlargements. Waldeyer's ring is more often involved in this disease than in Hodgkin's disease. As many as 40% of the patients have non-Hodgkin's lymphoma in the extranodal tissues. Constitutional symptoms are noted less frequently than in patients with Hodgkin's disease, and their presence suggests a poorer outlook.

Other Disorders.—Polymorphic reticulosis is a type of T-cell lymphoma characterized by destructive, ulcerative lesions in the upper respiratory tract. Eosinophilic granuloma is a benign condition most commonly involving the flat bones of the skull, in which accumulating histiocytes lead to bone resorption and a radiolucent lesion. A variety of benign reactive lymphoproliferative disorders may also be seen, including viral lymphadenopathy, toxoplasmosis, histiocytosis, a phenytoin reaction, and cat-scratch disease. Extramedullary plasmacytoma occurs in the head and neck region in 80% of cases.

▶ Lymphoproliferative disorders comprise a family of diseases that are seen with a confusing constellation of symptoms and signs. Accurate diagnosis may be difficult without open biopsy of the tumor itself (fine-needle aspiration is rarely adequate). New studies such as immunotyping, cytogenetic studies, cell proliferation measurements, and T- and B- cell gene-rearrangement studies may add information of value concerning a patient's diagnosis or prognosis.—B.J. Bailey, M.D., F.A.C.S.

Nasopharyngeal Carcinoma in the Young: A Combined M.D. Anderson and Stanford Experience

Ingersoll L, Woo SY, Donaldson S, Giesler J, Maor MH, Goffinet D, Cangir A, Goepfert H, Oswald MJ, Peters LJ (Stanford Univ; Univ of Texas MD Anderson Cancer Ctr, Houston)

Int J Radiat Oncol Biol Phys 19:881–887, 1990 10–33

Introduction.—Nasopharyngeal carcinoma accounts for only a fifth to a half of all primary nasopharyngeal cancers in children, compared with 85% in adults. The experience of 2 large cancer centers with the treatment and outcome of locally advanced nasopharyngeal carcinoma in children and young adults was reviewed.

Patients.—A group of 57 children and young adults (aged 4–21 years) was treated for nasopharyngeal carcinoma at the M.D. Anderson Cancer Center and Stanford University Medical Center from 1956 to 1988. There were twice as many boys as girls. A total of 43 patients had lymphoepithelioma, whereas 7 had undifferentiated neoplasms and 7 had SCC. Two patients had stage III disease and the rest had stage IV disease at presentation.

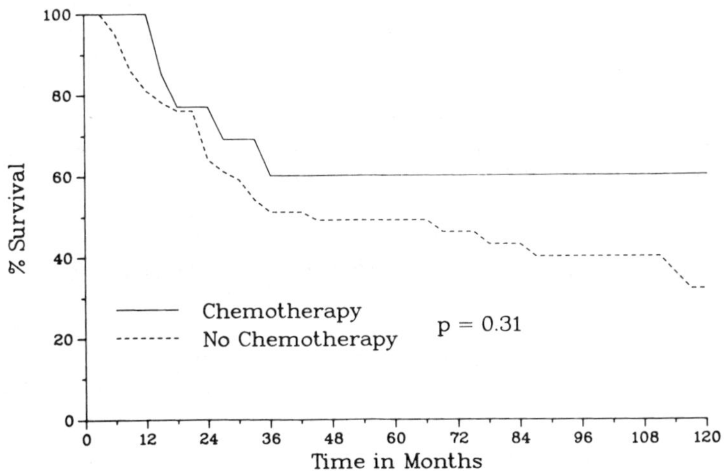

Fig 10–13.—The percentage survival of patients who received radiation therapy and adjuvant chemotherapy vs. those who received radiation therapy only. (Courtesy of Ingersoll L, Woo SY, Donaldson S, et al: *Int J Radiat Oncol Biol Phys* 19:881–887, 1990.)

Management.—All patients underwent primary radiotherapy. In addition, 14 had chemotherapy with combinations of dactinomycin, doxorubicin, bleomycin, cisplatin, cyclophosphamide, fluorouracil, methotrexate, and vincristine.

Outcome.—The median follow-up was 93 months. Twenty-six patients were alive. The actuarial survival rates at 5 and 10 years were 51% and 36%, respectively, and the corresponding disease-specific survival rates were 51% and 51%. The 5-year survival rate was 60% for 14 patients who had chemotherapy included in their treatment, compared with 50% for those patients who did not (Fig 10–13). After 42 months, there were no recurrences. Distant metastasis only occurred in 21 patients, locoregional metastasis only in 1, and both occurred in 5. Distant metastases occurred most often in bones, lungs, liver, and mediastinal lymph nodes. A significant number of long-term survivors had chronic treatment-related morbidity. The data trends suggested that prognosis was more favorable for girls, patients aged 15 years or younger, lymphoepithelioma or undifferentiated histologies, stages T3-4 NO-1 vs. T1-2 N2-3 vs. T3-4 N2-3, primary tumor doses of 65 Gy or greater, and patients receiving chemotherapy.

Discussion.—Nasopharyngeal carcinoma in children and young adults most commonly presents in advanced locoregional stages. However, the overall survival rates among the young are not significantly different from those of older adults. High-dose radiation therapy in children can be curative, but it is also associated with significant morbidity in long-term survivors.

▶ Although there is a higher frequency of advanced locoregional disease in children than there is in adults, the treatment outcome is nearly the same. Interestingly, patients who received a primary tumor dose of 65 Gy or more did better than the patients who received less than 65 Gy. Unfortunately, high-dose radiotherapy is associated with long-term complication rates. Neuroendocrine abnormalities, growth impairment, and fibrosis head the list of these complications.—B.J. Bailey, M.D., F.A.C.S.

Fibrosarcoma of the Head and Neck: The UCLA Experience

Mark RJ, Sercarz JA, Tran L, Selch M, Calcaterra TC (UCLA Med Ctr, Los Angeles)

Arch Otolaryngol Head Neck Surg 117:396–401, 1991 10–34

Background.—There have been few reports of the prognostic factors and optimal management for the rare lesion of fibrosarcoma. A series of 29 patients with fibrosarcoma of the head and neck was reviewed.

Methods.—The patients were seen during a 32-year period. There were 15 males and 14 females (median age, 35 years), including 9 children. The series excluded those patients with fibrous tumors that were

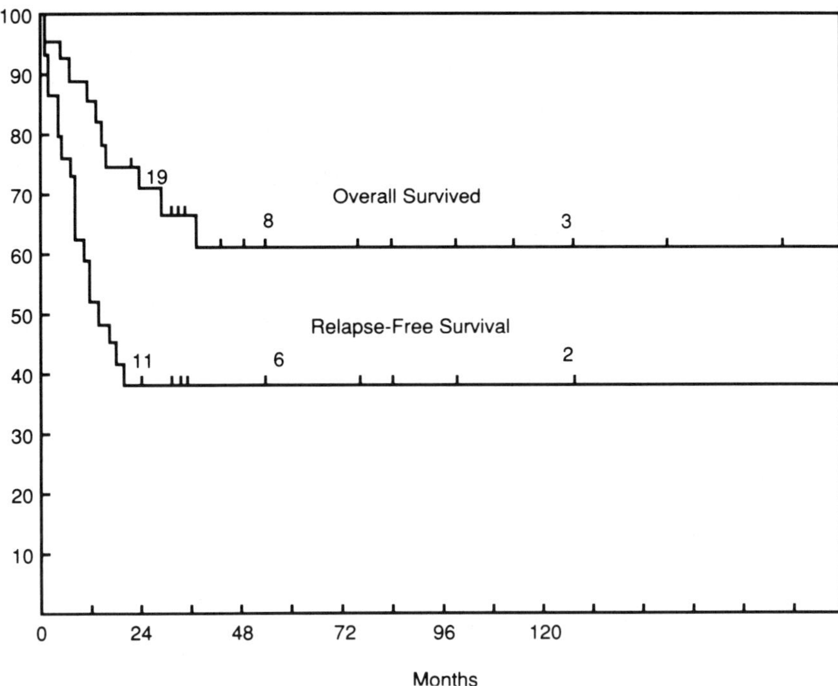

Fig 10–14.—Life-table showing survival in months from time of diagnosis. (Courtesy of Mark RJ, Sercarz JA, Tran L, et al: *Arch Otolaryngol Head Neck Surg* 117:396–401, 1991.)

distinguishable from fibrosarcoma. Treatment was individualized according to tumor size, location, extent of disease, and histological grade. There were 15 low-grade, 13 high-grade, and 1 unassigned lesion. The median follow-up was 66 months.

Results.—There was an absolute 5-year survival of 62%. Of the 17 patients who initially had only surgery, 5 with low-grade lesions achieved local control and long-term survival. Postoperative radiation was given in 5 cases because of positive surgical margins. Three of these patients, all of whom had low-grade lesions, achieved a disease-free state. Of the 6 patients who had primary radiation therapy, 4 received additional chemotherapy; 2 of the 6 were disease free after more than 5 years. Of the 12 patients with local recurrence, surgery with and without adjuvant therapy salvaged 5. Only 8% of the patients with high-grade lesions were ultimately rendered disease free, compared with 80% of those with low-grade lesions. Known positive surgical margins were present in 72% of the patients with local recurrence; 68% had high-grade lesions, tumors larger than 5 cm, or both. The median survival time was 152 months (Fig 10–14).

Conclusions.—The most important prognostic feature in these patients is tumor grade, followed by tumor size and status of the surgical margins. Surgery alone appears to be adequate for patients with low-grade lesions and adequate surgical margins. Adjuvant treatment is needed for those with high-grade lesions or positive surgical margins.

▶ Fibrosarcoma is a complex disease process that is seen in a variety of different ways in the head and neck. According to the observations of the UCLA series, surgery is the mainstay of treatment and is adequate therapy when the margins are free of tumor. However, it should be noted that in this series, only 8% of the patients with high-grade tumors were saved, whereas 80% of the patients with low-grade tumors survived. Residual disease was found at the surgical margins in 17 of 22 patients. Radiotherapy has been recommended as adjuvant therapy either when the surgical margins are positive or when a high-grade tumor is present.—B.J. Bailey, M.D., F.A.C.S.

Psychiatric Aspects of Head and Neck Surgery: I. New Surgical Techniques and Psychiatric Consequences

Bronheim H, Strain JJ, Biller HF (Mount Sinai Med Ctr, New York)

Gen Hosp Psychiatry 13:165–176, 1991 10–35

Introduction.—Although ear, nose, and throat (ENT) cancers comprise only 5% to 6% of all malignancies, they produce stress and anxiety that usually exceed those experienced by surgical patients. Facial mutilation is a common fear, and there may be alterations in taste, smell, chewing and swallowing function, vision, and hearing. The frequency of alcohol and tobacco use by these patients indicates that withdrawal states may be problematic. Despite the great stress and disfigurement, a large majority of patients have a satisfactory postoperative recovery.

Technical Advances.—Teflon injection can prevent aspiration after laryngectomy and improve vocal quality. Free flap transplant techniques may restore facial contour, occlusal relationships, and a functional denture-bearing surface. Carotid artery bypass combined with a myocutaneous pectoral flap can relieve pain in patients with persistent or recurrent cancer of the neck; it may also prolong life.

The Psychiatrist's Role.—Although the newer techniques have forestalled death, they have created a longer and more complicated rehabilitative process. The patients become quite regressed and helpless as their hospital stay lengthens. They may also become withdrawn and noncompliant because of depression or anxiety. Psychiatric efforts are necessary to help relieve distress and to enable the patient to engage fully in rehabilitative efforts.

▶ It is absolutely amazing to me that patients with head and neck cancer are able to cope with their malignancies and surgeries as well as they do. The diagnosis of "cancer" is an awesome event in the life of any individual. The impact ripples through the family and immediately turns plans, expectations, and relationships upside down. Next, the patient loses all control of his/her life when "specialists" begin to map out a plan of therapy in a somewhat paternalistic manner. Then comes the surgical experience with pain, strangling, coughing, and associated unpleasantries. To top it off, our procedures often affect appearance, speaking, chewing, swallowing, breathing, and other assorted bodily functions. Financial, social, job, and family worries are routine.

It is gratifying that our patients show such appreciation for our compassion and support when they are recovering. Things usually go well, all things considered; however, we must be alert to the occasional patient who needs heavy-duty psychiatric help. What sort of support system is available for your patients? Can you strengthen it and personalize it? It's worth a try.—B.J. Bailey, M.D., F.A.C.S.

Partial Laryngectomy After Irradiation Failure

Nichols RD, Mickelson SA (Henry Ford Hosp, Detroit)
Ann Otol Rhinol Laryngol 100:176–180, 1991 10–36

Introduction.—Limited carcinoma of the larynx can be treated with irradiation or partial laryngectomy. Historically, total laryngectomy was the only recommended salvage option in patients with failed radiotherapy because of a concern for complications associated with partial resection of the irradiated cartilage and the difficulty in assessing surgical margins.

Patients.—Between 1961 and 1988, 40 men and 3 women (aged 44–75 years) had partial laryngectomies after failed primary irradiation of the larynx for laryngeal carcinoma. The partial laryngectomies included 9 supraglottic, 3 endoscopic, and 31 vertical partial procedures. At diagnosis, 33 patients had stage I disease, whereas 6 had stage II, 1 had stage III, and 3 had stage IV disease. The interval between radiation therapy and tumor recurrence ranged from 1–191 months. Twenty-seven patients (65%) had tumor recurrences within 12 months, 32 (76%) within 24 months, and 3 (7%) were free of disease for more than 60 months before recurrence.

Results.—Twelve patients (28%) required total laryngectomy after partial laryngectomy because of disease recurrence. Five patients died with disease, 3 of whom had completion laryngotomies. The surgical margins were negative in 4 of the 5 patients who died with local disease. Of the remaining 38 patients, 29 had no evidence of disease, 4 died without laryngeal disease, 3 died with local disease, and 1 was living with disease. The status of 1 patient was considered indeterminate. The permanent sections of 6 patients showed positive margins. Frozen sections taken during operation had been negative in 5 of these patients. All 6 patients had recurrent or persistent disease. The 2-year determinant disease-free survival rate for stage I and stage II disease was 85%. The 3-year disease-free survival rate was 50% for stage III and stage IV disease.

Conclusion.—Partial laryngectomy can be done after irradiation failure, with a high expectation of cure and acceptable morbidity. Patients with positive margins should be considered for immediate completion laryngectomy.

► We agree entirely with the conclusion of Dr. Nichols' article, in which he states that partial laryngectomy is an appropriate approach for managing some patients with recurrent cancer after radiation therapy. Although the same caveats are present in salvage surgery as in primary surgery, strict adherence to the rules of exclusion is essential. The partial laryngectomy surgery must be adequate for the original laryngeal cancer, without regard to the apparent size of the recurrence. We have a strong preference for resecting the tumor and then obtaining frozen section margins from the patient side of the incision. We believe that this has improved the accuracy of our operative assessment of surgical adequacy. However, we agree that if there should be subsequent permanent section confirmation of a tumor at the resection margin, then completion laryngectomy is necessary and should be performed immediately.—B.J. Bailey, M.D., F.A.C.S.

Pediatric Thyroid Cancer

Sierk AE, Askin FB, Reddick RL, Thomas CG Jr (Univ of North Carolina)
Pediatr Pathol 10:877–893, 1990 10–37

Introduction.—Thyroid cancer is a relatively uncommon childhood cancer. Children with papillary thyroid carcinoma differ from adults with the same diagnosis in that the long-term prognosis is much more favorable for children, even in the presence of extrathyroidal disease in the neck. Recently, DNA flow cytometry of thyroid neoplasms has been used for obtaining additional prognostic information. Adults with papillary thyroid cancer have a poorer prognosis than pediatric patients, and a correlation of cellular DNA with clinical outcome does not appear to apply to pediatric patients. A review was made of the clinical and pathologic features of thyroid cancer in pediatric patients, using tissue from archival paraffin blocks for DNA flow cytometry.

Patients.—Between 1952 and 1987, thyroid cancer was diagnosed in 36 patients younger than 21 years of age. One patient was excluded from analysis. After reviewing the slides, the lesions in 4 patients were reclassified as benign. Of the remaining 31 patients, 27 (87%) had papillary carcinomas, 3 (10%) had well-differentiated follicular carcinomas with Hürthle cell change, and 1 (3%) had medullary carcinoma. All 16 patients with lymph node metastases at the time of diagnosis had papillary carcinoma.

Results.—The mean age at diagnosis was 16 years, and the follow-up ranged from 1–29 years. Of the 31 patients with confirmed thyroid cancer, 30 were alive and well at last follow-up (4 of them after therapy for recurrences). The only patient with a diagnosis of medullary carcinoma died 11 years after diagnosis. Flow cytometric study performed on tissue blocks obtained from 26 patients showed tumor aneuploidy in 8 of the 21 papillary carcinomas and in 2 of the 3 follicular carcinomas. The presence of aneuploidy did not correlate with the extent of disease at diagnosis or with clinical outcome.

Conclusion.—The findings of this study support those of previous studies that reported a favorable clinical outcome in pediatric patients with thyroid cancer.

Survival and Causes of Death in Thyroid Cancer: A Population-Based Study of 2,479 Cases From Norway

Akslen LA, Haldorsen T, Thoresen SØ, Glattre E (Univ of Bergen, Norway; The Cancer Registry of Norway, Oslo)

Cancer Res 51:1234–1241, 1991 10–38

Introduction.—Several previous studies have reported prognostic factors of thyroid cancer (TC). However, methodological problems such as the differences in the patient selection criteria between series and the changes in therapy over time plagued most of the studies. The major prognostic factors of TC were determined in a population-based study using data collected over a relatively short period of time by a single institution.

Methods.—From 1970–1985, 2,625 cases of clinically identified TC were reported to the Norwegian Cancer Registry. Patients in whom TC was diagnosed at autopsy or by death certificate (146) were excluded from this analysis. The 1,977 women and 648 men were observed from the time of diagnosis through 1985. The maximum follow-up was 16 years; the median follow-up was 48 months.

Findings.—Of the 2,479 patients with TC, 714 (28.8%) died during follow-up. Thyroid cancer was the main cause of death in 498 (69.7%) patients. Among the 216 patients who died of other main causes, TC was a contributing factor in 80 patients (11.2%). When only deaths from TC were considered, there were no sex differences in patient survival for any of the histological subtypes. However, the proportion of TC deaths increased with age. There were marked age effects for all histological groups except for anaplastic TC. Only 5 of the 498 patients who died of TC were younger than 35 years of age. None of these 5 patients had papillary TC, but the survival rate dropped significantly in patients older than 55 years with papillary TC. Marked differences were also observed between various histological types, even between papillary and follicular TCs when interactions were included. Tumor stage was the third strong predictor of TC deaths. Regional tumor spread and distant metastases were both associated with reduced survival. Survival was also reduced in patients with lymph node metastases.

Conclusion.—Age, histological type, and tumor stage are the 3 major prognostic factors in patients with TC.

11 Rhinology

The Sinusitis Cycle
Reilly JS (Birmingham, Ala)
Otolaryngol Head Neck Surg 103:856–862, 1990 11–1

Introduction.—The most common myths about sinusitis were reviewed, including the myth that chronic sinusitis always begins as an allergy and that chronic and recurrent acute disease is incurable.

Anatomy.—Computed tomography has contributed vastly to the current medical knowledge of sinusitis. The 3-dimensional images of the ethmoid sinus, which appears to be the most common site of acute disease, has led to an understanding of the predisposing factors in this condition. The maxillary and ethmoid sinuses serve as the more common

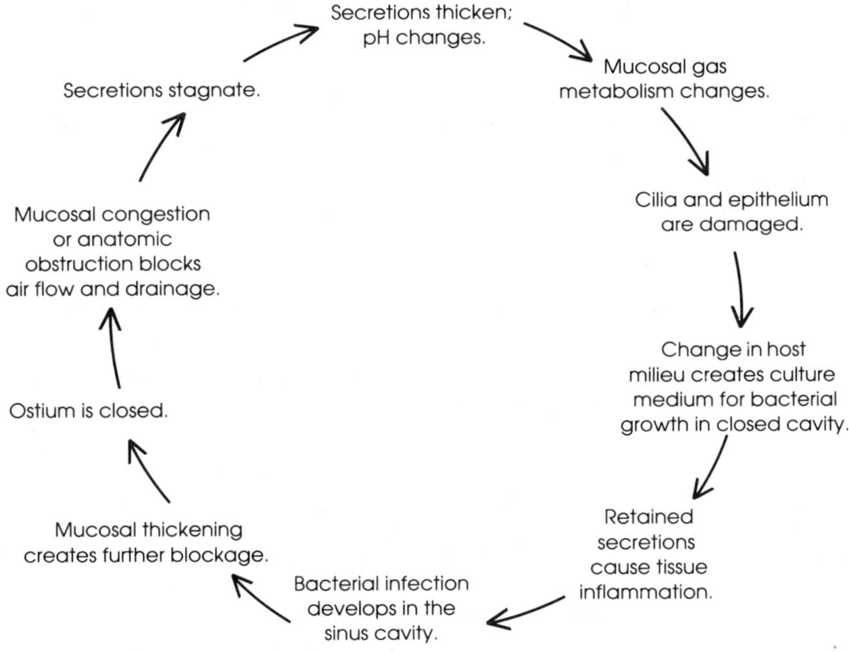

Fig 11–1.—The sinusitis cycle (after Draf W: *Endoscopy of the Paranasal Sinuses.* New York, Springer-Verlag, Inc, 1983). (Courtesy of Reilly JS: *Otolaryngol Head Neck Surg* 103:856–862, 1990.)

infection sites in children; the frontal and sphenoid sinuses may become infected more often in patients aged 8–18 years.

Pathophysiology.—Blockage of the sinus ostia appears to initiate acute sinusitis, which can lead to chronic sinusitis if not treated (Fig 11–1). To alleviate the cycle of chronic sinusitis, the ostia and ostiomeatal complex must be reopened and drained. Factors leading to the impairment of the patient's functional status include a reduction of the oxygen tension within the maxillary sinus; the patency and size of the maxillary, ethmoid, or frontal sinuses; the impairment of the sinus mucosa, and the cilia and granulocyte bactericidal function. Acute infection remains when mucosal damage has occurred. Chronic sinusitis usually occurs because of an anatomical derangement. Both aerobic and anaerobic bacteria have been found in infected sinuses. Beta-lactamase-producing organisms have been found in 25% of the sinus aspirates obtained from children with subacute maxillary sinusitis. The predisposing systemic factors for sinusitis include immune deficiency, cystic fibrosis, bronchiectasis, and immotile cilia syndrome. Predisposing local factors are viral infections, tumors or foreign bodies, barotrauma, cigarette smoke and other kinds of pollution, nasal polyps, deviated nasal septum, and overuse of topical decongestants.

Conclusion.—Clearing of the occlusion of the sinus ostia (which often initiates the sinusitis cycle), elimination of the ostial blockage, and keeping the ostial passages open to promote clearing of sinusitis are recommended.

Endoscopic and Computed Tomographic Findings in Ostiomeatal Sinus Disease

Jorgensen RA (Univ of California, Irvine)

Arch Otolaryngol Head Neck Surg 117:279–287, 1991 11–2

Background.—No organized method has been available for documenting the findings of nasal endoscopy and coronal CT sinus scanning.

Methods.—Findings from such studies were incorporated into 2 forms, the Nasal Endoscopy Exam Form and the Computed Tomographic Scan Findings form. Computerized graphics techniques were used.

Procedures.—The Nasal Endoscopy Exam Form (Fig 11–2) contains dotted lines that become solid as the pathologic findings are recorded. The CT form includes both coronal and axial views. Groups of pathologic features involving the individual paranasal sinuses, turbinates, and nasal septum are placed at the margins of the form. Both forms have lines at the bottom for listing pathologic findings.

Application.—These forms are chiefly used to organize and summarize clinical data, allowing a more precise diagnosis and optimal treatment planning. The diagrams can also be useful in training residents. They

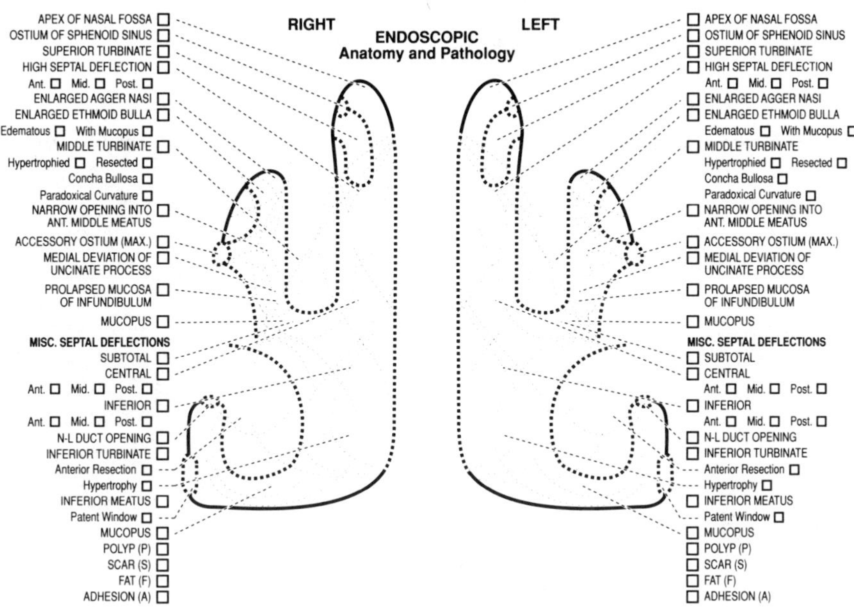

NASAL ENDOSCOPY

1. Neosynephrine 1/4%__, Xylocaine 4%__ was sprayed into Right__ Left__ nasal fossa.
2. Cocaine HCL 4% impregnated cotton pledgets were inserted into Right__ Left__ middle meatus.
3. Pontocaine HCL 2% impregnated cotton pledgets were inserted into Right__ Left__ inferior meatus.
4. Nasal endoscopy was performed: Right Side__ Left Side__
   2.7 mm. diameter 30 degrees__ 4 mm. diameter 30 degrees__ 4 mm diameter 0 degrees__
   2.7 mm. diameter 70 degrees__ 4 mm. diameter 70 degrees__ 4 mm diameter 120 degrees__
5. Afrin__, Neosynephrine, 1/ %__ into Right__ Left__ nostril for three (3) days.

ENDOSCOPIC DIAGNOSIS

RIGHT	LEFT
1. ____________________	1. ____________________
2. ____________________	2. ____________________
3. ____________________	3. ____________________
4. ____________________	4. ____________________
5. ____________________	5. ____________________

Fig 11–2.—Nasal endoscopy examination form. Diagram represents intranasal anatomy. Anatomical features are on either side. Procedure checklist is below diagram. At the bottom are numbered spaces for summarizing findings. (Courtesy of Jorgensen RA: *Arch Otolaryngol Head Neck Surg* 117:279–287, 1991.)

have proved helpful for communicating information to patients, other physicians, and insurance companies.

CT Evaluation of the Paranasal Sinuses in Symptomatic and Asymptomatic Populations

Calhoun KH, Waggenspack GA, Simpson CB, Hokanson JA, Bailey BJ (Univ of Texas, Galveston)

Otolaryngol Head Neck Surg 104:480–483, 1991 11–3

Introduction.—Coronal CT scanning is a widely used radiographic method for the evaluation of sinuses. The frequency of sinonasal abnormalities (e.g., concha bullosa, paradoxical middle turbinate, and septal deviation) on coronal CT scans is known in patients with sinus-related symptoms; however, it is not known in asymptomatic individuals.

Study Design.—A group of 100 consecutive coronal CT scans were compared with 82 consecutive scans performed for evaluation of orbital pathology, and the frequency of sinus abnormalities in symptomatic and asymptomatic populations was compared.

Results.—Radiographic sinus abnormalities occurred in more than 15% of the patients without sinus disease or symptoms. Nevertheless, the incidence of sinus abnormalities was significantly greater in patients with sinus disease (62%) than in the asymptomatic group. The patients with symptomatic sinus disease had a significantly greater incidence of septal deviation and concha bullosa than the asymptomatic group; however, the frequency of paradoxically curved middle turbinate was similar. Septal deviation was significantly associated with osteomeatal complex disease, anterior ethmoid disease, and posterior ethmoid disease, whereas concha bullosa was significantly associated with anterior ethmoid disease. Paradoxical turbinate was not associated with any sinus abnormalities.

Conclusion.—Coronal CT scanning of the paranasal sinuses can accurately delineate anatomical abnormalities and sinus disease. These findings suggest a causal relationship between concha bullosa or septal deviation and sinus disease.

▶ Abstract 11–1 is a succinct review article. We agree with the authors' conclusion that an improved understanding of the pathophysiology of sinusitis has provided some useful management guidelines. These guidelines emphasize that (1) sinus ostia occlusion initiates a cycle of events and produces acute sinusitis, which may, if untreated, progress to chronic sinusitis; (2) ostial occlusion promotes a sinus environment ideal for bacterial growth; and (3) opening the ostia and maintaining an open condition are the goals of all therapy.

Jorgensen (Abstract 11–2) provides excellent suggestions for a practical method of maintaining complete records of CT scan and endoscopic findings. Using the proposed diagrammatic forms allows a large volume of information to be summarized on a single page (where it can be maintained in the patient's chart).

The article by Calhoun et al. (Abstract 11–3) provides unique information on the incidence of septal and turbinate abnormalities in asymptomatic populations. Although it supports the association between septal deviation and concha bullosa with sinusitis, it fails to support a similar correlation between paradoxical turbinate and sinus disease. This point warrants further study.—B.J. Bailey, M.D., F.A.C.S.

Management of Sinusitis

Slavin RG (St Louis Univ, Mo)
J Am Geriatr Soc 39:212–217, 1991 11–4

Background.—Sinusitis, which is common in the elderly, is increasingly recognized as an important cause of morbidity. Its subtle clinical presentation requires a high index of suspicion; however, the results of therapy are gratifying.

Pathophysiology and Diagnosis.—Bacterial infection of the sinuses occurs when their self-cleaning mechanism is impaired. The most important factor in the development of sinusitis is patency of the ostia. Although systemic conditions may play a role, the most common predisposing factors are local, primarily viral upper respiratory infections and allergic rhinitis. A continuation of symptoms after a typical cold subsides is the most important clue in the diagnosis of sinusitis. The most common presenting signs are nasal obstruction, purulent postnasal drainage, chronic cough, hyposomia, sore throat, and unpleasant breath. Underlying sinusitis should be sought in patients with persistent cough and steroid-dependent asthma. Computed tomography is extremely helpful in making the diagnosis.

Medical Management of Sinusitis

1. Steam and Saline
   a. Prevents nasal crusting
   b. liquifies secretions
   c. mild decongestant effect
2. Decongestants—phenylpropanolamine, phenylephrine, oxymetazoline increase ostial diameter
3. Topical corticosteroids—beclomethasone, flunisolide
4. Mucoevacuants—guaifenesin, potassium iodide thin secretions aiding drainage
5. Antibiotics

(Courtesy of Slavin RG: *J Am Geriatr Soc* 39:212–217, 1991.)

Management.—Medical management of sinusitis seeks to increase the diameter of the maxillary ostium and promote mucociliary activity (table). Ampicillin or amoxicillin is the antibiotic of choice. Many bacteria responsible for sinusitis have become resistant to penicillin and cephalosporins. Two weeks of therapy is usually sufficient for acute disease, and 3 weeks or longer is usually sufficient for chronic disease. If there is no improvement after 1 month, surgery may be considered. A Caldwell-Luc operation or a more radical approach for pansinusitis may be used. Functional endoscopic sinus surgery is increasing in acceptance. It causes minimal trauma and allows conservative removal of diseased tissue. Appropriate management of underlying sinusitis often improves an associated asthmatic state.

Conclusions.—The diagnosis and management of sinusitis are discussed. It is hoped that less toxic and less expensive antibiotics will become available for the treatment of resistant organisms. In cases that are resistant to medical treatment, the availability of more definitive endoscopic surgery is promising.

Intracranial Complications of Paranasal Sinusitis: A Combined Institutional Review

Clayman GL, Adams GL, Paugh DR, Koopmann CF Jr (Univ of Minnesota; Univ of Michigan)

Laryngoscope 101:234–238, 1991 11–5

Introduction.—Intracranial complications of paranasal sinusitis (ICPS) include meningitis, subdural empyema, intracerebral and epidural abscesses, and rare cases of cavernous or superior sagittal sinus thrombosis. These complications always constitute true surgical and medical emergencies. To determine the incidence of ICPS, the records of patients treated for acute or chronic sinusitis during a 13-year period were reviewed.

Patients.—Between 1975 and 1988, a total of 649 patients was admitted with a primary diagnosis of acute or chronic sinusitis, and ICPS occurred in 24 (3.7%). The most frequent ICPS included frontal lobe abscess (46%), followed by meningitis (29%), subdural empyema (8%), cavernous sinus thrombosis (8%), and single cases of superior sagittal thrombosis and osteomyelitis of the frontal bone. Ten patients (42%) had possible contributing factors to the development of ICPS. Of the patients, 24% had a history of chronic sinusitis or allergic rhinitis. The patients received immediate systemic intravenous antibiotic therapy. Surgical treatment always included concurrent drainage or excision of the primary sinus disease and associated intracranial suppuration.

Findings.—The most common presenting signs and symptoms of ICPS were fever and headache. Although all patients with ICPS had clinical evidence of overwhelming acute infection, their white blood cell counts on admission were not indicative of the severity of their illness. Positive sinus cultures usually showed multiple organisms, but *Staphylococcus aureus* was the most common single organism isolated from intracranial abscesses.

Outcome.—Cavernous sinus thrombosis developed in 1 patient; this patient died. The patient also had chronic renal failure and mucormycosis of ethmoid-sphenoid origin. Eight patients (33%) had long-term morbidity, 4 had hemiparesis or hypesthesia, 3 had seizure disorders, 1 had decreased cognitive functioning, and 1 had residual cranial nerve deficits. Delayed surgical intervention correlated with the length of hospitalization and long-term morbidity. Computed axial tomography scanning was a most important laboratory examination in establishing the correct diagnosis of the ICPS.

► Slavin (Abstract 11–4) emphasizes the remarkable advances that have recently occurred in the diagnosis and management of sinusitis. Computed tomography scans, nasal endoscopy, and endoscopic sinus surgery have introduced new levels of sensitivity and accuracy into our management of patients with these disorders. Interestingly, he predicts an increasing incidence of β-lactamase-producing organisms as the offending agents in future years. He also makes a plea for cheaper, less toxic antibiotics to deal with these organisms (although it seems unlikely that the new and better agents will also be less expensive).

Intracranial complications of paranasal sinusitis should be suspected in any febrile patient with headache and/or lethargy (Abstract 11–5). Computed tomography scanning is highly effective in evaluating the sinuses and the CNS. In our opinion, aggressive antibiotic therapy should be initiated early (as soon as the diagnosis seems likely) and surgical intervention should be anticipated as very likely. Delays in surgical intervention predispose the patient to more serious long-term morbidity and an increased risk of a fatal outcome.—B.J. Bailey, M.D., F.A.C.S.

Middle Meatus Anstrostomy: Patency Rates and Risk Factors

Davis WE, Templer JW, Lamear WR, Davis WE Jr, Craig SB (Univ of Missouri, Columbia)

Otolaryngol Head Neck Surg 104:467–472, 1991 11–6

Introduction.—Functional endoscopic sinus surgery is an effective treatment for chronic sinus disease; however, the actual percentage of endoscopic middle meatotomies that remain patent over time and the various risk factors, (e.g., asthma, seasonal allergy, or polyp disease) are not well documented.

Setting.—A group of 200 consecutive patients with chronic sinusitis was closely followed during a 3-year period after functional endoscopic sinus surgery. A total of 310 middle meatotomies was performed, and patency was recorded using actuarial life-table methods.

Results.—The overall patency rate was 93.55%, and the actuarial patency rate of endoscopic middle meatotomy at 36 months was 87.47%. Fourteen (7.8%) patients had closure of the endoscopic middle meatotomy. The simultaneous presence of seasonal allergy and polyp disease was associated with an increased risk of closure (42.9%). The patency rate was significantly higher among patients who had middle turbinectomy (96.5%) compared with the total group. Of the patients who completed questionnaires at 1 year, 96% had improved or were asymptomatic after their procedures.

Conclusion.—The actuarial patency rate of endoscopic middle meatotomy at 3 years is significantly higher than the widely accepted 2-year closure rate of 30% of inferior meatus antrostomy. Seasonal allergy and polyp disease increases the risk of closure, whereas middle turbinectomy enhances patency of endoscopic middle meatotomy.

The Intranasal Ethmoidectomy: An Experience With 1,077 Procedures

Lawson W (Mount Sinai Med Ctr, New York)

Laryngoscope 101:367–371, 1991 11–7

Objective.—From 1974 to 1989, 1,077 intranasal ethmoidectomies (including 825 with sphenoid sinusotomies) were performed in 600 patients.

Technique.—The operative technique is a modification of the classical operation devised by Yankauer. The basic procedure was a total sphenoethmoidectomy, wherein the ethmoid labyrinth was completely exenterated and the sphenoid sinus was cannulated and opened.

Setting.—A subset of 90 patients who underwent 166 procedures was followed for an average of 3.5 years. The results of surgery were analyzed according to whether the disease was focal or diffuse, infectious or polypoid, and whether asthma was present.

Results.—The overall success rate was 73%. However, when analyzed based on the proposed classification, the success rate decreased significantly from 88% in nonasthmatic patients for focal and diffuse infectious and polypoid disease to 50% in asthmatic patients with this condition. The overall rate of significant complications was 1.1%.

Conclusions.—The presence of asthma is a biological modifier of surgical prognosis after intranasal ethmoidectomy. The proposed system of classification and staging of nasal disease, which is based upon disease type and extent and presence of asthma, should facilitate comparisons of surgical results.

▶ Although almost half of the patients with seasonal allergy and polyp disease had closure of the endoscopic middle meatotomy, the anstrostomy remained patent in almost all of the remaining patients. The authors of the study outlined in Abstract 1–6 suggest that it may be unwise to operate on allergic patients during the season of their symptoms or when there is evidence that their disease is not under good control. They emphasize that further studies are necessary to verify the wisdom of such a policy.

Along somewhat similar lines, Lawson (Abstract 11–7) observed surgical success rates of only 50% after intranasal ethmoidectomy in asthmatic patients, compared with success rates of 88% in nonasthmatic patients. He proposes that sinusitis may be encountered in either a localized or a generalized (biochemical/asthmatic disorder) manifestation, and that the distinction between the 2 forms is essential in counseling patients and developing effective management of plans.—B.J. Bailey, M.D., F.A.C.S.

Fatal and Other Major Complications of Endoscopic Sinus Surgery

Maniglia AJ (Case Western Reserve Univ)

Laryngoscope 101:349–354, 1991 11–8

Background.—Endoscopic sinus surgery is a rather novel technique that has become popular for the treatment of chronic sinus disease. Five patients with fatal and other major complications of endoscopic sinus surgery were studied.

Data Analysis.—Two patients had orbital complications. One had bilateral, permanent blindness caused by optic nerve injury, and the other had damage to the medial rectus muscle that resulted in permanent diplopia. The other 3 patients had intracranial complications. Of these, 2 had damage to the cribriform plate with brain injury and intracerebral hematoma. In 1 patient, the complication was recognized early with proper treatment and no residual neurological deficit. In the other patient, the surgeon was aware that he had introduced the scope too deeply intracranially (about 7–8 cm). On the spot neurosurgical consultation and CT scanning of the brain ruled out the need for intracranial intervention, and the injury was treated conservatively, similar to a closed head injury. The fifth patient had damage to the cribriform plate that resulted in extensive intracranial hemorrhage and death.

Discussion.—Even in the hands of experienced surgeons, major complications can occur with endoscopic sinus surgery. They are similar to those that occur with traditional intranasal sphenoethmoidectomy. Some complications are preventable, and knowledge of the anatomy and meticulous surgical technique is essential in preventing the occurrence of these complications. Endoscopic sinus surgery should be reserved for patients with lesser pathology and should be used with caution in patients with extensive pathology, especially if general anesthesia is selected. Good training and experience in traditional sinus surgery, as well as the ability to master other techniques, are beneficial before adopting this procedure.

Intracranial Complications of Transnasal Ethmoidectomy

Freije JE, Donegan JO (Dartmouth-Hitchcock Med Ctr, Hanover, NH)
Ear Nose Throat J 70:376–380, 1991 11–9

Introduction.—A transnasal approach to the ethmoid and sphenoid sinuses is an established approach for treatment of nasal polyposis and chronic sinusitis; however, serious intracranial complications may occur. The risks may be lower with modern endoscopic instrumentation.

Case 1.—Man, 71, underwent bilateral intranasal ethmoidectomies and sphenoidotomy for recurrent nasal polyps and sinusitis. He was confused postoperatively, and CT showed a large frontal hematoma and interhemispheric blood. Skull tomography demonstrated a defect in the roof of the ethmoid labyrinth. Later, air-fluid levels were present in the sphenoid sinus, and air was seen intracranially. Culture of CSF yielded *Staphylococcus aureus.* Although a fascial graft was placed to repair the frontal dural defect, hydrocephalus and pneumocophalus developed, requiring decompression.

Case 2.—Woman, 65, underwent bilateral revision intranasal ethmoidectomies for recurrent disease and bled briskly from the left nasal cavity. Intracranial hemorrhage and air were present postoperatively, and a frontal dural defect was repaired. Frontal lobectomy was required to gain access to the bleeding vessel. Reexploration was performed because of CSF leakage, and hydrocephalus necessitated subsequent shunt placement.

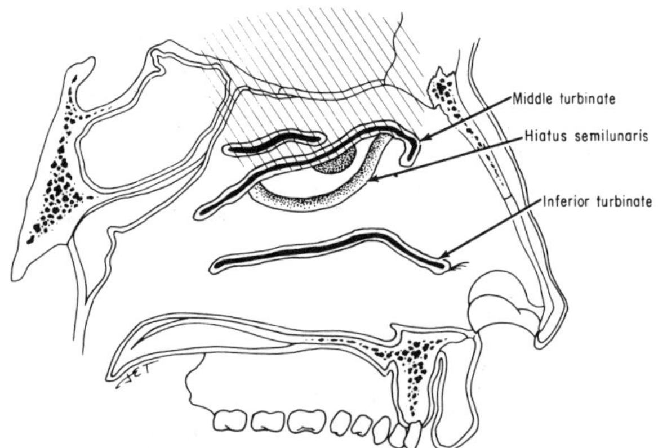

Fig 11–3.—Anatomy of a lateral nasal wall and ethmoid sinus: the shaded areas may be difficult to visualize during transnasal ethmoidectomy. (Courtesy of Freije JE, Donegan JO: *Ear Nose Throat J* 70:376–380, 1991.)

Discussion.—A thorough knowledge of the regional anatomy will enhance the surgical outcome in transnasal ethmoidectomy (Fig 11–3). The ethmoid roof and cribriform plate are vulnerable during intranasal ethmoid surgery. Modern radiographic methods also will help minimize the occurrence of complications. A dural defect may be repaired intracranially or extracranially.

Visual Loss Following Intranasal Anesthetic Injection

Savino PJ, Burde RM, Mills RP (Thomas Jefferson Univ; Albert Einstein Med Ctr, Bronx, NY; Univ of Washington)

J Clin Neuro Ophthalmol 10:140–144, 1990 11–10

Background.—Visual loss during nasal surgery is an uncommon occurrence. Most of the reported visual defects have occurred after injection of corticosteroids or other solutions containing particulate matter in the nasal cavity.

Patients.—Two men and 2 women had visual loss after nasal surgery. All had intranasal injection of anesthetic with epinephrine. None had injections of corticosteroids or particulate-containing solutions. The visual disorders included branch retinal artery occlusion, central retinal artery occlusion, anterior ischemic optic neuropathy, and posterior ischemic optic neuropathy. The visual defects persisted at follow-up.

Discussion.—Retinal and optic nerve ischemia with permanent visual defects may occur after intranasal injection of anesthetic with epinephrine. Transient ophthalmoparesis may accompany these visual defects. Vasospasm after submucosal injection (under pressure) of an anesthetic with epinephrine is postulated to be the cause of visual loss.

▶ Maniglia (Abstract 11–8) makes a strong plea for training and experience with traditional sinus surgery before undertaking endoscopic sinus surgery. He bases this view on the 5 cases of complications that he studied (2 orbital, 3 intracranial). Although we are not given sufficient information about this series (total number of patients having surgery, training and experience of the surgeons, etc.) to decide for ourselves, the point is well taken. Surgeons should proceed with the greatest degree of caution into unfamiliar territory, even though it may not be practical for all surgeons to learn traditional methods extensively before performing endoscopic sinus surgery.

Freije and Donegan (Abstract 11–9) remind us that traditional sinus surgery also carries a significant risk of serious complications. They echo the importance of a solid knowledge of the relevant surgical anatomy.

The injection of intranasal anesthetic agents carries some risk of temporary or permanent visual loss (Abstract 11–10). The exact mechanism by which this occurs continues to elude precise characterization, but every effort must be made to avoid an intravascular injection.—B.J. Bailey, M.D., F.A.C.S.

Nasal Polyposis as a Risk Factor for Hypertension

Granström G, Jacobsson E, Jeppsson P-H (Univ of Gothenburg; Mölndals Hosp, Sweden)
ORL 52:375–384, 1990 11–11

Objective.—Because of observations that patients with nasal polyposis often had arterial hypertension, the relationship between nasal polyposis and arterial hypertension was assessed.

Patients.—A total of 224 patients who underwent surgery for nasal polyposis between 1983 and 1988 was compared with a control group of 248 patients who were treated for cutaneous neoplasms of the nose.

Findings.—Arterial hypertension was diagnosed in 78 (34.8%) of the patients in the nasal polyposis group. Fifty patients had hypertension after the onset of nasal polyposis, and the mean interval between onset of nasal polyposis and onset of hypertension was 11.1 years. In 8 patients, the onset of hypertension occurred simultaneously with the onset of nasal polyposis. The remaining 20 patients had hypertension before the onset of nasal polyposis. Compared with the control group, the incidence of hypertension was significantly increased in the age groups older than 50 years. Twenty-eight (45.9%) of the patients with nasal polyposis for more than 10 years and 50% of the patients with the triad of nasal polyposis, asthma, and intolerance to acetylsalicyclic acid had hypertension. Improvement in blood pressure control was noted in 25% of the patients after operation.

Discussion.—In analogy with the knowledge that sleep apnea and snoring are etiological factors for arterial hypertension, long-standing nasal obstruction by nasal polyposis appears to be a factor for the development of arterial hypertension.

► Airway obstruction may lead to hypertension, whether the cause is tonsil/adenoid hypertrophy, sleep apnea, or obstructive nasal polyposis. It is interesting to note the low level of improvement (25%) in blood pressure after nasal polypectomy. This may suggest that this is commonly a multi-factorial situation.—B.J. Bailey, M.D., F.A.C.S.

Conservative Management of Epistaxis

Moñux A, Tomás M, Kaiser C, Gavilán J (La Paz Hosp, Autonomous Univ, Madrid)
J Laryngol Otol 104:868–870, 1990 11–12

Objective.—There are no uniformly accepted criteria for the management of epistaxis. The clinical usefulness of conservative management of this condition was assessed retrospectively.

Treatment-Results.—Between June 1983 and January 1988, a total of 340 patients with epistaxis was hospitalized. The mean age of the patients was 56.5 years (range, 13–93 years). The procedures performed included nasal packing in 94.7%, withdrawal of previous packing in 2.6%, cauterization in 3%, and surgery in .3%. The mean hospitalization time was 5.6 days, with 82.9% of the patients hospitalized for less than 7 days. Blood transfusion was not necessary in 89.7% of the patients. One patient died of an unrelated cause.

Conclusion.—This retrospective study supports the clinical usefulness of conservative management of epistaxis. Nasal packing is a highly effective treatment and has the advantage of easy placement and removal. Its main inconvenience is the discomfort to the patient.

Intranasal Balloon Catheters: How Do They Work?

McGarry GW, Aitken D (Glasgow Royal Infirmary, Scotland)

Clin Otolaryngol 16:388–392, 1991 11–13

Introduction.—Various intranasal balloon catheters are used to treat nasal bleeding; however, the way in which they work is not well appreciated. Manufacturers' drawings show the balloons neatly filling the nasal cavity or precisely occluding the nasal appertures, but the complexity of internal nasal anatomy makes this an unlikely picture.

Objective.—Radiographic methods were used to determine the configuration of 3 frequently used intranasal balloons within the noses of 4 human cadavers. The devices assessed included the Epistat nasal catheter, the Simpson Plug, and the Brighton Balloon (Fig 11–4).

Findings.—The Epistat and Simpson devices were too long for the average nasal cavity, even before inflation. The Epistat did not conform closely to the contours of the nasal cavity; it tended to inflate along the

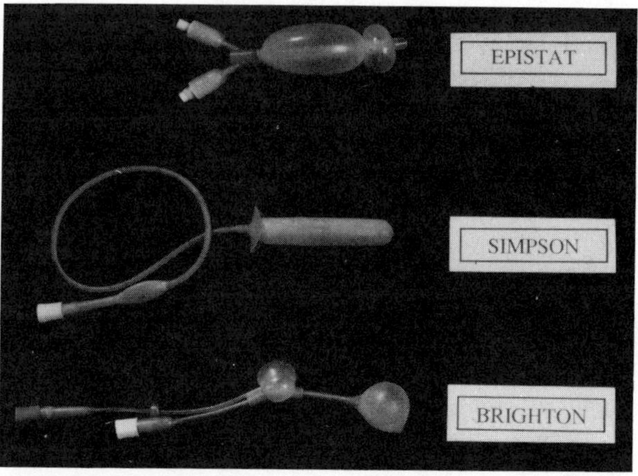

Fig 11–4.—Illustration showing the 3 devices investigated. (Courtesy of McGarry GW, Aitken D: *Clin Otolaryngol* 16:388-392, 1991.)

inferior part of the cavity. The Simpson also did not "fill" the nasal cavity, but tended to inflate along the line of the inferior meatus. The Brighton came closest to what is claimed for it, closing off the anterior nares effectively.

Summary.—Nasal balloon catheters are a useful aid for treating posterior epistaxis. However, a more reliable and safe device needs to be developed. Caution is necessary when using high inflation volumes in unconscious patients.

▶ This study from Spain (Abstract 11–12) emphasizes that a high percentage of the patients who are hospitalized with epistaxis may be managed successfully by conservative (medical) methods. The results are more supportive of medical management than are most reports in the literature, and no explanation for this is provided. One explanation might be that the patients who are hospitalized in the United States might be bleeding more seriously; however, there may be other related factors. In any event, the goal in this population of patients is to differentiate those who may be managed conservatively from those who require surgical treatment. This is preferable to picking one form of treatment vs. the other and then trying to build a case to defend it.

The article on the use of intranasal balloons for controlling epistaxis (Abstract 11–13) is quite informative. Several myths concerning the mechanism of action of these devices are exploded by careful clinical observation. The authors provide some valuable suggestions for improving future balloon designs.—B.J. Bailey, M.D., F.A.C.S.

12 Reconstructive Surgery

The Surgical Anatomy of the Scalp

Tolhurst DE, Carstens MH, Greco RJ, Hurwitz DJ (Academic Hosp, Leiden, The Netherlands; Univ of Pittsburgh)
Plast Reconstr Surg 87:603–614, 1991 12–1

Objective.—Twelve fresh head specimens from 6 cadavers were dissected, 3 after injection of colored Microfil into the external carotid artery and its branches. Special attention was given to the loose connective tissue beneath the galea and above the cranial periosteum and to the temporalis fascia.

Layers of the Scalp.—The galea strictly refers to the aponeurotic part of the musculoaponeurotic layer. It is a dense sheet of fibrous tissue between the occipitalis and frontalis muscles. The subgaleal fascia is often called the "loose areolar layer". It consists of loose areolar and fibrous tissue that becomes progressively thicker as it descends over the temporoparietal regions on both sides of the ear. The temporoparietal fascia is the most superficial fascial layer beneath the subcutaneous fat. The subgaleal fascia is well developed in the temporoparietal region, where it is supplied by branches of the superficial temporal artery.

Clinical Implications.—The subgaleal fascia is readily separated from the overlying galea, leaving a thin sheet of well-vascularized tissue. Flaps may be designed on the branches of the major arteries. Such flaps have been used to recontour the cheek, cover aural cartilage, reconstruct the retroorbital and frontal sinus region, and provide eyelid tissue.

Flap Dynamics

Dzubow LM (Univ of Pennsylvania)
J Dermatol Surg Oncol 17:116–130, 1991 12–2

Introduction.—In flap surgery, the first decision to be made is whether to use a flap at all. A fusiform side-to-side closure has the advantages of simplicity and minimal complications. If there is insufficient skin looseness to close the lesion in this way, or if cosmetic boundaries would be violated, a flap may be better.

Advancement Flaps.—An advancement flap allows one to change the scar location. A classic advancement flap does not reduce the closure tension that would be created by a similar fusiform closure, and it is no more mobile. With inadequate undermining, a newly seated flap may become bunched up (the trap door phenomenon). Nevertheless, the advancement flap is the method of choice for flaws involving the forehead and eyebrow.

Rotation Flaps.—A rotation flap is indicated when there is a need to redirect and redistribute wound closure tension. The shape and site of the flaw are changed by creating a secondary defect in a site where closure can be attained with less tension. This flap can reduce but not eliminate tension at the primary closure site. Scars may seem out of proportion to the size of the original flaw. Lateral upper lip wounds, cheek defects, and flaws of the nasal tip are well dealt with by rotation flaps.

Transposition Flaps.—A transposition flap can use loose skin from a site distant from the primary defect. An almost strain-free closure of the primary site is possible with this flap. The flap rotates freely around a pedicle that is more narrow than that of the rotation flap; however, its geometric design tends to produce more conspicuous scars than the latter. Although the popular rhombic (Limberg) flap is the same size as the flaw it corrects, restraint by the pedicle prevents a tension-free placement. Rotational restriction can be reduced by making the flap slightly longer than the diameter of the circular defect. All transposition flaps require wide undermining at donor and recipient sites to avoid the trap door effect. The most common complication is the appearance of tension in unexpected locations. The geometric scars may also be difficult to orient aesthetically. Transposition flaps are advantageous in an area of relatively taut skin, such as the side of the nose, that is located near an area of loose skin, such as the cheek.

Subcutaneous Island-Pedicle Flaps.—These generally triangular flaps achieve maximum mobility at the expense of vascular input. They are created by eradicating peripheral epidermal-dermal attachments. The pedicle is either deep or lateral to the flap. Lateral pedicles may be single (for pivotal movements) or double, and a central deep pedicle allows straight advancement. Preserving the vasculature of the fatty connecting pedicles and avoiding damage to branches of the facial nerve are the crucial factors in flap survival. Although the trap door effect is a common complication, it tends to improve spontaneously. The flap is useful when a donor site with plenty of well-vascularized fat, such as the cheek, can be used. Defects of the lips and side of the nose may be repaired in this way.

Summary.—The defect size, shape, and site determine the cosmetic boundaries affected and the strain created by wound closure. The characteristics of tissue in the vicinity of the defect determine which flaps would be appropriate.

▶ These 2 articles (Abstracts 12–1 and 12–2) emphasize the importance of a detailed understanding of the basic science principles upon which our clinical practice is based. As Dr. Edgerton points out in his comment after the article on surgical anatomy of the scalp, "It is always a delight to see surgeons directing attention to precise details of anatomy. This is clearly the scientific bedrock of all good surgery." In the study outlined in Abstract 12–1, the authors make an attempt at standardization of terminology and identification of the important features of the subgaleal layer of fascia. Their anatomical investigations, as well as the physiological research of Dr. Dzubow (Abstract 12–2), enhance our understanding of the indications and the limitations of flap reconstructive techniques in the head and neck.—B.J. Bailey, M.D., F.A.C.S.

The Free Scapular Flap for Head and Neck Reconstruction

Sullivan MJ, Carroll WR, Baker SR, Crompton R, Smith-Wheelock M (Univ of Michigan Med Ctr)

Am J Otolaryngol 11:318–327, 1990 12–3

Background.—The surgical removal of large head and neck carcinoma lesions can result in extensive bone and soft tissue defects. Microsurgery free tissue transfer techniques can allow the reconstructive surgeon to avoid some of these complications. Three years of experience with the free scapular flap in 36 consecutive patients undergoing cutaneous and osteocutaneous reconstruction of the head and neck were evaluated.

Methods.—Between June 1986 and August 1989, 36 patients (aged 27–83 years) received a free scapular flap in the reconstruction of head and neck defects. The cutaneous scapular flap was used in 5 patients, whereas the osteocutaneous flap was used in 31. The primary neoplasm in most of these patients was squamous cell carcinoma.

Technique.—The free scapular flap was harvested from the patient; it was usually designed to meet the soft tissue requirements of the particular defect. The cutaneous paddles, which were sometimes harvested simultaneously with the flap, were raised above the deep fascia over the infraspinatus muscle. Continued dissection of the blood vessels requires that the branching vessels be carefully ligated with vascular clips. The required bone length must be carefully measured along the later scapular border. The overlying infraspinatus muscle was incised to the periosteum and 3 cm medial to the lateral scapular border (Fig 12–1). For the osteocutaneous flap, the donor defect was closed by reattaching the teres muscles' origins to the rest of the scapula border with nonabsorbable sutures. Postoperative care included 4–5 days of shoulder immobilization after harvesting the flap and gradual postoperative shoulder exercises to regain range of motion. Patients received a set series of exercises before hospital discharge that were reinforced by home physical therapy.

Findings.—Of the 36 patients, 33 had a successful reconstruction and 34 patients demonstrated solid bony unions. No complications occurred in the 5 patients undergoing cutaneous scapular flap reconstruction, and all patients regained full shoulder function and range of motion. Minor surgical complications were observed in 28% of the patients with the

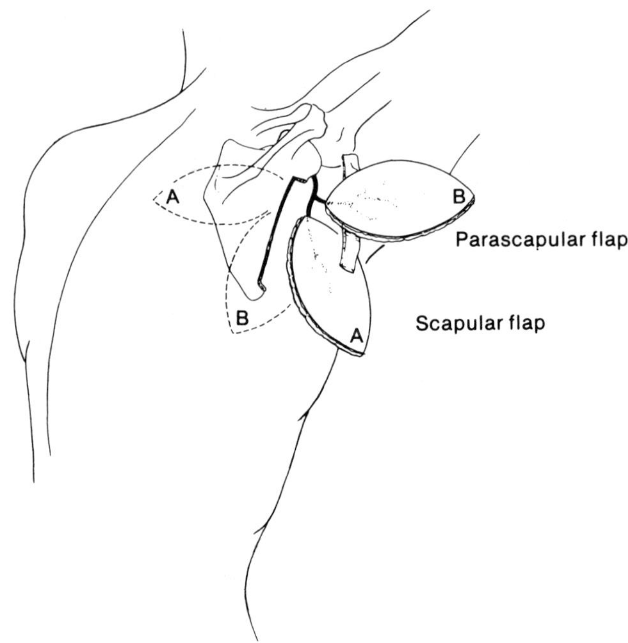

Fig 12–1.—Osteocutaneous scapular flap pedicled by the circumflex scapular vessels. From Baker SR, Sullivan MJ: *Arch Otolaryngol* 114:267–277, 1988. (Courtesy of Sullivan MJ, Carroll WR, Baker SR, et al: *Am J Otolaryngol* 11:318–327, 1990.)

scapular flap reconstruction. All patients had a decreased scapulohumeral function from the scapular osteocutaneous flap harvesting.

Conclusions.—These findings indicate that the free scapular flap offers a reliable and highly vascularized reconstruction material for large head and neck defects.

Treatment of Chronic Facial Palsy by Transplantation of the Neurovascularized Free Rectus Abdominis Muscle

Hata Y, Yano K, Matsuka K, Ito O, Matsuda H, Hosokawa K (Kagawa Med School, Kagawa, Japan)

Plast Reconstr Surg 86:1178–1189, 1990 12–4

Introduction.—The surgical treatment of chronic facial palsy attempts to provide symmetrical voluntary facial movement, muscle tone, and involuntary facial movement. It also attempts to restore the sphincter function of the orbicularis oris and orbicularis oculi muscles. Recent advancements in microsurgery have made dynamic muscle transplantation with facial nerve control innervation possible, confering a more natural appearance on the patient. Data were reviewed on 2 patients who underwent cross-face nerve grafting and neurovascularized free rectus abdominis muscle transplantation.

Technique.—The operation is performed in 2 stages: cross-face nerve grafting and muscle transplantation. In the cross-face nerve grafting procedure, a portion of the sural nerve (approximately 20 cm) is collected from the patient's leg and sutured to the transected branches of the facial nerve. The sural nerve, thus connected to the facial nerve, is passed through a subcutaneous tunnel in the superior upper lip to the preauricular part of the affected side. Muscle transplantation is performed using 1 segment of the rectus muscle with its maximum length of vessels and nerves. The graft is then reversed with one end fixed to the temporozygomatic suture and the other end split into 3 parts and inserted into the upper lip, the corner of the mouth, and the lower lip.

Case 1.—Man, 30, had a hematoma develop after intracranial bleeding in a traffic accident 10 years earlier. The hematoma was removed twice; however, right hemiparesis and left facial palsy developed. Cross-face nerve transplantation was performed, followed 1 year later by free rectus abdominis muscle transplantation. The grafted muscle began to move 6 months after transplantation. Muscle insertions were adjusted 6 months after movement started. An electromyogram showed that the contractile power of the grafted muscle was 4 times stronger than that of the zygomatic major on the nonaffected site.

Case 2.—Man, 37, had right paresis and left facial palsy that resulted from an intracranial hemorrhage related to hypertension that developed 8 months earlier. Although the patient recovered uneventfully from the surgery, a massive hematemesis developed. The patient died of heart failure shortly thereafter.

Conclusions.—The rectus abdominis muscle served as a suitable donor for the muscle transplantation in this procedure. This muscle offers 4 advantages: (1) simultaneous surgical teams can work together with the supine patient; (2) it provides long nerves and vessels; (3) it is flat and has tendinous intersections suitable for anchoring sutures; and (4) it possesses the appropriate force and distance of contraction.

A Biochemical Study of Acute Ischemia in Rodent Skin Free Flaps With and Without Prior Elevation

Angel MF, Mellow CG, Knight KR, Coe SA, O'Brien BMcC (St Vincent's Hosp, Melbourne)

Ann Plast Surg 26:419–426, 1991 12–5

Background.—Elevation of a vascular island flap 24 hours before an ischemic insult significantly increases flap survival in rodents. Recent studies have demonstrated decreased blood thromboxane levels with prior flap elevation compared with acutely ischemic flaps. Whether prior elevation causes other biochemical changes that could be beneficial for flap survival, was determined.

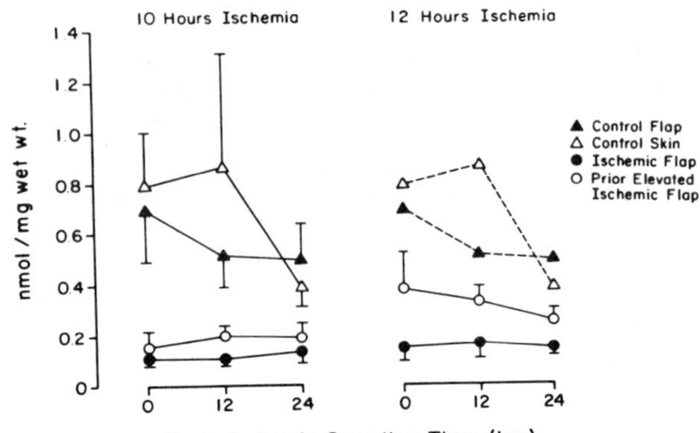

Fig 12–2.—Adenosine triphosphate (ATP) levels: there is a significant difference for treatments ($P < .025$) but not for reperfusion time by analysis of variance (ANOVA). The ATP levels after 12 hours of ischemia were significantly greater in prior elevated ischemic flaps compared with acutely ischemic flaps ($P < .05$). The ATP levels, however, for prior elevated flaps were significantly less ($P < .01$) than control flaps for both ischemia times. (Courtesy of Angel MF, Mellow CG, Knight KR, et al: *Ann Plast Surg* 26:419–426, 1991.)

Methods.—Rat epigastric flaps, with or without prior elevation, were subjected to either 10 or 12 hours of acute ischemia. Biopsy specimens were taken at 0, 12, and 24 hours after reperfusion, and the tissue levels of adenosine triphosphate, superoxide dismutase, xanthine oxidase, and edema were measured.

Findings.—Significantly more flaps survived acute ischemia when the flaps had undergone prior elevation, compared with ischemic flaps (100% vs. 67% at 10 hours and 67% vs. 8% at 12 hours of acute ischemia). After 12 hours of ischemia, both adenosine triphosphate levels and edema were significantly less in the acutely ischemic flaps than in the previously elevated flaps (Fig 12–2), whereas superoxide dismutase and xanthine oxidase did not change significantly.

Discussion.—Prior elevation of a flap before an ischemic insult increases flap survival. It is not clear whether the increased tissue level of adenosine triphosphate in prior elevated flaps is a result of increased tissue viability. Prior elevation does not affect the free radical mechanisms; however, it improves flap survival despite increased edema.

▶ The extensive defects in the head and neck that occur after cancer excision or trauma continue to provide an important challenge to the reconstructive surgeon. The past 2 decades have seen enormous advances in the successful use of various pedicled flaps; however, all of these flaps are limited by an important degree of morbidity at the donor site and the mechanical restrictions of their pedicles. Although free flaps have been relatively slow to emerge as major instruments for reconstruction, it appears that their role is increasing. Leading head and neck cancer services are now using free flap reconstruction much more extensively than they did 5 years ago. These 3 articles (Abstracts 12–3, 12–4, and 12–5) review head and neck reconstruction using free flaps in a general manner and the use of free muscle flaps to rehabilitate the paralyzed face. Abstract 12–5 reports a favorable effect on free flap survival with prior elevation, and it describes the advantages achieved from a biochemical perspective. Although this step is not routinely used, further experience and reports from other investigators may lead us to reconsider the matter of prior elevation as a standard part of this technique.—B.J. Bailey, M.D., F.A.C.S.

An Improved Technique for Development of the Pectoralis Major Myocutaneous Flap

Marx RE, Smith BR (Univ of Miami)

J Oral Maxillofac Surg 48:1168–1180, 1990 12–6

Background.—Axial pattern myocutaneous flaps have replaced skin-subcutaneous flaps for soft tissue reconstruction of the oral cavity and upper neck because of greater predictability, improved functional and morphological results, and their ability to place vascular and cellular tissue into a bed better able to support bony reconstruction. The pectoralis major myocutaneous flap is the most commonly used flap for soft tissue reconstruction of the oral cavity.

Technique.—The technique involves removal of a strip of muscle (including the overlying skin) along the oblique course of the pectoral branch of the thoracoacromial artery. The muscle is divided just medial to the axilla to extend the arc of rotation toward the recipient site without damaging the axillary artery and vein. The flap is passed through a tunnel prepared in the neck and is placed in the recipient site.

Results.—The procedure was used in 33 men and 21 women. A total of 51 donor wounds and 51 recipient wounds healed without complication. The 6% recipient site and 6% donor site complication rate appeared to be unrelated to age, sex, radiation, or previous surgery. This technique resulted in only a 1.9% incidence of necrosis of all or part of the skin paddle and no necrosis of the underlying muscle. The low necrosis rate may be related to the inclusion of nearly the entire muscle and more of its vascular supply in construction of the flap.

Discussion.—This approach to the pectoralis major myocutaneous flap maintains better vascular inflow and outflow tracks and provides a more tension-free closure than other approaches do. These advantages make this modification of the procedure more versatile and reliable.

The Lower Trapezius Island Musculocutaneous Flap Revisited: Report of 45 Cases and a Unifying Concept of the Vascular Supply

Urken ML, Naidu RK, Lawson W, Biller HF (Mount Sinai Med Ctr, New York)
Arch Otolaryngol Head Neck Surg 117:502–511, 1991 12–7

Background.—Because it offers thin, pliable tissue and a long arc of rotation to reach almost any head and neck defect, the lower trapezius island musculocutaneous flap (LTIMF) is a valuable tool in head and neck reconstruction. However, high failure rates and questions about the reliability of the vascularity have appeared. An experience with 45 reconstructions using the LTIMF was reviewed.

Methods.—The flaps, which were used during an 11-year period, were used to address a wide variety of head and neck defects. They were used most often to resurface cutaneous defects of the lateral skull and neck in 13 and 17 cases, respectively. They were also used for defects of the

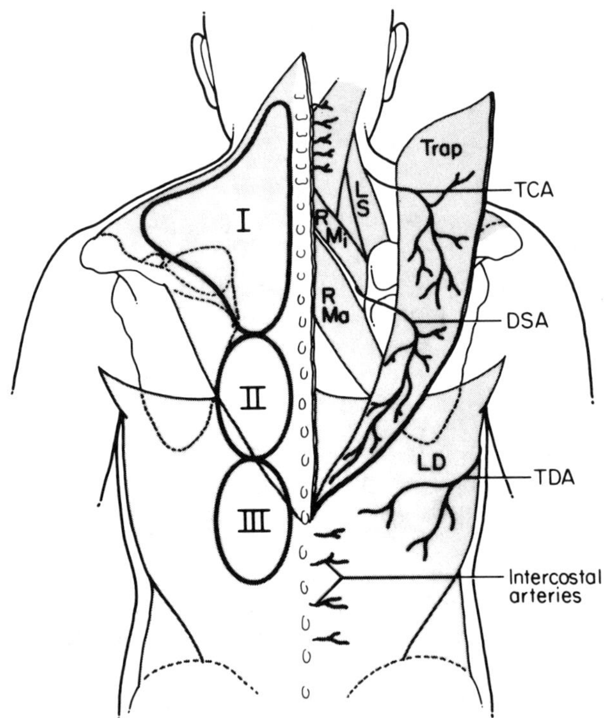

Fig 12–3.—*Abbreviations: LS,* levator scapulae muscle; *RMi,* lesser rhomboid muscle; *RMa,* greater rhomboid muscle; *TDA,* thoracodorsal artery. The approximate boundaries of the angiosomes of the trapezius muscle *(Tr).* The upper angiosome *(I)* is supplied by the transverse cervical artery *(TCA),* whereas the lower angiosome *(II)* is supplied by the dorsal scapular artery *(DSA).* The angiosome inferior to the Tr *(III)* overlies the latissimus dorsi muscle *(LD)* and is supplied by the intercostal arteries. (Courtesy of Urken ML, Naidu RK, Lawson W, et al: *Arch Otolaryngol Head Neck Surg* 117:502–511, 1991.)

lower third of the face in 7 cases, for defects of the middle and upper thirds of the face in 4 cases, and for defects of the oral cavity and pharynx in 4 cases. Ipsilateral neck dissection preceded use of the LTIMF in 16 patients. All patients underwent the same technique of flap harvest; the dorsal scapular artery was never preserved, and the rhomboid muscles were not included with the trapezius muscle.

Results.—One patient, a 74-year-old man who had undergone total laryngopharyngectomy and gastric pull-up, died of sepsis from a perforated duodenal ulcer 2 weeks after flap harvest; this was the only postoperative death. There were 2 other major complications: 1 complete loss in an elderly woman who had undergone a previous ipsilateral neck dissection and 1 loss of the distal portion of the trapezius flap in a patient with a large buccal carcinoma. Three minor complications occurred because of a loss of less than 20% of the cutaneous paddle. The overall complication rate was 13%, with 5 of 6 complications occurring in patients who had undergone previous neck dissection. Complications at the donor site were relatively minor. Although shoulder function was disturbed, this was well tolerated.

Conclusions.—Use of the LTIMF is a valuable technique in head and neck reconstruction. The incidence of major and minor flap loss can be low, despite the controversy surrounding the flap's reliability when it is based solely on the transverse cervical pedicle. A variety of observations on the viability of the cutaneous portion of the flap may be explained by the angiosome model of Taylor et al. (Fig 12–3).

The Pedicled Extended Serratus Anterior Myocutaneous Flap for Head and Neck Reconstruction

Inoue T, Ueda K, Hatoko M, Harashina T (Saitama Med Ctr, Saitama Med School, Japan)

Br J Plast Surg 44:259–265, 1991 12–8

Introduction.—A new "extended" serratus anterior myocutaneous flap has been designed for head and neck reconstruction.

Technique.—The extended myocutaneous flap is designed by fasciocutaneous extension anteriorly and inferiorly from the 6th to 8th slips of the serratus anterior muscle (Fig 12–4). The vascular pedicle includes the serratus branch of the thoracodorsal artery and vein.

Outcome.—The extended serratus anterior myocutaneous flaps were used for various types of head and neck reconstruction in 11 patients. The largest flap obtained was 10 × 22 cm, and the longest vascular pedicle was 22 cm. The results were satisfactory.

Discussion.—The extended serratus anterior myocutaneous flap is superior to conventional flaps for head and neck reconstruction. It provides a long pedicle that allows reconstruction without microvascular an-

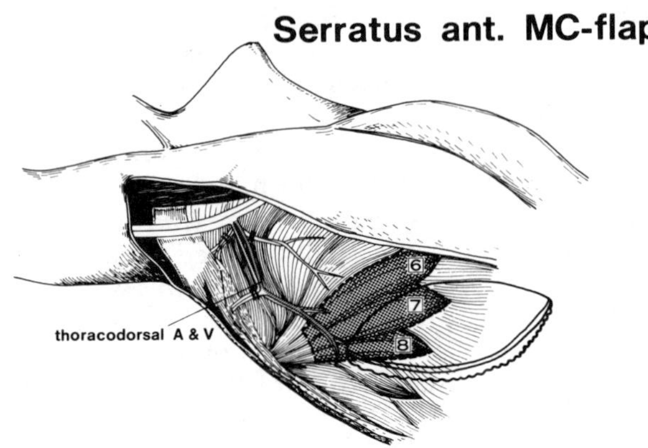

Fig 12–4.—A diagram of the extended serratus anterior myocutaneous flap. (Courtesy of Inoue T, Ueda K, Hatoko M, et al: *Br J Plast Surg* 44:259–265, 1991.)

astomosis in nearly all cases. There is little postoperative functional loss at the donor site because the flap uses only a small amount of the serratus anterior muscle and the long thoracic nerve is preserved. The donor site is located in a covered area and can be closed primarily. The procedure requires no postural change during surgery.

▶ In the study by Marx and Smith (Abstract 12–6), the authors, who are oral surgeons, report that they are achieving superior results because they include a larger muscle component in the pectoralis major myocutaneous flaps when reconstructing patients. Most of their cases involve osteoradionecrosis, and they describe having a partial loss of the skin paddle in only 1 of 54 patients. Although it may be true that including a larger muscle component is advantageous, it is important to remember that larger muscle components were common in the early 1980s, when this flap was just being popularized. It is more likely that their results are superior because they are using much smaller skin paddles than those used in the series with which they are comparing their results. Also, since the early 80s, much has been learned about the limitations of size and sight that are relevant to skin paddle survival with this flap. It might be wise to await confirmation of these findings before returning to the use of large, bulky muscle components.

The LTIMF is an excellent flap for head and neck reconstruction, even though it carries a somewhat higher implication rate than the pectoralis major myocutaneous flap. Abstract 12–7 is an elegant study; its authors conclude that the skin-muscle flap should not be extended below the inferior border of the scapula if optimal results are to be achieved. They also emphasize the advantages of this flap: its long arch of rotation and the thin, pliable tissue layer that is available for reconstruction. It is the authors' flap of choice for the reconstruction of lateral skull defects.

The study from Japan by Inoue et al. (Abstract 12–8) describes a "new flap" for which its authors have considerable enthusiasm. They describe 5 cases from a series of 11 patients; however, they do not provide such key information as specific indications for the use of this flap, morbidity, complications, or contraindications. In addition, they provide no comparison with other flaps to document the superiority that they claim. Although it is an interesting concept, further reports might be necessary to confirm whether the level of enthusiasm is justified.—B.J. Bailey, M.D., F.A.C.S.

The Frontonasal Flap: Utility for Lateral Nasal Defects and Technical Refinements

Wee SS, Hruza GJ, Mustoe TA (Washington Univ, St Louis, Mo)
Br J Plast Surg 44:201–205, 1991 12–9

Background.—Use of the extended glabellar or frontonasal flap has been described mainly for the repair of defects of the central tip of the nose. With further refinements, this flap can improve the cosmetic result, as well as extend its usefulness to both large defects and, in combination with other flaps, lateral defects. The frontonasal flap was used in 27 patients.

Technique.—The flap is designed as an inverted "V" in the glabella, not extending above the brow (Fig 12–5). Flap elevation is in the thin subcutaneous plane along the lateral nose; to avoid a stairstep deformity, the flap does not go beneath the nasalis until the midline. Rather than merely advancing it in V-Y fashion, the flap can be rotated nearly 90 degrees. To avoid a standing cone and allow a short glabellar scar, the procerus and glabellar subcutaneous tissue are extensively removed. A nasolabial, rotation advancement, transposition, or island nasalis flap may be used in combination with the frontonasal flap. Early dermabrasion at 6 weeks is beneficial.

Patients.—A group of 27 patients was treated during a 5-year period. There were 19 women and 8 men, ranging in age from 31 to 92 years. Except in 1 case of skin-graft deformity, the resection margin was controlled by Mohs micrographic surgery. The smallest defect measured 1.2

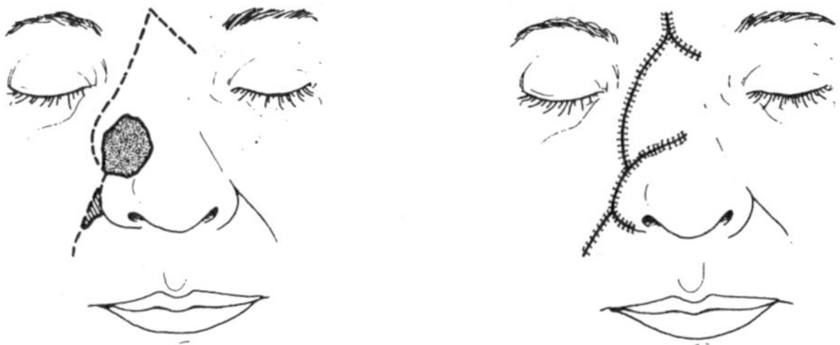

Fig 12–5.—The extended glabellar flap can be rotated down into a lateral defect *(dark area)* combined with a cheek advancement rotation along the nasolabial fold with excision of the standing cone along the alar crease *(hatched area)*. The resulting nostril asymmetry is minimal and improves with time. (Courtesy of Wee SS, Hruza GJ, Mustoe TA: *Br J Plast Surg* 44:201–205, 1991.)

$\times$ 1.2 cm and the largest 4 $\times$ 3 cm. At 1 month - 5 years, all flaps survived with no tumor recurrences and generally excellent cosmetic results. Standing cone deformities were revised at the time of dermabrasion in several patients. Occasionally, deviated alar cartilage and nasal humps were also dealt with at this time.

Conclusions.—The frontonasal flap is a useful technique for repairing relatively large defects of the lower, upper, lateral, and central nose. The flap may be combined with other flaps to resurface large defects. Early dermabrasion improves the scars in sebaceous skin.

Modified Nasolabial Transposition Flap Provides Vestibular Lining and Cover of Alar Defect With Intact Rim

Robinson JK, Horan DB (Northwestern Univ Med School, Chicago)

Arch Dermatol 126:1425–1427, 1990 12–10

Introduction.—Desiccation, infection, and/or necrosis often accompany the placement of nasolabial flaps into through and through nasal defects without alignment of the flap. Wound contraction with unacceptable retraction of an intact alar rim can occur. The need to align all these facial components is still controversial. The use of a modified nasolabial transposition flap to cover the alar defect with intact rim was reviewed in 1 patient.

Case Report.—Woman, 77, was seen with several basal cell carcinomas, 1 of which was located on the left nasal ala. Resection of this carcinoma resulted in a perforation wound (3.10 $\times$ 2.5 cm). A nasolabial flap of sufficient size was designed to repair the external cover and vestibular lining (Fig 12–6).

Technique.—The flap was incised and raised, and the secondary defect underwent closure. The distal tip of the distal flap formed the new vestibular lining. After defatting and thinning, the 3-mm distance that was originally considered was found to be too long; it was then reduced to 2 mm. The distal flap was inset using 4 buried sutures of Vicryl, with the last buried suture securing the deepithelialized strip to the subcutaneous tissue of the ala at the medial section of the defect. A deep periosteal buried suspension suture was then inset from the flap base to the periosteal rim of the nasal notch of the maxilla. The remainder of the proximal flap was secured by interrupted skin sutures.

Results.—At postsurgery follow-up, the patient showed healing with slight epidermal necrosis of the vestibular lining at the flap's tip. The flap eventually healed without retraction of the alar rim. Five months after the first operation, the flap was debulked. Then the standing cone of skin around the flap's turning point was excised and the alar crease was refined.

Implications.—These results indicate that, after the edema resolves, a second procedure can restore the definition of the cheek-nose concavity

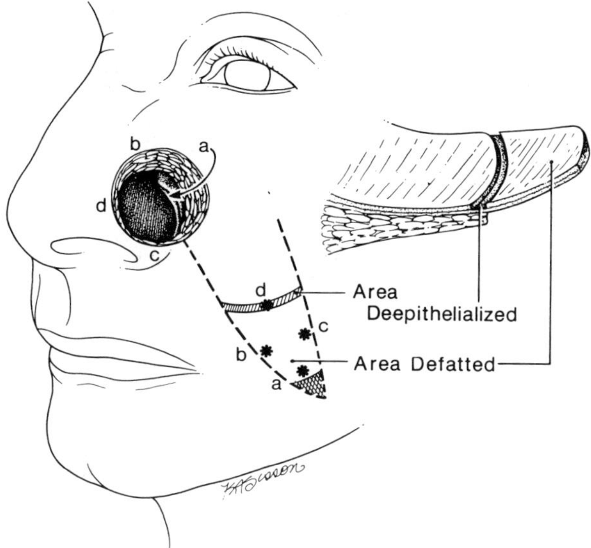

Fig 12–6.—Planning the nasolabial transposition flap included an estimate of the region of the flap that will be deepithelialized. This was marked on the flap by the 2 central parallel curved lines. The flap tip was rounded to conform to the defect in the vestibular mucosa. The lateral incision extended from the arrow to the tip **(left).** Placement of the 4 internal buried sutures was marked by *a, b, c,* and *d* **(right)** (Courtesy of Robinson JK, Horan DB: *Arch Dermatol* 126:1425–1427, 1990)

in the older patient. This series of small and subtle modifications allows the surgeon to use the nasolabial transposition flap to repair the vestibular lining and cover in a single operation while causing fewer complications.

An Alternative for Nasal Tip Reconstruction: The Bilateral Rotation Flap

Greenbaum SS, Greenbaum CH (Thomas Jefferson Univ, Philadelphia)
J Dermatol Surg Oncol 17:455–459, 1991 12–11

Background.—Many of the skin tumors that dermatologic surgeons treat are located on the nose. A significant proportion of these tumors are on the nasal tip, which is notoriously difficult to reconstruct. A bilateral rotation flap that may be useful in some cases for nasal tip reconstruction was assessed.

Patients.—Patients with a basal cell carcinoma on the nasal tip were treated. Each patient had relatively little skin that could be borrowed laterally from either side; however, each had some excess tissue proximally on the bridge of the nose extending into the glabella.

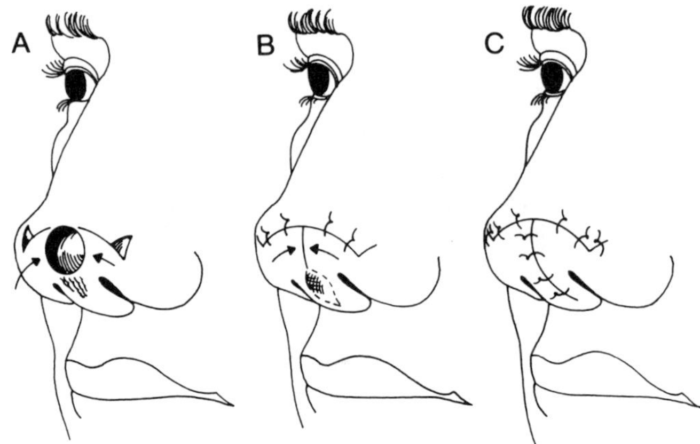

Fig 12–7.—A, proposed bilateral rotation flap. Note the location of the anticipated standing-cone deformity and Burow's wedge resections. **B,** rotation flaps sutured in place. **C,** completed repair after removal of the standing-cone deformity. (Courtesy of Greenbaum SS, Greenbaum CH: *J Dermatol Surg Oncol* 17:455–459, 1991.)

Technique.—A random-pattern local flap was chosen for closure, and a bilateral rotation flap was chosen to both fill in the defect with similar skin and permit closure of the secondary defect with the excess tissue located more superiorly on the nose. The flaps were then drawn and cut (Fig 12–7).

Conclusions.—The bilateral rotation flap appears to be a good option for nasal tip repair. Three advantages of this option are that similar skin is used to cover the defect, a minimum of cosmetic units are violated, and many of the incision lines are camouflaged in junctions of cosmetic units. Although multiple incisions are made, the overall length of each is minimal. Another advantage is that the nasal tip is not displaced from its normal, midline position. Patients with small- to medium-sized nasal tip defects should be considered candidates for this procedure.

Intraoral Reconstruction With the Nasolabial Island Flap: A Modified Technique

Garatea J, Buenechea R, Bescos C, Gonzalez E, Bassas C (Hosp Valle de Hebrón, Barcelona, Spain)

J Craniomaxillofac Surg 19:119–122, 1991 12–12

Background.—The traditional nasolabial flap for reconstruction of intraoral defects has some limitations, including the necessity for a 2-stage procedure, a paucity of available skin, the presence of hair-bearing skin in males, and the relatively difficult insetting of a wide cutaneous pedicle. A modification of the nasolabial technique is proposed to increase the amount of skin available in the donor area.

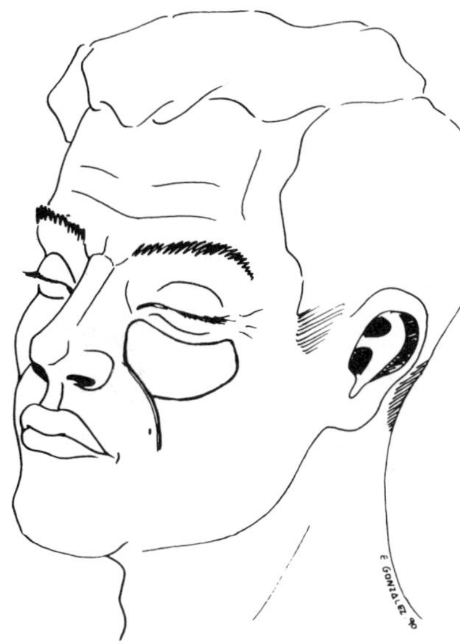

Fig 12–8.—Island incised with a relieving incision. (Courtesy of Garatea J, Buenechea R, Bescos C, et al: *J Craniomaxillofac Surg* 19:119–122, 1991.)

Technique.—The hairless skin under the lower eyelid is designed extending lateral to the nasolabial fold in a circular fashion. The island is incised with a relieving incision (Fig 12–8). The flap is raised, and the pedicle is dissected through a relieving incision along the nasolabial fold to obtain sufficient length that ensures easy insetting (Fig 12–9). The flap is then brought into the mouth through

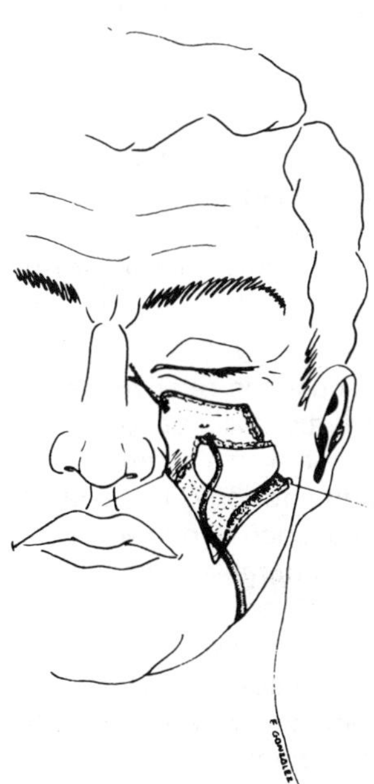

Fig 12–9.—Flap raised and pedicle dissected through the relieving incision. (Courtesy of Garatea J, Buenechea R, Bescos C, et al: *J Craniomaxillofac Surg* 19:119–122, 1991.)

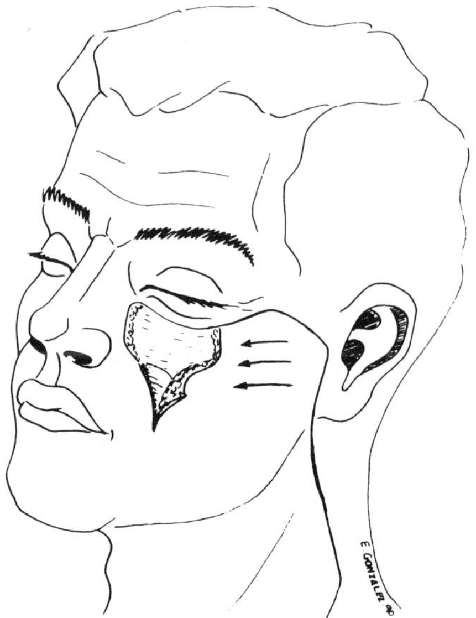

Fig 12–10.—Donor defect closure with a check rotation flap. (Courtesy of Garatea J, Buenechea R, Bescos C, et al: *J Craniomaxillofac Surg* 19:119–122, 1991.)

a tunnel in the buccal area and is sutured into the intraoral defect. The donor defect is closed by a cheek rotation flap (Fig 12–10).

Outcome.—The nasolabial island flap was performed in 3 patients with oral cancer. The lesions were 2–3 cm in diameter and were located in the buccal mucosa in 2 patients and in the posterior maxilla in the third patient. The only sequel was an upper lip palsy without loss of mouth sealing and salivary drooling, and both were a result of extensive tumor excision.

Conclusion.—The nasolabial island flap provides greater availability of hairless skin for intraoral reconstruction in a 1-stage fashion. The longer pedicle permits greater versatility, and oral defects of moderate size can be repaired. This method does not permit simple closure of the donor defect; this is achieved with a cheek rotation flap.

▶ These 4 abstracts (Abstracts 12–9 — 12–12) discuss the relatively small defects in and around the nose that require reconstruction using a local flap. The paper by Wee et al. (Abstract 12–9) reviews the use of the extended glabellar flap to reconstruct a defect located laterally and inferiorly. The authors point out that the alternatives to be considered are a bilobed flap or a precise midline flap. The extended glabellar frontonasal flap is durable, reliable, and versatile. It should be part of the reconstructive surgeon's armamentarium.

The modified nasolabial transposition flap is reviewed in the form of a single case report (Abstract 12–10). It is advantageous because it allows a single stage reconstruction of a through and through defect involving the nose. The drawbacks to this approach are that it lacks cartilaginous support (which may be important in the region of the nasal valve) and that scar contracture is somewhat more problematic with this type of reconstruction. In addition, the surgeon must be cautious regarding excessive thickness and must take appropriate measures to avoid hair growth within the nasal cavity.

The article describing the use of bilateral rotation flaps in the reconstruction of nasal tip defects less than 1.5 cm in diameter is interesting (Abstract 12–11). Although this appears to be a reliable and satisfactory approach, defects of this small size can often be managed using a small full-thickness skin graft obtained from the postauricular or superclavicular regions.

Along the same lines, the abstract on intraoral reconstruction with the nasolabial island flap (Abstract 12–12) describes an elegant solution to a relatively simple problem. In many instances, a skin graft is entirely adequate to repair a mucosal, intraoral defect. Taken as a group, these 4 abstracts provide an interesting review of this general type of reconstruction.—B.J. Bailey, M.D., F.A.C.S.

Oromandibular Reconstruction Using Microvascular Composite Free Flaps: Report of 71 Cases and a New Classification Scheme for Bony, Soft-Tissue, and Neurologic Defects

Urken ML, Weinberg H, Vickery C, Buchbinder D, Lawson W, Biller HF
(Mount Sinai Med Ctr, New York)

Arch Otolaryngol Head Neck Surg 117:733–744, 1991 12–13

Background.—The restoration of normal oral function after ablative surgery or trauma relies on various factors, including the reconstruction of complex osseous, dental, and soft tissue anatomy. A variety of classification schemes have been proposed for segmental mandibular defects. A series of patients who underwent reconstruction using microvascular composite free flaps was reviewed, and a new classification scheme was proposed for bony, soft tissue, and neurological defects.

Methods.—A total of 71 patients underwent oromandibular reconstruction. The new classification system was applied in the description of the mucosal and cutaneous defects of each case (Figs 12–11 and 12–12).

Results.—The overall flap success rate was 94%. Of the patients, 97% had mandibular reconstruction with free vascularized bone flaps. Implant-borne dental prostheses were used to rehabilitate 15 patients, and 16 patients had primary repair of discontinuity defects of the inferior-alveolar nerve using a variety of nerve grafts.

Conclusions.—The vascularized composite free flaps can clearly be transferred to the oral cavity with a high degree of consistency and an acceptable complication rate. The primary oromandibular reconstruction is now so refined that it can be offered to virtually any patient who must undergo ablative surgery for oral carcinoma.

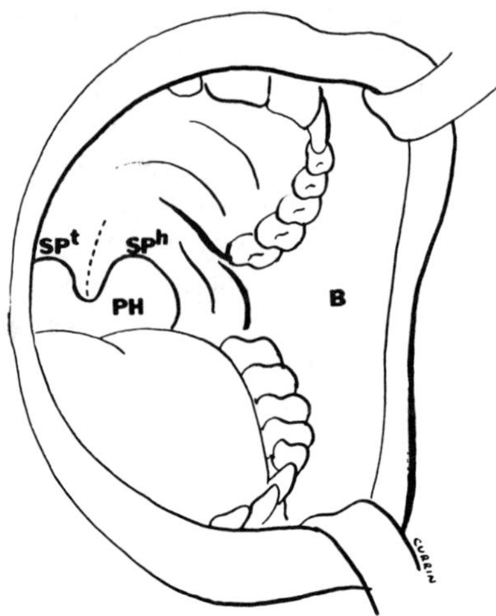

Fig 12–11.—*Abbreviations: B*, buccal defect of the oral cavity; *SP*ʰ, hemi-defect of the soft palate; *SP*ᵗ, total defect of the soft palate; *PH*, pharyngeal defect. Classification of the mucosal defects of the oral cavity. The pharyngeal defects are further divided into posterior and lateral. (Courtesy of Urken ML, Weinberg H, Vickery C, et al: *Arch Otolaryngol Head Neck Surg* 117:733–744, 1991.)

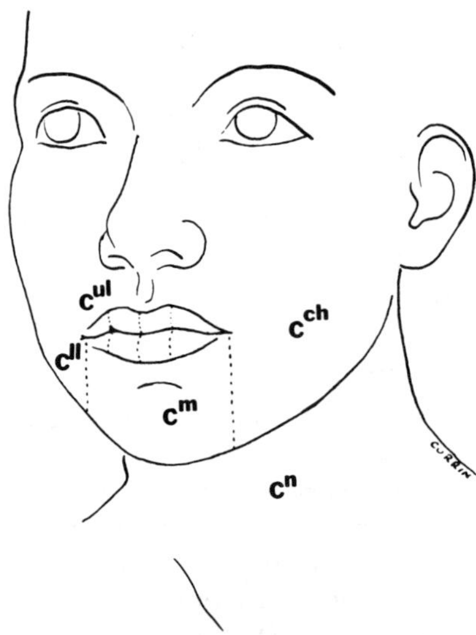

Fig 12–12.—*Abbreviations:* C^{ch}, cutaneous defects of the cheek; C^{n}, of the neck; C^{m}, of the mentum; C^{ul}, of the upper lips (¼, ½, ¾, and total); C^{ll}, of the lower lips (¼, ½, ¾, and total). Classification of cutaneous defects. (Courtesy of Urken ML, Weinberg H, Vickery C, et al: *Arch Otolaryngol Head Neck Surg* 117:733–744, 1991.)

Mandible Reconstruction With Vascularized Bone Grafts: A Histologic Evaluation

Hoffman HT, Harrison N, Sullivan MJ, Robbins KT, Ridley M, Baker SR (Univ of California and VA Med Ctrs, San Diego; Univ of Michigan; Univ of South Florida)

Arch Otolaryngol Head Neck Surg 117:917–925, 1991 12–14

Background.—There is disagreement about the best method to reconstruct mandibular bone defects. To date, there has been no histological assessment of bone healing after mandible reconstruction with vascularized human bone grafts.

Methods.—Four patients who required surgical removal of their reconstructed mandibles were studied. The serial sections through both the decalcified graft and the junction between mandible and graft were assessed.

Findings.—A failed scapular bone graft that had been wrapped in a pectoralis major myocutaneous flap for salvage demonstrated markedly resorbed but viable bone after pedicle thrombosis. A fibrous union to the native mandible was also noted. An iliac osteocutaneous bone graft and 2 scapula osteocutaneous grafts that healed with continuity of healthy bone between the graft and the mandible were characterized by viable vascularized grafts without signs of ongoing resorption.

Conclusions.—The histological assessment of these 4 reconstructed mandibles permitted observations about bone graft survival, bone union, and bone circulation as they occur clinically. A continued critical look at mandible reconstruction using vascularized bone grafts is needed to optimize treatment for patients who require this reconstructive surgery.

Double Lumen Free Jejunal Transfer for Reconstruction of the Entire Floor of Mouth, Pharynx and Cervical Oesophagus

Jones NF, Eadie PA, Myers EN (Univ of Pittsburgh)

Br J Plast Surg 44:44–48, 1991 12–15

Introduction.—The preferred technique for reconstruction of the hypopharynx and cervical esophagus is free jejunal transfer. In patients who require total glossectomy and laryngopharyngectomy, there is a large discrepancy between the superior pharyngeal defect and the lumen of the free jejunal transfer. A technique was developed to prevent postoperative fistulae at the proximal anastomosis in patients with large superior pharyngeal defects.

Case Report.—Man, 34, had extensive oropharyngocutaneous fistula and recurrent T4N0M0 squamous cell carcinoma of the base of the tongue. Radiotherapy failed, and the fistula measured 9.5 × 7 cm. Total glossectomy, resection of the floor of the mouth, and bilateral modified radical neck dissections were performed for palliation. The defect had an anterior-posterior dimension of 7.5 cm,

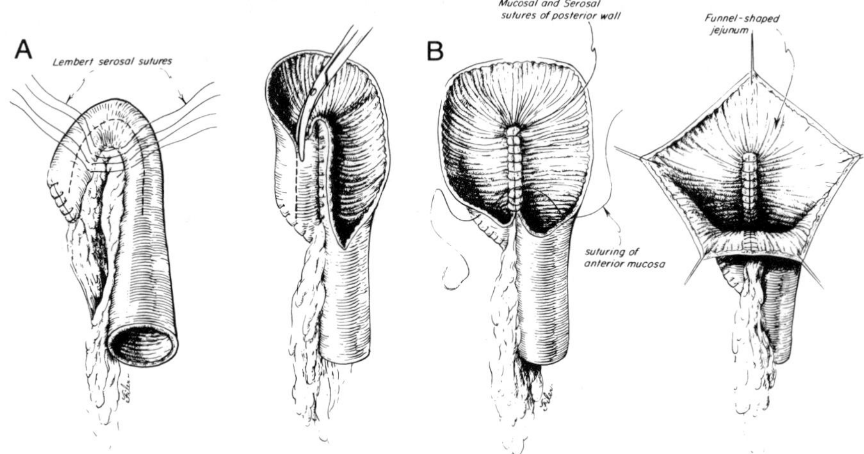

Fig 12–13.—A diagrammatic representation showing prefabrication of an inverted J-shaped jejunal funnel. (Courtesy of Jones NF, Eadie PA, Myers EN: *Br J Plast Surg* 44:44–48, 1991.)

with its superior margin extending from the cervical fascia posteriorly along the bare lingual surface of the mandible to the symphysis of the mandible. An inverted J-shaped jejunal funnel, extending from the symphysis of the mandible anteriorly and the posterior nasopharynx superiorly to the remnant of the cervical esophagus at the sternal inlet, was used to reconstruct the defect (Fig 12–13). The distal jejunum and cervical esophagus were anastomosed end to end. The mesenteric vein was anastomosed to the left internal jugular artery and the superior mesenteric artery was anastomosed to the left facial artery. Pectoralis major flaps were used to cover the jejunum and reconstruct the neck soft tissue defect. The patient began a liquid diet 12 days after surgery and gained 30 pounds during the next 3 months.

Conclusion.—The use of an inverted J-shaped jejunal funnel to enlarge the proximal stoma of a free jejunal transfer overcomes the size discrepancy in patients with large superior pharyngeal defects, thereby preventing postoperative fistulae at the proximal anastomosis. This technique allows reconstruction of the entire floor of the mouth, pharynx, and cervical esophagus in patients with extreme conditions.

▶ These 3 papers (Abstracts 12–13, 12–14, and 12–15) provide an excellent overview of the major reconstructive dilemmas involving the oral cavity. The philosophical dilemma that is almost always present is whether to perform a major, expensive, time-consuming reconstruction in a patient who is at a very high risk for recurrence of cancer. A positive accomplishment during the past 2 decades has been the improvement of reconstructive techniques that have allowed for more extensive tumor resection with wider margins. There is general concurrence that anterior mandibular defects should be reconstructed because of the esthetic and functional problems that accompany loss of the mandibular arch anteriorly.

The second article (Abstract 12–14) emphasizes the lingering unanswered questions regarding graft survival, bone resorption, bone fixation, and circulation within nonvascularized bone grafts. Obviously, the ability to reconstruct the mandible without using a vascularized graft would have many advantages. Unfortunately, the successes that have been reported in animal series and in some human series are rarely achieved by most of us.

The third article (Abstract 12–15) is a case report that provides excellent details on the reconstruction of a large defect involving the floor of the mouth, pharynx, and cervical esophagus. The authors have a strong preference for free jejunal transfer in this situation, and they present an excellent case to support their conclusions.—B.J. Bailey, M.D., F.A.C.S.

A Regional Approach to Reconstruction of the Upper Lip

Zitelli JA, Brodland DG (Pittsburgh)

J Dermatol Surg Oncol 17:143–148, 1991 12–16

Background.—In reconstruction of the upper lip, preservation of function and appearance is difficult. Lip reconstruction with local flaps was evaluated, and the type of repair within the various cosmetic subunits of the lip examined (Fig 12–14).

Methods.—Two hundred cases of upper lip defects were reviewed. For each defect, the location, size, depth, and type of closure was recorded. The cases were evaluated for trends in management.

Results.—In 20% of the cases, second-intention healing was chosen; it was limited to all superficial wounds or deeper wounds in the concave area. Grafts, most useful in defects on the philtrum, were chosen in 6% of cases. Skin flaps were the most useful repair, with local flaps accounting for 74% of cases. Advancement flaps were used in 80% of these

FLAPS FOR LIP RECONSTRUCTION

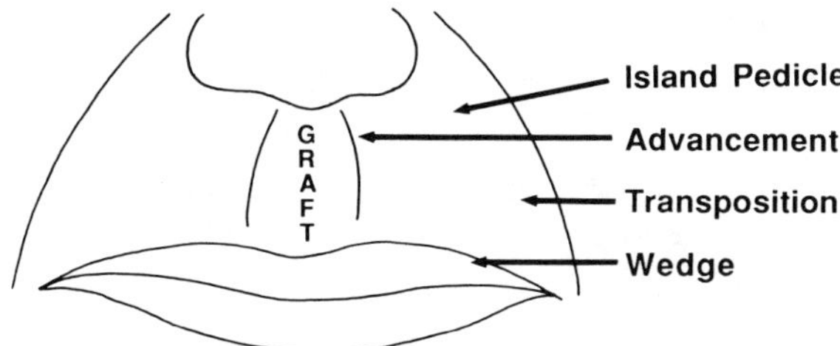

Fig 12–14.—Good cosmetic and functional results are predictable within different subunits of the upper lip when repaired with the methods illustrated in the text. (Courtesy of Zitelli JA, Brodland DG: *J Dermatol Surg Oncol* 17:143–148, 1991.)

cases, with tissue advanced horizontally from the lateral lip and cheek. A primary fusiform closure was the simplest form of advancement flap. For wounds less than 10 mm, the free margin was usually displaced only 1 or 2 mm, and it returned to normal within a few weeks. Extreme lengthening was a modification of the fusiform close, and wedge closure was used as a modification of the primary closure. Of the remaining flaps, 10% were transposition flaps and 10% were island-pedicle flaps. The transposition flaps were used to repair defects of the lateral lip near the commissure. The island-pedicle flap was especially useful for defects of the superior corner of the upper lip near the junction of the melolabial fold and ala. It was also used for large lesions near the midline involving both vermilion and skin.

Conclusions.—Most defects of the upper lip are repaired surgically using local flaps, especially variations of advancement flaps. The subunit location of the wound guides the choice of flap.

Propeller Flap for Reconstruction of the Tubercle of the Upper Lip

Yoshimura Y, Nakajima T, Yoneda K (Fujita Health Univ, Aichi, Japan)

Br J Plast Surg 44:113–116, 1991 12–17

Introduction.—Primary repair of the bilateral cleft lip commonly produces a whistling deformity of the upper lip that appears to be related to the tissue deficiency of the original prolabium.

Repair.—The upper lip tubercle may be reconstructed by designing 2 opposing transposition flaps, 1 on either side of the upper lip (Fig 12–15). Each flap is rotated 180 degrees. The resulting dog-ear formation near the pivot point of the flap helps add volume to the central part of the red lip.

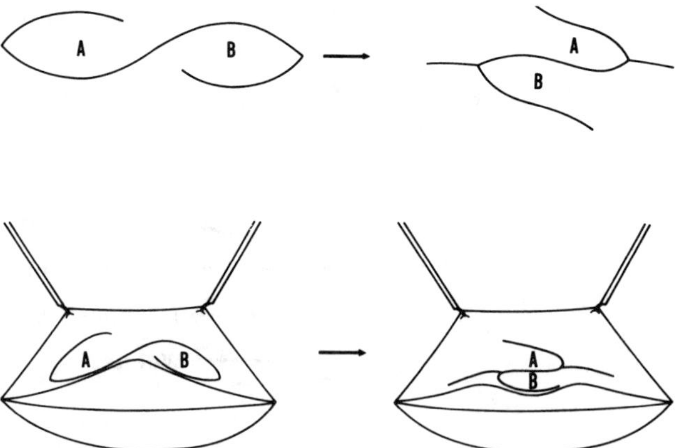

Fig 12–15.—Schematic drawings of the "propeller flap" procedure. (Courtesy of Yoshimura Y, Nakajima T, Yoneda K: *Br J Plast Surg* 44:113–116, 1991.)

Discussion.—The propeller flap technique takes advantage of the relative abundance of tissue in the lateral portions of the red lip. The proportion of the upper and lower lips is maintained. Ten patients who underwent this procedure had satisfactory results and no complications. In cases with a shallow oral vestibule, the propeller flap method may be combined with V-Y advancement.

▶ In the article by Zitelli and Brodland (Abstract 12–16), the authors describe the tendency of the upper lip to be prone to postoperative complications. They list hematoma, infection, hypertrophic scar, increased wound contracture, and other complications as being more likely to occur in the upper lip than in the lower lip. They proceed to provide a rational system for reconstruction based on the site and depth of the defect, and they provide a few, relatively short-term, illustrative cases. It would be of great interest to have them study a more extensive series with longer follow-up to substantiate the conclusions they present in this article.

Yoshimura et al. (Abstract 12–17) describe the use of a propeller flap for reconstruction of a tubercle in the mid portion of the upper lip. This might be necessary after trauma, tumor excision, or cleft lip repair. The technique of creating 2 propeller-shaped flaps and then rotating them to the midline provides bulk and creates a central lip tubercle by creating intentional dog-ear defects at the midpoint of the upper lip. Although the technique is intriguing, one wonders if the same result might be achieved using bilateral V-Y advancement flaps.—B.J. Bailey, M.D., F.A.C.S.

Tracheal Stenosis: A Study of 100 Cases

Maggi G, Ardissone F, Cavallo A, Oliaro A, Scappaticci E, Giobbe R (Univ of Turin, Italy)

Int Surg 75:225–230, 1990 12–18

Background.—The effectiveness of various treatments of tracheal stenosis was determined. Thirty-four neoplastic and 66 nonneoplastic tracheal stenoses were reviewed at the University of Turin from 1959 to 1989.

Methods.—The causes of the 66 nonneoplastic stenoses were varied (table); 58 were located at the cervical level and 8 were at the thoracic level. Before 1974, 6 patients were fitted with rigid prostheses. Later, 12 were treated using silicone T-tube stents. Circumferential resection with end-to-end anastomosis was performed on 28 patients. Of the 34 neoplastic stenoses, 2 squamous epithelium carcinomas were inoperable and 8 underwent endoscopic resection and radiotherapy. Two were treated by circumferential resection with end-to-end anastomosis. One patient with cystic adenoid carcinoma underwent laryngectomy and cervical resection of the trachea with definitive tracheotomy; 3 underwent circumferential resection with end-to-end anastomosis; 2 underwent circumfer-

Causes of 66 Nonneoplastic Stenoses

Post-intubation	32	(48.8%)
Post-tracheotomy	21	(31.8%)
Malacia	4	(19.8%)
Tuberculosis	3	
Post-surgical	2	
Trauma	1	
Post X-ray therapy	1	
Osteoplastic tracheotomy	1	
Idiopathic chronic tracheitis	1	

(Courtesy of Maggi G, Ardissone F, Cavillo A, et al: *Int Surg* 75:225–230, 1990.)

ential resection and definitive tracheotomy; and 3 underwent wedge resection. Benign neoplastic lesions were treated with simple endoscopic resection in 5 cases and wedge resection in 1 case. One patient with sarcomatous-type lesions, 1 with a metastatic lesion, and 5 with thyroid carcinoma were treated by definitive tracheotomy and complementary therapy.

Results.—The results were good in 81% of the resections for nonneoplastic stenoses. One patient who underwent resection for adenoid cystic carcinoma died after 2 years with metastases; the other 2 were alive after 10 years. Two patients who received tracheal resection for epidermoid carcinomas died after 3 and 4 years with metasteses. Use of T-tube treatment for inflammatory tracheal stenosis was satisfactory in only a third of the cases.

Conclusions.—The trachea is a high-risk area for surgery. Preoperative study and preparation are critical in obtaining favorable end results, and the surgical technique must be extremely precise. It can be concluded that the complex back-up needs of tracheal surgery make it advisable to seek out the few centers that offer the best possible chances for patients requiring such procedures.

Experimental Studies on an Artificial Trachea of Collagen-Coated Poly(L-Lactic Acid) Mesh or Unwoven Cloth Combined With a Periosteal Graft

Ike O, Shimizu Y, Okada T, Ikada Y, Hitomi S (Kyoto Univ, Japan)
ASAIO Transactions 37:24–26, 1991 12–19

Background.—Infection and air leakage are the major problems occurring in the early postoperative period after tracheal replacement using a prosthesis. The design and use of a new kind of artificial trachea composed of biodegradable materials such as poly(L-lactic acid) mesh or unwoven cloth coated with collagen were evaluated. This type of trachea allowed for reconstruction of the respiratory airway by self-regeneration without retaining the prosthesis at the replacement site, thereby reducing the incidence of infection in an animal model.

Materials.—The artificial trachea was made from a mesh or unwoven cloth composed of poly(L-lactic acid) with an average molecular weight of 86,000 daltons. The mesh was coated with dry collagen that had been, enzymatically extracted from pig skin and purified so that it was more than 90% pure collagen. These materials were then sutured into a tubular shape for use.

Methods.—Male rabbits (body weight range, 1,600–3,600 g) underwent 3 types of surgery: group A animals had a piece of periosteum sutured around the cervical trachea of the same rabbit; group B animals had a window-shaped defect in the cervical trachea patched using autologous periosteum; and group C animals had the artificial trachea sized to fit in place of the cervical trachea, with the natural trachea introduced into the artificial trachea and the artificial trachea sutured around this site.

Findings.—No infections occurred in groups A and B, and no air leakages were observed in groups B and C. The group A animals demonstrated ossification of the grafted periosteum at 3 weeks postimplantation. Group B animals showed a well-epithelized (by ciliated columnar epithelium similar to respiratory mucosa) internal surface of the cervical trachea at 2 weeks postsurgery. The group C rabbits had cartilage produced around the artificial trachea from the grafted periosteum but no ossification or epithelization. When unwoven cloth was used, all animals died of pneumonitis related to material collapse within 11 days of implantation.

Conclusions.—These findings suggest that formation of bone rings around the trachea can be expected using this material and technique. They also indicate that this procedure can be a useful surgical treatment for tracheomalacia or bronchomalacia.

▶ These 2 studies (Abstracts 12–18 and 12–19) reflect the continuing international interest in reconstructive techniques that can improve the success rate for correcting tracheal stenosis. The study from Italy (Abstract 12–18) emphasizes the importance of allowing tracheal lesions to mature before undertaking reconstruction; it also emphasizes the important role played by long-term stenting in these patients. The article from Japan (Abstract 12–19) describes several attempts to use an artificial trachea of collagen-coated poly mesh with periosteal grafts. Although long-term success was not possible in this study, the ability to achieve ossification outside a tracheal prosthesis would be a major step in achieving tracheal support.—B.J. Bailey, M.D., F.A.C.S.

The Use of Periosteal Flaps in Scalp and Forehead Reconstruction

Terranova W (Med Univ of South Carolina, Charleston)

Ann Plast Surg 25:450–456, 1990 12–20

Background.—Flaps of periosteum or pericranium can be raised successfully for scalp and forehead reconstruction. This technique was used in 8 patients with small to moderate scalp and forehead defects with exposed bone.

Patients.—Of the patients, 4 had excision of squamous cell carcinoma, 3 had removal of basal cell carcinoma, and 1 had a scalp avulsion injury. There was a history of severe arteriosclerotic cardiovascular disease in 3 patients, and 3 others were heavy smokers.

Case 1.—Man, 55, had insulin-dependent diabetes mellitus and multiple facial skin cancers that were removed. The glabellar defect resulting from the removal of a recurrent basal cell carcinoma was repaired using a flap of periosteum centered over the contralateral supraorbital and supratrochlear vessels covering the bone (Fig 12–16). The patient had minimal contour deformity and no displacement of the eyebrows.

Case 2.—Man, 70, had severe arteriosclerotic cardiovascular disease and then an infiltrating squamous cell carcinoma developed with perineural invasion. After surgical removal of the carcinoma, the patient had a 7-cm defect that was repaired using 2 periosteal flaps (Fig 12–17). The repair site had good color match, acceptable contour, and no disturbance of the hair line 4 months after surgery.

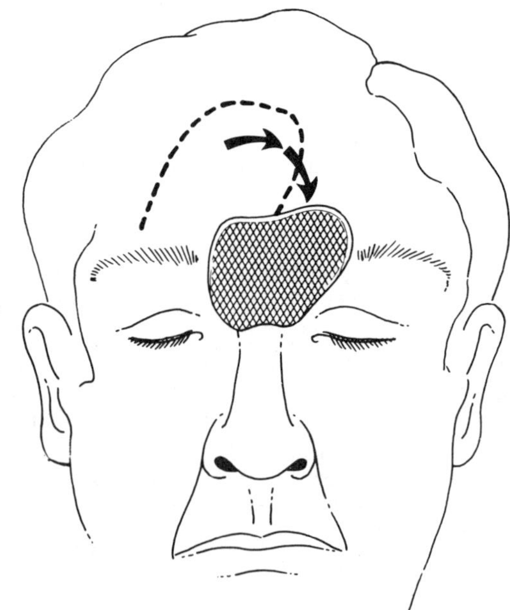

Fig 12–16.—A 3 × 4-cm flap of periosteum was transposed to cover the exposed bone of a glabellar defect. (Courtesy of Terranova W: *Ann Plast Surg* 25:450–456, 1990.)

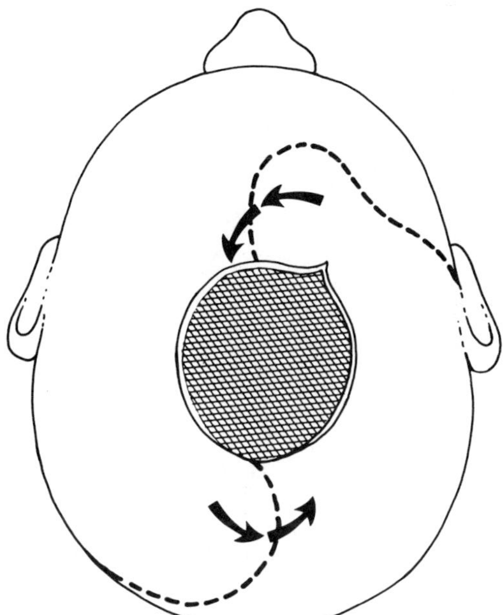

Fig 12–17.—A, a 7-cm diameter defect, with bone exposed, resulted after frozen-section controlled excision (nose is in upper right corner). **B,** bilateral 7 × 12-cm transposition flaps of periosteum covered the exposed bone. (Courtesy of Terranova W: *Ann Plast Surg* 25:450–456, 1990.)

Results.—No patient demonstrated any breakdown during the follow-up period. Although mild contour deformity did occur, the cosmetic results were acceptable because of appropriate color match and no need for additional incisions. They were also acceptable because anatomical landmarks, such as the eyebrows and the hairline, were not altered.

Conclusion.—Periosteal flaps work well enough in skin grafting to cover exposed bone. Although there are other options to repair these defects, periosteal flaps have the advantages of a variety of acceptable positioning (anterior, anterolateral, and posterolateral), easy and rapid dissection, and minimal blood loss.

Recontouring of the Lateral Forehead Using the Temporalis Muscle

Hallock GG (Allentown Hosp; Lehigh Valley Hosp Ctr, Allentown, Penn)

Ann Plast Surg 27:21–26, 1991 12–21

Background.—An obvious forehead depression often develops posterior or superior to the lateral orbital rim after lateral upper or midface blunt trauma. Recontouring of the lateral forehead using the temporalis muscle was assessed.

Procedure.—The temporalis muscle is a type III muscle with a dominant blood supply from the anterior and posterior deep temporal branches of the internal maxillary artery (Fig 12–18). The surgeon uses existing scars or a preauricular incision extending vertically onto the scalp to visualize the superficial temporal

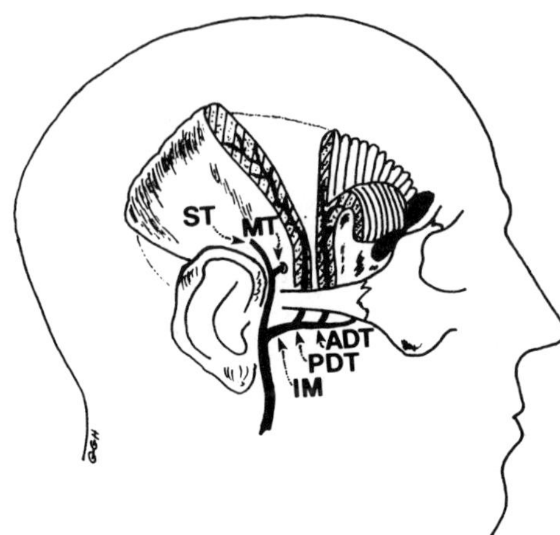

Fig 12–18.—*Abbreviations: ST,* superficial temporal; *MT,* middle temporal; *IM,* internal maxillary; *PDT,* posterior deep temporal; *ADT,* anterior deep temporal arteries. Pertinent vascular anatomy of the temporalis muscle. Temporalis muscle may be split in the coronal plane (as demonstrated by elevation of the posterior lobe) or sagittally between the deep and superficial origins (as depicted in anterior portion). The *shaded area* represents the forehead defect to be recontoured. (Courtesy of Hallock GG: *Ann Plast Surg* 27:21–26, 1991.)

vessels and fascia. If the temporoparietal fascia flap is intact, then it will suffice to fill most lateral forehead depressions. However, if it is not intact, the deep temporal fascia is entered starting posteriorly along the superior temporal line. When the muscle appears reasonable, the surgeon elevates only the portion needed for advancement. Subperiosteal dissection is done to protect the deep arteries and nerves. Conspicuous hollows in the temporal fossa are minimized by advancing the entire muscle forward, only the posterior part, or a sagittal split. Proper muscle insetting is achieved through percutaneous pullout sutures anterior to the perimeter of the defect.

Conclusions.—For patients with contour deformities of the lateral forehead, transposition of noncutaneous local vascularized autogenous tissues is associated with few risks and minimal donor-site morbidity. If the temporoparietal fascia is not available for this procedure, then the temporalis muscle itself is an excellent option.

▶ These 2 studies (Abstracts 12–20 and 12–21) deal with forehead reconstructive techniques and the use of local tissue in specific types of repair. The paper by Terranova (Abstract 12–20) documents the usefulness of periosteum/pericranium in the reconstruction of forehead cranial defects and in covering exposed bone. This step is important to prevent osteomyelitis or local bone necrosis, and it is often vital in the prevention of postoperative infection and CSF leak.

The paper by Hallock (Abstract 12–21) stresses the utility and durability of the temporalis muscle in the reconstruction of lateral forehead defects. Forward rotation of the temporalis muscle is facilitated by its anatomical configuration (a broad expansive muscle that narrows down to a vascular base anteriorly and inferiorly). When appropriate, this technique provides reliable, single-stage reconstruction.—B.J. Bailey, M.D., F.A.C.S.

Gold Weight Lid Load as a Secondary Procedure

Liu D (Henry Ford Hosp, Detroit)
Plast Reconstr Surg 87:854–860, 1991 12–22

Background.—The use of the gold weight lid load was evaluated in the treatment of a paralyzed eyelid. Because the gold implant procedure is simple to perform, the technique is recommended to correct a variety of different types of eyelid problems (Fig 12–19). Three cases of gold weight lid load implants were reviewed.

Case 1.—Woman, 32, had a post right acoustic neuroma resection that led to a lateral tarsorrhaphy of the right eye in 1983. In 1989, after 2 other recommendations for gold implant procedures, the patient underwent an opening of the tarsorrhaphy and the placement of a 1.4-g implant to obtain the desired results. The patient continues to use a Lacrisert.

Case 2.—Woman, 44, underwent excision of a left acoustic neuroma and insertion of a silicone encircling band. Six months later, the band eroded via the conjunctiva. This was removed, requiring the patient to undergo a Gunderson flap and a lateral tarsorrhaphy that produced unacceptable eye appearance. After tarsorrhaphy release, 2.2 g of gold were implanted to completely close the left eye.

Case 3.—Woman, 52, had an acoustic neuroma removed from her right eye; this procedure was followed by a tarsorrhaphy. After release of the tarsorrhaphy, a 1.6-g weight was implanted to achieve a normal, acceptable appearance.

Conclusions.—The outcomes of the gold weight implant technique in these 3 patients suggest that more than 1 gold implant may be necessary to obtain the desired results in specific cases. The gold weight lid implant provides protection of the cornea by achieving complete lid clo-

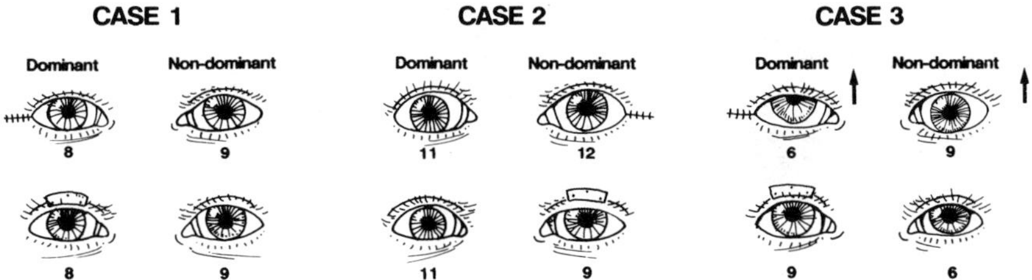

Fig 12–19.—Preoperative palpebral fissures (with tarsorrhaphy or silicone band intact) (**upper row**). Postoperative palpebral fissures (with gold implant) (**lower row**). By Hering's law of equal innervation, there is additional innervation to both upper eyelids when the vision in the dominant eye is interfered with by the eyelid. A postoperative drop of the fellow eye is anticipated. (Courtesy of Liu D: *Plast Reconstr Surg* 87:854–860, 1991.)

sure and simulating blink without causing a functional or cosmetic ptosis. Very little additional effort is required to achieve these beneficial results.

Lower Eyelid Repair Utilising Triangular Skin Flaps With Subcutaneous Pedicles

Destro MWB, da Silva AL, Speranzini MB (Univ of Minas Gerais Med School, Univ of Taubaté, São Paulo, Brazil)

Br J Plast Surg 44:363–367, 1991 12–23

Background.—The use of triangular skin flaps with a central subcutaneous pedicle for the repair of small facial lesions is a simple technique that yields good results. A series of patients underwent surgery for lesions of the lower lid. The lesions were repaired by a triangular flap with a subcutaneous pedicle with or without a chondromucosal graft of nasal septum.

Methods.—A group of 54 patients underwent 55 procedures. The lower lid defect was reconstructed with a triangular flap alone in 39 cases. In 16 cases, a chondromucosal graft of the nasal septum was done along with the triangular flap procedure (Fig 12–20).

Results.—The results were good in 94.5% of the repairs, satisfactory in 3.6%, and poor in 1 case. The lower lid could be repaired in all cases.

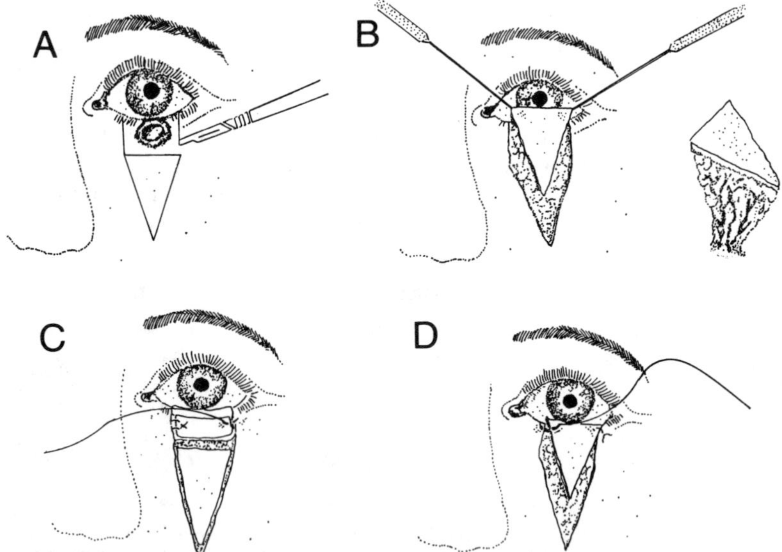

Fig 12–20.—A, excision of the lesion and outline of the triangular flap. **B,** advancement of the sliding flap. **C,** suture of the chondromucosal graft. **D,** suture of the triangular flap. (Courtesy of Destro MWB, da Silva AL, Speranzini MB: *Br J Plast Surg* 44:363-367, 1991.)

The complications related to lid function included edema in 10 cases during the immediate postoperative period. During the late postoperative period, slight ectropion occurred in 3 cases, epiphora in 2, moderate ectropion in 1, and reduction of the lid margin in 1. The lower lid complications were cosmetic in 4 cases, resulted from the neoplastic defect in 4, and resulted from the donor area of the chondromucosal graft in 1. Function was restored completely in all but 1 patient because of ectropion that resulted from partial loss of the chondromucosal graft caused by infection.

Conclusions.—This technique is feasible for the simplest to the most complex repairs in different areas of the lower lid. The procedure can be done using local anesthesia, and the use of the triangular flap with flaps from other facial areas enables repairs of larger regions.

▶ These 2 articles (Abstracts 12–22 and 12–23) provide an excellent update of the specific approaches to eyelid rehabilitation that we encounter in practice. Abstract 12–22 deals with facial paralysis and emphasizes the value of gold weight procedures in eye protection. When everything goes well, the gold weight lid load procedures result in the patient having the ability to close the eye at will, the eye closing during sleep, and the restoration of the ability to blink (with only a minimal ptosis from the weight). We have found that this approach provides excellent cosmesis and lid function. When other measures have failed and eye protection is suboptimal, this is a very good option.

Abstract 12–23 deals with the reconstruction of a lid defect, and the authors report excellent results using a triangular advancement flap that is moved into a rectangular lower lid defect in a V-Y repair. This technique is simple and can be performed with the patient under local anesthesia. We agree with the authors that this approach is preferable to using upper lid tissue, and that it provides a stable eyelid margin with a good match of skin color and texture.—B.J. Bailey, M.D., F.A.C.S.

The Use of Tissue Expansion in Nasal Reconstruction

Reifen E, Freeman JL (Mount Sinai Hosp, Toronto; Univ of Toronto)

J Otolaryngol 20:5–9, 1991 12–24

Introduction.—The forehead flap may not provide adequate tissue for nasal reconstruction, and an unsightly donor site deformity remains. Tissue expansion can be used to gain large flaps for large defects. The technique and 3 cases were reviewed.

Technique.—In the first stage of reconstruction, a large expander (usually a 250–300 cc expander) is placed through a coronal incision posterior to the hairline. When the coronal incision has healed, subsequent expansion is continued at weekly intervals for 3–6 weeks, as needed. In the second stage of reconstruction the expander is removed and advanced into the defect.

Results.—In 1 patient with recurrent basal cell carcinoma of the nasal dorsum, a midline glabellar flap was designed with satisfactory result. Another patient underwent both partial rhinectomy for carcinoma of the tip of the nose and insertion of an expander in the first stage. A midline glabellar flap was used with acceptable result; however, necrosis of the tip caused some columellar retraction. Sufficient tissue expansion was achieved in both patients during a 5-week period. A third patient had resection of a malignant fibrohistiocytoma of the left nasal cavity and insertion of the expander in the first stage. The midline glabellar flap was used for lining, a Converse scalping flap was used for coverage, and the expanded forehead skin was mobilized medially to close the midline defect. Recovery was complicated by infection.

Conclusion.—Tissue expansion seems to offer reasonable solutions for the problems of nasal reconstruction. It provides extra flap length, offers better flap survival, and allows for better donor site closure. Its disadvantages include the prolonged reconstruction period, the temporary forehead deformity, and the poor result when used for total nasal reconstruction because of contraction and distortion of the nasal shape.

Immediate Versus Chronic Tissue Expansion

Machida BK, Liu-Shindo M, Sasaki GH, Rice DH, Chandrasoma P (Los Angeles County/Univ of Southern California Med Ctr, Huntington Mem Hosp, Pasadena, Calif)

Ann Plast Surg 26:227–232, 1991 12–25

Introduction.—Tissue expansion, which was developed more than 30 years ago, has become a useful procedure in reconstructive surgery. However, functional and cosmetic deformities are associated with buried expanders and remote valves. Load cycling is a method of incrementally elongating skin immediately without the use of expanders. Another immediate expansion technique, intraoperative expansion, is an outgrowth of the principles used in the 2 previous methods. These 3 techniques were compared.

Methods.—The gain in surface area, increase in arc length of the flap, flap viability, and histological changes associated with each technique were studied in a guinea pig model.

Observations.—The group that underwent chronic expansion, which included booster and nonbooster expansions, had a 137% increase in surface area (or a 52% increase in the arc length of the flap). Intraoperative expansion produced a 31% increase in surface area (or a 15% increase in the arc length of the flap). An almost negligible amount of skin increase was observed in the load-cycled group. Immediate postexpansion stretchback was associated with all 3 methods. Despite the elevated pressures that occurred during expansion, flap viability was not hindered by any of the techniques.

Conclusion.—Chronic tissue expansion still produces the greatest amount of skin increase, compared with other techniques. Intraoperative expansion is effective mainly in limited expansions of small defects.

► Nasal reconstruction is often extremely challenging because of the need for a large amount of skin and the constraints regarding donor site scarring and deformity (see Abstract 12–24). The precise midline forehead flap, although useful for small defects, may be deficient for the repair of an extensive nasal deformity. Tissue expansion provides a workable solution to many of these problems; however, there are drawbacks in the form of appearance when the expander is in place, including expander migration, hematoma, infection, and skin necrosis. In spite of these problems, expansion is quite useful in many cases because it provides more skin and a higher survival rate (because of the delay) while limiting the cosmetic deformity.

Study of immediate/intraoperative tissue expansion has not yet determined whether the increased surface area and arch of rotation are "apparent" or "real" (Abstract 12–25). Stretchback has been shown to return expanded tissue virtually back to its original dimensions very rapidly. This seems to be a greater disadvantage than was initially described.—B.J. Bailey, M.D., F.A.C.S.

Transplantation of Purified Autologous Fat: A 3-Year Follow-up Is Disappointing

Ersek RA (Southwest Texas State Univ)

Plast Reconstr Surg 87:219–227, 1991 12–26

Introduction.—Although transplantation of autologous fat has been attempted previously, it has recently received attention because of the refinements in liposuction technique. The results of transplantation of autologous fat were reviewed.

Methods.—While patients were under local anesthesia with sedation, fat was harvested from convenient areas, rinsed, and purified. It was then reused in 3 patients. The fat was used to raise acne pits in 1 patient; to correct a scar depression on the anterior calf in another; and to correct burn scar depressions on the forehead in a third patient. All patients were informed of the experimental nature of the procedure.

Results.—Good immediate results were seen in all 3 patients; however, these were short lived. Although injections were repeated in 2 patients, the depressions reappeared after 3 years in 1 and after 1 year in another. Both patients insisted that there was an improvement when compared with the presurgical condition.

Conclusion.—Of 41 patients surveyed, 15 responses were received, and only 3 patients were satisfied with their results. They were never charged for the procedure or the postoperative visits, and there were no postoperative complications. It was concluded that very little, if any, autologous fat survives in a new environment. This substance does not fulfill the criteria required of an inexpensive, nonallergic, injectable bulking material used in reconstructive surgery.

▶ The idea of transplanting autologous fat is certainly intriguing, and there is an acute need for a reliable means of filling defects of all sizes. The authors suggest that approximately 10% of the fat cells injected into acne pits survive for more than 2 years. The temporary nature of the improvement obtained by autologous fat transplantation continues to be a major obstacle to the general acceptance of this technique by reconstructive surgeons.—B.J. Bailey, M.D., F.A.C.S.

Team Approach to Total Auricular Reconstruction

Kesselring UK, de Goumoens R (Centre de Chirurgie Plastique, Lausanne, Switzerland)

Ann Plast Surg 26:299–305, 1991 12–27

Background.—Reconstructive ear surgery is a challenging procedure that requires precise planning and consideration of the patient's individuality. If surgery of the middle ear will improve the patient's hearing, reconstructive surgery is coordinated with intervention in the middle ear during the second session of reconstruction. Total auricular reconstruction was undertaken using a team approach.

Technique.—The procedure is usually begun between the ages of 7 and 10 years. Cartilage is harvested from the contralateral thorax side (using the seventh

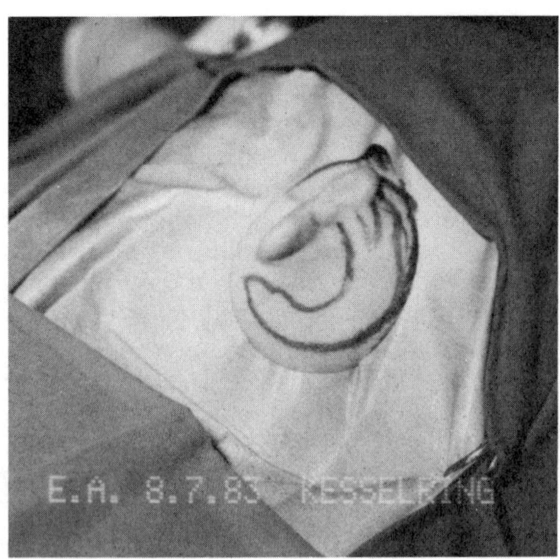

Fig 12–21.—The receiving pocket is created as superficially as possible and follows, in its circumference, the outline of the prepared implant. (Courtesy of Kesselring UK, de Goumoens R: *Ann Plast Surg* 26:299-305, 1991.)

and eighth rib), and a film template or cast from the normal ear is essential. Without endangering the cutaneous vascularization, the receiving skin is created as superficially as possible (Fig 12–21). Thinner skin will cling better to the cartilage mold. A small vacuum drain, left for at least 48 hours, accentuates the contours. Petrolatum gauze is packed gently into the convolutions; this, along with a lightly compressing cotton dressing, immobilizes the graft. In the second session, the retroauricular area is generously undermined and a crescent-shaped area of the mastoid is denuded to give access to the ear, nose, and throat surgeon. An external auditory canal is drilled from the mastoid and the ossiculoplasty is performed. At the same time, the plastic surgeon harvests the full-thickness skin graft in the inguinal region. The retroauricular area is grafted with 2 separate halves; the graft is harvested generously to provide a small portion for the lining of the auditory canal. Nonabsorbable sutures are used, except in the crease (where resorbable material is used). To prevent stenosis, the linear auditory canal graft is cut to join in a Z-like imbrication. The graft is glued to the bone, the meatus is packed with antibiotic-soaked cotton, and the retroauricular grafts are packed with iodine gauze. A third session, consisting of various refinements and touch-ups, is often done using local anesthesia.

Conclusions.—Simultaneous performance of middle ear surgery during the second session is an optimal procedure for total auricular reconstruction. It allows the plastic surgeon to work with unscarred tissue and provides unobstructed access for the ear, nose, and throat surgeon.

▶ The authors provide an excellent description of a 3-stage technique for total auricular reconstruction. Appropriately, they pay tribute to the accomplishments of Burt Brent, whose work during the past 2 decades has set the standards for total auricular reconstruction.—B.J. Bailey, M.D., F.A.C.S.

The Tongue Flap: Placement and Fixation for Closure of Postpalatoplasty Fistulae

Argamaso RV (Albert Einstein College of Medicine)
Cleft Palate J 27:402–410, 1990 12–28

Introduction.—Oronasal fistulas may affect 21% to 22% of all patients who undergo cleft palate repair. Surgeons have used the lingual flaps as a convenient and effective method for obliterating both large and small palatal fistulas. Tongue flaps were used in 6 patients with fistulas resulting from cleft palate surgery.

Technique.—After anesthesia via a nasoendotracheal tube, the patient's head is positioned in hyperextension and the palate is fully exposed. The mucoperiosteum is elevated toward the fistula and reflected from the hard palate to view the entire defect. A transverse incision on the palatal flap proximal to the rim of the fistula creates a sling for the suspension of the tongue pedicle. A bite block is used instead of the Dingman mouth gag to manage the tongue flap. A suture is

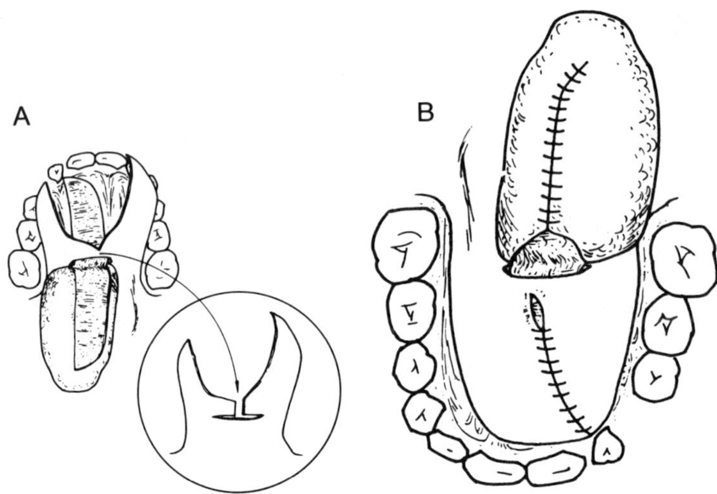

Fig 12–22.—A, palatal flaps have been elevated, and tongue flap has been passed above sling and occupies its position on nasal side. Inset depicts division of sling, if necessary, to accommodate pedicle. **B,** closure of tongue donor site and midline approximation of palatal flaps (closure is incomplete). (Courtesy of Argamaso RV: *Cleft Palate J* 27:402–410, 1990.)

placed at the distal end of the tongue flap and pulled through to lead it over the sling to the fistula. Each half of the sling is draped under and sutured to the underside of the pedicle (Fig 12–22). The nasal mucosa may become attenuated; however, as long as the tongue flap covers the nasal side, this defect will heal in 2 to 3 weeks. Only fluids can be taken by mouth for the first week, followed by a soft diet until regular food can be eaten. The next stage, the transection and inset of the pedicle, occurs between the second and third postoperative week. The bite block is again used. An incision is made at the entry site of the pedicle into the palate to allow the proximal stump to be enclosed.

Findings.—The operative sites on both the palate and the tongue should heal by the third or fourth week. The slight narrowing of the tongue that follows gradually improves over time. Six consecutive patients had palotoplasties performed elsewhere and were seen as late referrals or "salvage cases". All 6 had complete fistula closure and appeared well at follow-up as much as 2 years later. The inhospital stay averaged 2½ days for the first stage of the procedure and a half day for the second stage.

Conclusions.—Patients have had a favorable response to this operative procedure. Medical team members, including those involved with dental restoration and speech rehabilitation, also approved of the functional and aesthetic results achieved by this technique.

▶ Although this technique has been described in regard to cleft palate fistulas after cleft palate repair, it is also a useful option for repairing the palate after cancer excision or trauma. The general concept of using the remaining posterior rim of the palatal mucosa as a sling is very important. This step appears to add significantly to the success rate of the procedure by overcoming the tendency of the flap to pull away.—B.J. Bailey, M.D., F.A.C.S.

13 Facial Plastic Surgery

The Extended Subperiosteal Face Lift: A Definitive Soft-Tissue Remodeling for Facial Rejuvenation

Ramirez OM, Maillard GF, Musolas A (Johns Hopkins Univ, Baltimore; Lausanne Univ, Switzerland; Hosp Gen Manual Gea Gonzales, Mexico City)

Plast Reconstr Surg 88:227–238, 1991 13–1

Background.—Psillakis' subperiosteal face lift has been criticized for not producing more dramatic improvements than conventional brow and face lift procedures. This approach has also been associated with a significantly high incidence of nerve damage. Anatomical findings and surgical modifications that significantly improved both the safety and the clinical results of the subperiosteal face lift were reviewed.

Technique.—Extensive interconnected subperiosteal dissection that included the entire zygomatic arc was used (Fig 13–1). This permitted

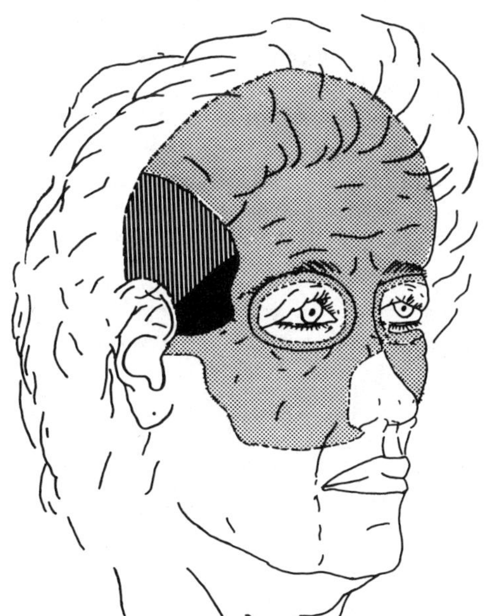

Fig 13–1.—The different areas of the extensive subperiosteal dissection are interconnected. This includes the entire zygomatic arch and part of the periorbita. Laterally, observe the dissection deep to the temporal fascia. (Courtesy of Ramirez OM, Maillard GF, Musolas A: *Plast Reconstr Surg* 88:227–238, 1991.)

better repositioning of the deep soft tissues of the entire upper face, most of the midface, and, indirectly, key structures of the lower face. The upward pull of the muscles of the cheek and mouth produced an elevation of the corner of the mouth that positively affected the smiling mechanism, oral frowning, and the jowls. Dissection deep to both layers of the temporal fascia reduced the risk of injury to the frontalis nerve. The temporal fascia was used as a lifter and an anchoring element of the entire cheek-perioral soft tissues rather than the periorbital fibrofatty tissues, thereby reducing the risk of damage to the frontal and zygomatic branches of the facial nerve.

Results.—These modifications, which were used in 28 patients, produced a high rate of patient satisfaction. There were no complications with regard to nerve injury. In an earlier series of 60 patients, in whom the Psillakis or Tessier approach was used, the nerve damage rates were 11 percent and 20 percent, respectively.

Conclusions.—In some cases, the subperiosteal face lift compares favorably to other techniques, because it is not as difficult or unsafe as had been believed.

▶ In his comment on this article, Dr. Ortiz-Monasterio points out that the search for better and longer lasting results in facial rejuvenation has presented a fascinating problem to the plastic surgeon. This particular article emphasizes 2 main points: (1) the anatomical relationship of the frontalis branch of the facial nerve and (2) the quality of the results that can be achieved using this technique. This is a formidable surgical procedure, and it should not be performed by the inexperienced facial surgeon. Neither is it indicated in all patients. The key issue of whether the results achieved are superior or more lasting than those that can be accomplished with other techniques is not answered by this particular paper. Long-term follow-up in larger numbers of patients is needed.—B.J. Bailey, M.D., F.A.C.S.

How to Obtain Symmetry in a Unilaterally Cleft Nose: A New Technique

Gubisch W (Stuttgart, Germany)
Eur J Plast Surg 13:241–246, 1990 13–2

Deformity.—Asymmetry of the nasal vestibules is the most conspicuous feature of the unilateral cleft nose. The alar cartilage on the cleft side is usually distorted and displaced, causing the appearance of a sunken overhanging nasal ala. The dome is flattened and lowered, and the nostril sill is often deficient. Internally, the anterior border of the cartilaginous septum is subluxed to the noncleft side. In addition, the septum is always dislocated toward the cleft side, and the lower concha on the noncleft side is always hypertrophied.

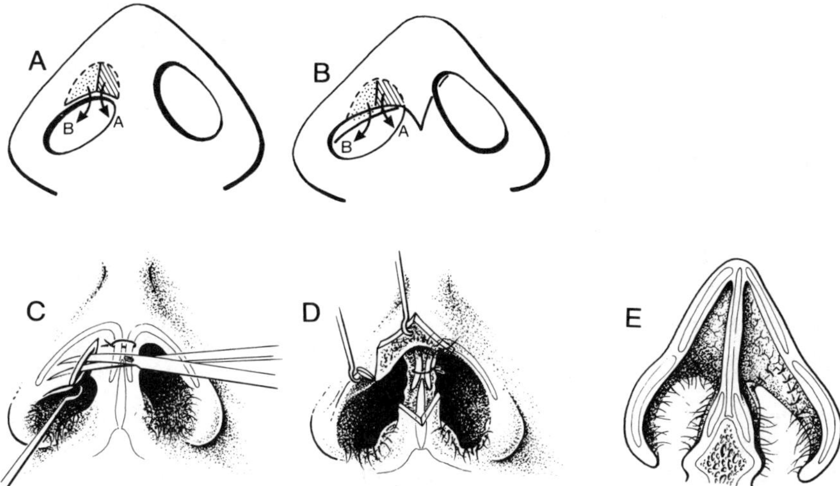

Fig 13–2.—The technique of ala correction by a closed (**A**) or open approach (**B**). *A,* columella pedicled flap for lengthening of the columella; *B,* ala pedicled flap for lifting the free margin of the ala wing to the height of the opposite side. The redundant skin of the vestibule will become trimmed. *Dashed line* indicates incision for open approach. **C–E,** the sutured flaps from an endonasal view. (Courtesy of Gubisch W: *Eur J Plast Surg* 13:241–246, 1990.)

Techniques.—The first step in correcting cleft node deformity is an alveolar bone graft. After the entire deformed septum is removed, the deformed cartilaginous part is straightened by means of a scratch cut. The reconstructed septum is then replanted between the mucosal leaves. A submucous resection of the inferior turbinate on the noncleft side can reduce the concha without affecting the mucosa. The nasal tip is then corrected, and the overhanging alar cartilage is shortened near the front edge. A cartilage graft is often desirable to optimize the projection of the nasal tip. A rotation flap pedicled on the columella and a second pedicled inversion flap on the alar edge can provide a symmetrical nasal vestibule (Fig 13–2). Any resulting gap between the 2 flaps may be covered by the surplus vestibular skin. The silicone foils provide a splint for the desired alar position and prevent hematoma formation.

Discussion.—This technique produces a natural rounding that is cosmetically optimal. Good results have been achieved in 118 patients.

▶ The fact that there are so many techniques for correcting cleft palate nasal deformities supports the conclusion that this is a complex problem and that no single procedure is universally applicable or superior. The type of operation performed is controversial, and there is an equivalent amount of controversy regarding the timing of these procedures. Some have advocated repairing the alar deformity at the time of the primary procedure in an attempt to avoid developmental deformities during childhood. The authors prefer to delay the nasal repair until much later, and they show illustrative cases involving young adults. We share their enthusiasm for utilizing the open reconstructive approach and agree with their emphasis on septal deformity correction as 1 of the keys to a satisfactory result.—B.J. Bailey, M.D., F.A.C.S.

The Effect of Carbon Dioxide Laser Surgery on the Recurrence of Keloids

Norris JEC (St Luke's/Roosevelt Hosp Ctr, New York)
Plast Reconstr Surg 87:44–53, 1991 13–3

Background.—Seven males and 16 females (age range, 5–72 years) who were treated with carbon dioxide laser excision of keloids from 1984 to 1987 were studied retrospectively.

Patients.—A total of 37 keloids was found in 29 anatomic sites; they ranged in size from 1 to 30 cm in diameter. Twelve patients had undergone previous surgery, and only 1 had undergone radiation therapy. Steroids were used intraoperatively in 10 patients. Most of the wounds were permitted to heal by secondary intention; they healed in 3½–14 weeks. The wounds on the earlobes, abdomen, and neck healed faster than those on flat surfaces such as the sternum, back, and upper arm.

Results.—One patient, who received intraoperative steroids, experienced no recurrence. Nine patients experienced keloid recurrence suppressed with steroids. Five patients who were treated with intraoperative steroids and 7 who were not treated in this manner experienced failure of the carbon dioxide laser treatment.

Discussion.—Carbon dioxide laser excision alone fails to suppress keloid growth or recurrence. Although laser excision of a keloid temporarily retards collagen synthesis, it must be supplemented by repeated laser impaction or by frequent steroid injections.

► Argon and carbon dioxide laser treatment of hypertrophic and keloid scars has been proposed since the late 70s. Recently, we have had the opportunity to learn of Dr. Fred Stucker's success with and enthusiasm for carbon dioxide laser treatment in the management of keloid scars. We have used this technique in a series of patients at the University of Texas Medical Branch, and our results have been very encouraging. We agree with the author of this paper that either repeated laser treatments or long-term steroid injections are necessary to prevent keloid occurrence in many of these patients.—B.J. Bailey, M.D., F.A.C.S.

Comparative Study of Dermabrasion, Phenol Peel, and Acetic Acid Peel

Ersek RA (San Marcos, Tex)
Aesthetic Plast Surg 15:241–243, 1991 13–4

Background.—The phenol chemical peel can be very beneficial in the treatment of pigmented lesions and fine facial wrinkles. Various concentrations of acetic acid achieve essentially the same result. Dermabrasion has long been used to remove skin blemishes, fine wrinkles, and scars. These modalities were compared for superficial surface surgery of the skin.

Methods.—The patient was a 36-year-old woman with a benign congenital blue nevus of the skin. Six areas of her face and forehead were treated by dermabrasion, bichloracetic acid, and classic phenol peel. The results were assessed at 6 months.

Results.—Each method was nearly equal in the depth of penetration and the quality of skin on healing (Fig 13–3). Dermabrasion seemed slightly more efficient in removing pigment. The patient's forehead and cheeks were therefore treated with dermabrasion followed by a chemical peel. When acetic acid touch-up was attempted in the dermabraded

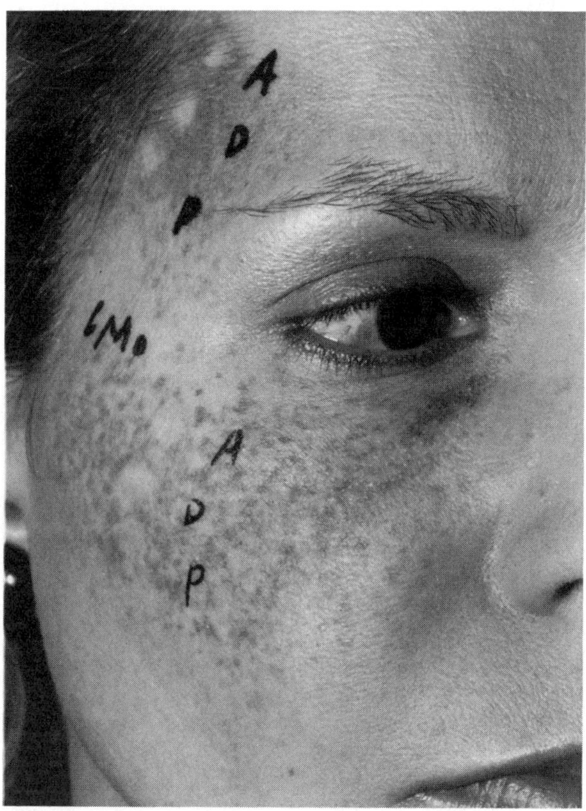

Fig 13–3.—Six months after testing several sites with different methods of pigmentation removal, including bichloracetic acid (*A*), dermabrasion (*D*), and phenol (*P*). All 3 sites show reasonable results. (Courtesy of Ersek RA: *Aesthetic Plast Surg* 15:241–243, 1991.)

area, full-thickness burns occurred. These burns resulted in thick scarring that took many months to heal.

Conclusions.—The depth of treatment and the results seem approximately equal for these 3 modalities. Once an area has been treated, the effects are long-lasting. Any subsequent treatment must be done with great care to prevent a summation of the effect and full-thickness loss of skin.

▶ The author emphasizes that the mechanism of action of cauterization and coagulation has already been well described for chemical peels and dermabrasion. If dermal appendages such as hair follicles, sweat glands, and some dermis can be preserved, then the patient can regenerate a smooth new skin surface. We have been particularly pleased with the acetic acid peel during recent years, and we believe that it is generally safer and just as effective as the phenol peels. When used appropriately, these techniques can provide dramatic improvement in the appearance of these patients.—B.J. Bailey, M.D., F.A.C.S.

14 Pediatric Otolaryngology

Evaluation of Epiglottoplasty as Treatment for Severe Laryngomalacia

Marcus CL, Crockett DM, Davidson Ward SL (Children's Hosp, Los Angeles; Univ of Southern California)

J Pediatr 117:706–710, 1990 14–1

Introduction.—Laryngomalacia is the most common cause of congenital stridor. Although the disorder is usually benign and self-limiting, severe laryngomalacia may be associated with life-threatening complications, including upper airway obstruction and cor pulmonale. Although there have been several reports of clinical improvement after epiglottoplasty, the improvements have not been objectively evaluated. Polysomnography was performed before and after epiglottoplasty to document changes in gas exchange and other physiological measurements that resulted from the operation.

Methods.—Six infants (mean age, 9.4 months) who had been referred for epiglottoplasty because of clinically severe laryngomalacia and stridor underwent polysomnography as part of the preoperative evaluation. Four patients had life-threatening episodes of airway obstruction. Of these, 2 had required tracheal intubation, and 1 had required cardiopulmonary resuscitation. Two children had failure to thrive and 2 had cor pulmonale. Polysomnography was performed during a daytime or evening nap.

Findings.—All 6 patients had obstructive sleep apnea, 4 had hypoxemia, and 4 had hypoventilation. At operation, 3 patients were found to have anteromedial collapse of the aryepiglottic folds and cuneiform cartilages into the laryngeal inlet. The other 3 patients had anteromedial collapse of the mucosa overlying the arytenoid cartilages. All 6 patients had varying degrees of a long, tubular, redundant epiglottis that contributed to laryngeal inlet obstruction. There were no surgical or postoperative complications. All 6 children showed clinical improvement immediately after operation. Repeat polysomnography performed a mean of 2.8 months after epiglottoplasty revealed residual mild episodes of obstructive apnea in 2 patients and mild hypoventilation and desaturation in 1 patient. None of the children experienced further life-threatening events or required further hospitalization after undergoing epiglottoplasty.

Conclusion.—Epiglottoplasty is safe and effective as a surgical treatment in selected patients with severe laryngomalacia.

▶ The authors report success in managing severe laryngomalacia using a new technique, epiglottoplasty. Other articles have referred to similar techniques as "supraglottic trimming" or "anterior epiglottopexy". More information will be forthcoming as the procedure is performed and evaluated more broadly, and such reports should clarify the specific indications and details of surgery. Long-term follow-up of these patients will be needed to confirm that there are no late problems such as supraglottic stenosis and to verify that this is as useful as it appears to be.—B.J. Bailey, M.D., F.A.C.S.

Infant Tracheotomy—Endoscopy and Decannulation

Benjamin B, Curley JWA (Royal Alexandra Hosp for Children, Sydney, Australia)

Int J Pediatr Otorhinol 20:113–121, 1990 14–2

Introduction.—The indications for the use of tracheotomy in young children have recently changed, partially because of the survival of premature infants of low birth weight. It has been suggested that some infants may become physiologically and psychologically dependent on the tracheotomy. The results of tracheotomy in infants 24 months of age or younger were evaluated.

Methods.—The records of 73 infants who had undergone a tracheotomy during a 10-year period were retrospectively reviewed. Of the infants, 19 were premature. Laryngoscopy and bronchoscopy were performed before the tracheotomy in all infants. The first tube change and a follow-up endoscopic examination were conducted with the infants under general anesthesia 7–10 days after the initial procedure. The decannulation procedure was performed when the patient had a clear airway, after treatment of any granulations or suprastomal collapse at the tracheotomy site; this usually occurred 24–48 hours after endoscopy and under general anesthesia.

Results.—At the end of the study, 49 patients had undergone decannulation, 38 within 12 months and 11 after 12 months; 15 subjects continued with the tracheotomy. Six infants died soon after the tracheotomy procedure of causes not related to this operation, and 3 patients were lost to follow-up. Suprastoma collapse from a flap of anterior tracheal wall cartilage located above the stoma was found in 10 patients at endoscopy. Of these 10 patients, 5 were treated with a nasotracheal tube for internal support of the flap or by placement of a suture during endoscopy (Fig 14–1). The initial attempt at decannulation was not successful in 15 infants; however, decannulation was successful on the second procedure in all but 1 infant. Nine children experienced complications.

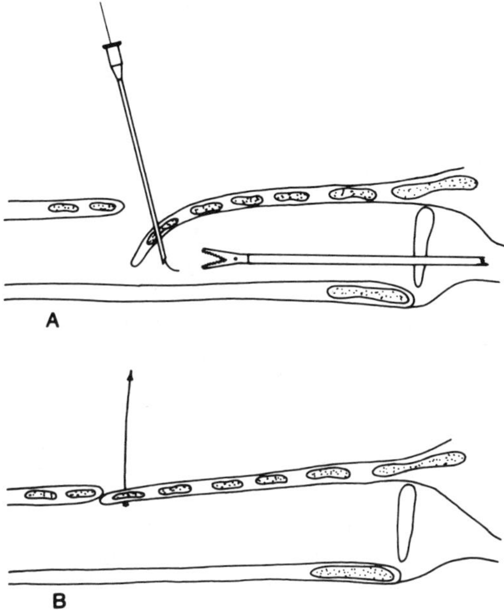

Fig 14–1.—Placement of a suture to elevate the obstructing anterior tracheal wall causing suprastomal collapse. **A,** the suture passes through a 21-gauge needle and is retrieved by forceps to be withdrawn through the oral cavity to be knotted. **B,** the suture is drawn out, the needle is removed, and the knotted end of the suture elevates the obstructing flap. It is sewn to the skin of the neck. (Courtesy of Benjamin B, Curley JWA: *Int J Pediatr Otorhinolaryngol* 20:113–121, 1990.)

Implications.—Unexplained dependence on the tracheotomy did not occur in this patient population. Tracheotomy appears to be a safe procedure for both the short and long term for infants in this age group. Decannulation should be based on clinical readiness and endoscopic assessment.

▶ Decannulation after prolonged tracheotomy may be problematic. Endoscopy is recommended 24–48 hours before decannulation to determine whether there is an adequate airway. Of particular interest is the endoscopic placement of a suture that serves to elevate the anterior tracheal wall (if it tends to collapse into the airway). The safety and utility of this approach to decannulation are impressive.—B.J. Bailey, M.D., F.A.C.S.

CO_2 Laser Excision of Pediatric Airway Lesions

Bagwell CE (Univ of Florida)

J Pediatr Surg 25:1152–1156, 1990 14–3

Introduction.—For the treatment of life-threatening pediatric airway lesions, the carbon dioxide (CO_2) laser offers endoscopic visualization, precise tissue destruction, and minimal local inflammation and subsequent edema. Between 1986 and 1988, 96 laser procedures were performed for excision of airway lesions in 26 children aged 1 day–20 years. Most patients were younger than 2 years of age.

Setting.—Laser excisions were performed via bronchoscopy in 23 patients and via microlaryngoscopy in 3. The airway lesions consisted of 3 main types: 6 mass lesions, 8 cases of granulation tissue, and 12 stenoses.

Results.—Treatment of the airway lesions required from 1 to 8 procedures (mean, 2.8), excluding 1 patient with congenital long-segment tracheal stenosis who required 24 laser excisions of recurrent tracheal granulation tissue. Most of the lesions responded to 1 or 2 laser treatments. There were no episodes of hemorrhage or perforation secondary to laser use. Use of the laser simplified treatment of the lesion in 21 patients (81%). Little or no benefit from laser endoscopy was evident in the remaining 5 patients, including 3 with cystic hygroma that affected the laryngeal structures and soft tissues of the neck and 2 patients who had a recurrence of their subglottic stenosis that initially responded to laser excision. Two of the other 6 patients with subglottic stenosis were cured after a single laser excision; another 2 were cured after laser procedures to establish a lumen followed by cartilage interposition procedures. The other 2 patients remained tracheostomy dependent because of underlying tracheomalacia in 1 and glottic narrowing from preexisting traumatic fusion of the posterior arytenoids in the other.

Conclusion.—The CO_2 laser provides significant benefits and minimal risks in the management of pediatric airway lesions. It should be considered as an adjunctive or complementary procedure in the treatment of obstructive airway lesions of infants and children.

▶ This article reviews the safety and efficacy of CO_2 laser treatment of pediatric airway lesions. Few complications are reported, and the authors emphasize that, in many instances, the laser procedures are adjunctive or complementary in association with other surgical approaches.—B.J. Bailey, M.D., F.A.C.S.

Laryngeal Morphology in Sudden Unexpected Death in Infants

Harrison DFN (London)

J Laryngol Otol 105:646–650, 1991 14–4

Background.—The physiological changes that occur in infants who have attacks of prolonged expiratory apnea have not been well documented. Epidemiological studies indicate that between 8% and 20% of infants who die sudden, unexpected deaths have previously had cyanotic attacks. Therefore, laryngeal morphology was examined in infants who died of sudden infant death syndrome (SIDS).

Methods.—A total of 104 larynges removed from infants who died of SIDS was examined histologically. Twenty larynges from age-matched control infants were also studied. The SIDS babies were aged 28–392 days; the control infants, 92–114 days. The mean weights at death were 5,744 g in SIDS infants and 5,100 g in control infants.

Results.—In 35% of the SIDS larynges from infants aged 2–4 months, excessive amounts of subglottic submucosal glandular tissue had reduced the available airway by more than half. This airway reduction was more than 60% in 30% of these infants.

Conclusions.—Although this study suggests that hyperplasia of the subglottic mucous glands is 1 cause of fatal hypoxia in infants dying of SIDS, it does not provide guidance for establishing which infants are at high risk in most cases.

► As he has done many times before, Professor Harrison has provided a new perspective on a poorly understood clinical entity. Careful histological evaluation of 104 larynges from infants dying of SIDS revealed the presence of excessive subglottic submucosal glandular tissue in more than one third. There may be increased viscosity of the secretions from these glands, in addition to the marked airway restriction they cause. Sudden infant death syndrome is probably a multifactorial disorder, and it is also possible that neurological dysfunction and/or inflammatory changes are present in other individuals.—B.J. Bailey, M.D., F.A.C.S.

Management of Epistaxis in Children

Ruddy J, Proops DW, Pearman K, Ruddy H (Birmingham Children's Hosp, Birmingham, England; Regional Radiation Physics and Protection Dept, Birmingham, England)

Int J Pediatr Otorhinolaryngol 21:139–142, 1991 14–5

Objective.—Epistaxis is a common problem in childhood. The effectiveness of an antiseptic nasal cream carrier (Naseptin ICI) containing chlorhexidine and neomycin in a white base was compared with that of chemical cautery with silver nitrate in the treatment of childhood epistaxis.

Study Design.—Forty-eight patients (aged 3–14 years) with at least 1 nose bleed in the previous month and a history of repeated epistaxis were randomly assigned to treatment with either Naseptin cream applied to both nostrils twice daily for 4 weeks or cautery with 75% silver nitrate under local anesthesia.

Results.—A total of 50% of the children treated with Naseptin cream and 54% of those treated with chemical cautery had no nose bleed during the 8-week follow-up period; the difference between the groups was not significant. The failure rates were high but comparable in both groups. Those children who had cautery complained of pain during the procedure. There were no adverse reactions to Naseptin cream.

Conclusion.—The use of antiseptic nasal cream alone is as effective as chemical cautery in the treatment of epistaxis in children. Antiseptic nasal cream should be the first line of treatment in childhood epistaxis.

► The authors propose that antiseptic cream should become the first line of treatment for recurrent mild epistaxis in children. Their suggestion is supported by a comparative study that is interesting but flawed. There was no control group with observation, and first aid (probably the most common treatment in the general population) was not administered. The parameters for entering patients into the study, other forms of cautery, and associated inflammatory and infectious diseases were not mentioned. Also, the manner in which cautery was used is absent from the report.—B.J. Bailey, M.D., F.A.C.S.

Underdiagnosis and Undertreatment of Chronic Sinusitis in Children

Richards W, Roth RM, Church JA (Children's Hospital of Los Angeles; Kaiser Permanente Med Ctr, Orange County, Calif)

Clin Pediatr 30:88–92, 1991 14–6

Purpose.—There has been a marked increase in the number of children referred for treatment of worsening respiratory allergy who are subsequently found to have sinusitis. The case reports of 34 misdiagnosed children were reviewed retrospectively.

Antibiotic Therapy

Drug	Outcome: Successful	Outcome: Unsuccessful
Erythromycin/ sulfisoxazole	4	2
Cefaclor	12	0
Amoxicillin clavulanate	12	0
Cefixime	1	1
Amoxicillin	4	2
Trimethoprim/ sulfamethoxazole	1	1
Cephalexin	0	1

Note: Successful outcome refers to the number of patients who ultimately responded to the antibiotic. *Unsuccessful outcome* refers to the number of patients who failed initial treatment with the antibiotic.

(Courtesy of Richards W, Roth RM, Church JA: *Clin Pediatr* 30:88–92, 1991.)

Patients.—The 34 children ranged in age from 9 months to 11 years, and they had been referred with the chief complaint of worsening allergy. Most of the children had a history of severe cough, nasal congestion, and constant or frequently recurrent colds and rhinorrhea. The mean duration of symptoms was 6 months (range, 1–14 months). None of the children had previously undergone sinus radiography, nor had the diagnosis of sinusitis previously been suggested.

Findings.—Initial physical examination revealed that a significant number of children had edematous or erythematous nasal tubules with purulent or mucoid nasal secretions. A total of 21 children also had otitis media or serous otitis media. After the removal of cerumen from the external ear canal, several children were found to have unsuspected otitis media. Sinus radiographs were obtained in 24 patients; they were interpreted as positive in 22 patients. The diagnosis of sinusitis in the other 2 patients and in the 10 patients for whom sinus radiographs were not obtained was based on clinical findings. Fifteen patients had a past history of asthma, and another 6 patients were misdiagnosed with asthma, probably because of noisy upper airway breathing and transmitted rhonchi. The asthma symptoms increased in 12 of the 15 patients during the time they had sinusitis. Although all children were eventually cured by appropriate antibiotic therapy (table), earlier diagnosis and appropriate therapy would have shortened the course of their illness.

Conclusions.—The diagnosis of chronic sinusitis should always be suspected in children with cold-like symptoms and cough that persists for more than 10 days, particularly if they also have otitis media. Early diagnosis and appropriate antibiotic therapy can significantly reduce the significant morbidity associated with this common disorder.

► This is an interesting report of observations regarding chronic sinusitis in children. It provides an excellent review of both the range of symptoms that children are seen with and the difficulty involved in diagnosis. Treatment is characterized by a 3–4 week course of cefaclor or amoxicillin clavulante in most patients, with a general pattern of success. The important message to take away from this study is that children with complaints of cough, congestion, and purulent rhinorrhea that persist for more than 10 days should be looked upon with a high index of suspicion.—B.J. Bailey, M.D., F.A.C.S.

Long-Term Results of Submandibular Duct Transposition for Drooling

Burton MJ, Leighton SEJ, Lund WS (Radcliffe Infirmary, Oxford, England)

J Laryngol Otol 105:101–103, 1991 14–7

Background.—Excessive drooling is a frequent occurrence in patients with cerebral palsy and other forms of cerebral dysfunction. Apart from requiring frequent changes of clothing or wearing of a bib, drooling promotes social isolation and can lead to skin maceration.

Results of Submandibular Duct Transposition

	Immediately post-operatively	Now
Crysdale criteria		
Excellent	9	10
Good	5	4
(Good to Fair)	1	2
Fair	1	0
Poor	1	1
Total	17	17
Bailey and Wadsworth criteria		
Much better	17	14
Better	3	4
No change	0	2
Worse	0	0
Total	20	20

(Courtesy of Burton MJ, Leighton SEJ, Lund WS: *J Laryngol Otol* 105:101–103, 1991.)

Methods.—The long-term outcome of submandibular duct transposition was studied in 20 drooling children (aged 3–18 years) who were operated on between 1984 and 1987 for drooling associated with neurological dysfunction.

Findings.—All patients improved initially, and only 3 deteriorated during a mean follow-up of 3½ years (table). Several caregivers reported that drooling was worse during upper respiratory tract infection or when the child did not concentrate properly.

Conclusion.—Submandibular duct transposition is often an effective means of controlling drooling in children with neurological dysfunction. Morbidity is limited.

▶ Drooling can be a serious problem in the lives of children with neurological dysfunction and those who care for them. In this series of patients, submandibular duct transposition succeeded in reducing the amount of drooling. The fact that there was minimal morbidity associated with the procedure is of equal importance.—B.J. Bailey, M.D., F.A.C.S.

Abscesses of the Neck in Infants and Young Children: A Review of 112 Cases

Hawkins DB, Austin JR (Los Angeles County–Univ of Southern California Med Ctr, Los Angeles)

Ann Otol Rhinol Laryngol 100:361–365, 1991 14–8

Background.—Abscesses of the neck are fairly common in young children. A series of 112 children (aged 5 years and younger) with cervical abscesses was reviewed to evaluate the cause, bacteriological findings, and clinical courses of these abscesses.

Patients.—The patients were seen during a 7½-year period. Of the patients, 93% were younger than 4 years of age, and 46% were younger than 12 months of age. A total of 84% of the patients was Hispanic. The abscess site was the lateral neck in 93% of cases and the anterior triangle in 87%; all of the latter were high in the neck. The abscesses ranged in diameter from 2 to 10 cm, and only 52% were definitely fluctuant when they were drained. The white blood cell count was between 10,000 and 20,000 in 57% of the patients. Of the abscesses, 107 developed in areas of cervical adenitis; 91 of these were unilateral and responded to drainage and antibiotics. All but 3 of the patients were hospitalized, for a range of 3–28 days. All but 4 of the patients underwent incision and drainage, although some had 1 or more needle aspirations beforehand.

Outcome.—The most common finding on culture was *Staphylococcus aureus,* which was found in 39% of the cases, followed by group A β-hemolytic streptococci in 17% of the cases (table). Unusual abscesses, including infected congenital cysts, cat-scratch disease, or mycobacterial abscess, were found in 14% of the cases. There was 1 case of necrotizing infection with group A streptococci and anaerobic streptococci. A total of 104 patients received intravenous antibiotics; a penicillin derivative, usually an antistaphylococcal penicillin, was used in 94% of these pa-

Results of Abscess Culture

Bacteria	*No. of Patients*
Staphylococcus aureus alone	44
Staphylococcus aureus in combination	3
Group A β-hemolytic *Streptococcus*	15
Group A *Streptococcus* in combination	4
Atypical mycobacteria	
Mycobacterium avium	5
Mycobacterium intracellulare	2
Unidentified	1
Anaerobic bacteria	
Anaerobic *Streptococcus*	1
Microaerophilic *Streptococcus*	1
Peptostreptococcus	1
Hemophilus influenzae, not type B	1
Various others cultured in combination with above	7
No growth	29

(Courtesy of Hawkins DB, Austin JR: *Ann Otol Rhinol Laryngol* 100:361–365, 1991.)

tients. More than 1 incision and drainage procedure was required in 8 cases, and airway intervention was required in 2.

Conclusions.—In children with cervical abscesses, most cases respond well to appropriate intravenous antibiotic therapy, incision, and drainage. The work-up of these abscesses, which are particularly common in very young children, includes a complete blood count, chest radiograph, and blood culture if pyrexia is present.

▶ Cervical abscesses occur most often between the ages of 6–12 months. There is usually a history of recent upper respiratory infection, fever, and white blood cell elevation. Of special interest in this report were the 4 children who were managed with needle aspiration and antibiotic therapy. Efforts should be made to find a treatment that is effective without surgical incisions for drainage.—B.J. Bailey, M.D., F.A.C.S.

The Use of Biopsy in the Evaluation of Pediatric Nasopharyngeal Masses

Burkey B, Koopmann CF, Brunberg J (Univ of Michigan Hosp)
Int J Pediatr Otorhinolaryngol 20:169–179, 1990 14–9

Introduction.—Pediatric nasopharyngeal tumors are rare. The differential diagnosis includes a small but diverse group of benign and malignant tumors. Juvenile nasopharyngeal angiofibroma (JNA) is the most common of the benign tumors. Because JNA has such characteristic clinical, angiographic, and CT findings, many authors suggest that routine biopsy for histological confirmation is not essential. In some cases, however, the use of diagnostic biopsy for nasopharyngeal masses is valuable.

Case Report.—Boy, 6 years and 9 months of age, was examined locally because of headaches. He was healthy except for a 2-year history of seasonal rhinitis and intermittent epistaxis. Sinus films were abnormal, and he was started on antibiotic therapy for sinusitis. Ophthalmological examination revealed complete left ophthalmoplegia, and he was referred to this institution. Examination revealed a deep red submucosal nasopharyngeal mass on the left side, complete left ophthalmoplegia, decreased left visual acuity at 20/400, hypesthesia in the left trigeminal nerve distribution, a 20 dB conductive left hearing loss, and ipsilateral middle ear effusion. Computed tomography scanning revealed an enhancing mass in the left nasopharynx, the pterygopalatine fossa, and in the infratemporal fossa with destruction of the posterior wall of the maxillary sinus and the lateral pterygoid plate. Angiography revealed a hypervascular lesion. The differential diagnosis was angiofibroma or possible rhabdomyosarcoma. The patient underwent preoperative embolization, which resulted in an 80% decrease of the tumor blush on angiography. A left transantral biopsy of the tumor performed 48 hours later confirmed the diagnosis of embryonal rhabdomyosarcoma. Bone scan and abdominal CT were negative. Chest CT revealed multiple bilateral pulmonary metastases. The patient was classified as stage IV parameningeal rhabdomyosarcoma and was started on chemotherapy and radiation therapy to the whole brain and the primary site.

Conclusion.—Although the lesion clinically and radiographically resembled JNA, pretreatment biopsy confirmed a highly malignant and metastatic neoplasm. The correct diagnosis thus averted inappropriate and possibly morbid surgical excision.

Management of Tracheobronchial Foreign Bodies in Children: An Update

Healy GB (The Children's Hosp, Boston)
Ann Otol Rhinol Laryngol 99:889–891, 1990 14–10

Introduction.—Tracheobronchial foreign bodies remain an important cause of morbidity and mortality in children. A review was made of the appropriate use of diagnostic studies and management of tracheobronchial foreign bodies in children.

Discussion.—The management of tracheobronchial foreign bodies involves a coordinated team effort that includes a radiologist, an anesthesiologist, and an endoscopist. Neck and chest radiographs, obtained both during the expiratory and inspiratory phases, are basic in evaluation of these patients. If fluoroscopy is not feasible, decubitus films of the chest should be attempted. The image intensifier may be used for foreign bodies that have migrated to the periphery of the lung. Before extraction, the endoscopist and anesthesiologist should carefully evaluate the pertinent radiographs and characteristics of the suspected foreign body. The endoscopist should have a complete selection of appropriate endoscopes (including a full range of rigid and flexible laryngoscopes, bronchoscopes, and esophagoscopes) and a wide selection of extraction forceps, including magnets. Telescopic forceps are suited for teaching situations, and they provide an accurate means of extracting specific foreign bodies. With the child under general anesthesia, a complete examination of the aerodigestive tract should be performed. Extraction with rigid instrumentation is the method of choice. The anesthesiologist must be alerted before actual extraction to make sure that the level of anesthesia is of sufficient depth to avoid laryngospasm as removal occurs. Once the object is removed, the airway is reinspected to rule out the possibility of other foreign objects.

Conclusion.—Refinement of radiologic, anesthetic, and endoscopic techniques allows the relatively safe and reliable removal of foreign bodies from the aerodigestive system. However, endoscopic expertise is necessary.

15 General Otolaryngology

Nasal and Oral Flow-Volume Loops in Normal Subjects and Patients With Obstructive Sleep Apnea

Shepard JW Jr, Burger CD (Mayo Clinic and Found, Rochester, Minn)

Am Rev Respir Dis 142:1288–1293, 1990 15–1

Background.—To test the hypothesis that limitations to airflow through the nasopharyngeal ventilatory pathway would correlate with the severity of obstructive sleep apnea (OSA), 14 obese men with a mean age of 56 years and clinically suspected OSA were studied along with 14 nonobese, healthy, age-matched control subjects. The role of nasal and oral flow-volume loops (FVLs) was assessed in evaluating patients with OSA.

Methods.—Overnight polysomnography and spirometry were performed, and both nasal and oral FVLs were obtained with controls in the seated upright position and patients in both upright and supine positions. Oral and nasal airflow were monitored, as well as the thoracoabdominal movement, ECG activity, electroencephalographic activity, arterial oxyhemoglobin desaturization and electrooculographic activity. Apneas and hypopneas per hour of sleep were reported as the apnea plus hypopnea index.

Results.—Oral upright data for patients with OSA showed significantly decreased forced vital capacity (FVC) and increased upper airway resistance. Expiratory flow rates at 25% and 50% of VC were significantly higher in patients than in controls. Nasal upright data indicated that nasopharyngeal resistance during inspiration increased in both groups. The differences between nasal and oral FVLs for controls and for patients in upright and supine positions were matched at total lung capacity (Fig 15–1). In normal subjects, the airflow was limited during inspiration but not during expiration with both nasal and oral FVLs. In patients with OSA, both inspiratory and expiratory flow limitation indicated nondistensibility in the nasopharyngeal ventilatory pathway. Changing to a supine position reduced the expiratory but not the inspiratory flow rate. Reductions in the area under the flow-volume loop correlated with the severity of hypoxemia and hypercapnia.

Conclusions.—Patency of the nasopharyngeal ventilatory pathway is an important determinant of sleep-disordered breathing. The functional

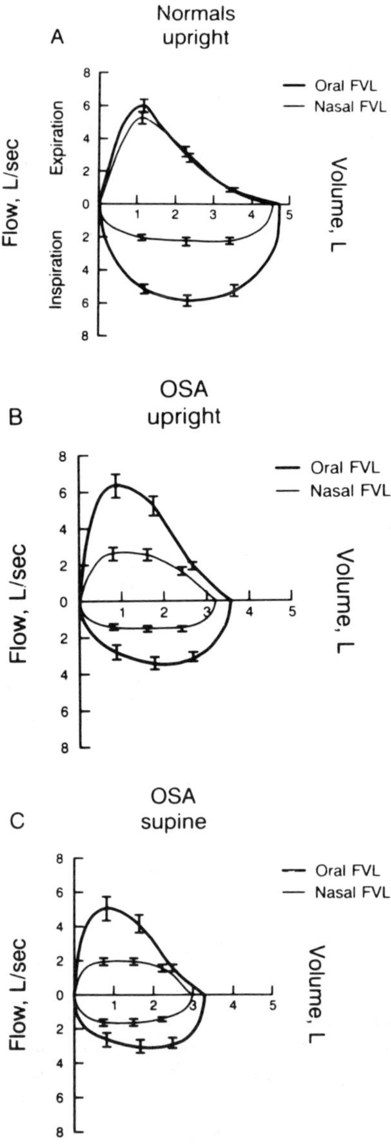

Fig 15–1.—**A,** nasal and oral flow-volume loops obtained in 14 normal male control subjects in seated upright position. Data are mean ± standard error of mean. **B,** nasal and oral flow-volume loops obtained in 14 male patients with obstructive sleep apnea in seated upright position. Data are mean ± standard error of mean. **C,** nasal and oral flow-volume loops obtained in 14 male patients with obstructive sleep apnea in supine position. Data are mean ± standard of mean. (Courtesy of Shepard JW Jr, Burger CD: *Am Rev Respir Dis* 142:1288–1293, 1990.)

capacity of the ventilatory pathway to accommodate airflow is easily evaluated with nasal FVLs.

Snoring (I): Daytime Sleepiness in Regular Heavy Snorers
Guilleminault C, Stoohs R, Duncan S (Stanford Univ)
Chest 99:40–48, 1991 15–2

Background.—In chronic heavy snorers, complaints of fatigue, tiredness, and/or excessive daytime sleepiness (EDS) often lead to the suspicion of obstructive sleep apnea syndrome (OSAS). However, clinical investigation may not demonstrate OSAS or any other valid explanation for the EDS. Fifteen chronic heavy snorers were investigated to assess the relationship between snoring and EDS.

Methods.—The subjects were men (mean age, 44 years; mean body mass index, 21.9 kg/m^2). All had a respiratory disturbance index (RDI) below 5 and good nocturnal oxygen saturation. Monitoring was done for several nights both with and without a tight-fitting facial mask, pneumotachometer, esophageal balloon, and nasal continuous positive airway pressure (CPAP) measurement. After 2 baseline nights and the second CPAP night, the Multiple Sleep Latency Test (MSLT) was administered. Short EEG arousals during nocturnal sleep were determined, and the relationship between the arousals, esophageal pressure (Pes) nadir, and airflow decrease was investigated. The relationships between reporting of decreased daytime alertness and MSLT results and between MSLT results and frequency of EEG arousals were determined.

Results.—The esophageal pressure nadir increased significantly with abrupt decrease in flow leading to EEG arousals. Nasal CPAP with positive end-expiratory pressure (PEEP) of 3–8 cm of H_20 led to better overall oxygenation, reduction of RDI, and reduction of arousal index, confirming that the patients had a partially obstructed upper airway during sleep. Nasal CPAP also improved mean MSLT significantly, despite the absence of pathologic baseline MSLT findings. Negative correlations were noted between mean RDI and MSLT, arousal index and MSLT, and PEEP and MSLT; positive correlations were noted between PEEP and lowest SaO_2 and PEEP and mean MSLT.

Conclusions.—Some regular heavy snorers without OSAS may be at risk of decreased daytime alertness. An increase in short EEG arousals may be an indication of this risk; the arousals appear to be a consequence of increased upper airway resistance. The long-term effect of this increased resistance on the well being of regular snorers should be investigated further.

► Attention has been heavily focused upon the oropharyngeal and hypopharyngeal regions in most studies of patients with OSA. During sleep, however, the nasopharynx is the primary ventilatory pathway. Shepard and Burger (Abstract 15–1) found that inspiratory and expiratory airflow was decreased in patients with OSA (but not in controls) and that there was a high correlation between the flow-volume loop measurements and the apnea hypopnea index during sleep studies. If confirmed, this would provide a simpler and less costly screening test for OSA. Because obese patients were not included in this study, we are not able to assess the relative contributions of such important patient variables as airway anatomy, tissue distensibility, and obesity. Given the complexity of this disorder, it is likely that there are several subgroups within the total OSA population and that the etiology of the clinical presentations may be different.

In a study from Stanford (Abstract 15–2), Guilleminault evaluated an interesting group of patients who are heavy snorers but who do not have OSA according to standard tests. The study population did not spontaneously report excessive daytime somnolence as a significant complaint. On close examination, several measures of disturbed sleeping patterns were believed to be important causal factors that may correlate with decreased daytime alertness. This type of study is difficult to interpret because of the subjective nature of the daytime symptoms; however, its implications are quite important. Clinicians should become more aware of these subtle decreases in daytime alertness and their possible association with chronic heavy snoring.—B.J. Bailey, M.D., F.A.C.S.

The Surgical Management of Chronic Parotitis

Arriaga MA, Myers EN (Univ of Pittsburgh; Eye and Ear Inst, Pittsburgh)
Laryngoscope 100:1270–1275, 1990 15–3

Introduction.—Recurrent painful enlargement of the parotid gland with accompanying purulent sialorrhea characterizes chronic parotitis. Conservative medical and mechanical treatment usually help the patient, but complications such as abscesses or fistulas may require surgery. In the past, parotidectomy was almost always avoided in the treatment of parotitis because of the potential for injuring the facial nerve. An experience with the use of parotidectomy in managing chronic parotitis was reviewed retrospectively.

Methods.—The records of all patients who had parotidectomies between 1979 and 1989 were studied. The follow-up data for these patients were collected by chart review and telephone interviews. Indications for surgery included frequent infections despite aggressive medical therapy, complications such as abscesses or fistulas, recurrent parotitis, and patient comfort. The technique for parotidectomy comprised a standard preauricular incision to an upper cervical neck crease. The main trunk of the facial nerve was usually identified by the anterior border of the sternocleidomastoid muscle, the mastoid tip, the bony external auditory meatus, and the cartilaginous pointer of the external auditory meatus.

Results.—Between 1979 and 1989 a total of 308 parotidectomies was performed; 16 of these were total parotidectomies for chronic parotitis. Before total parotidectomy, 3 patients had had incomplete surgical treatments. Preoperative imaging was found to aid the surgery. Eight patients had underlying disease conditions: 3 had Sjögren's disease and 5 had pathologically confirmed sialolithiasis. In the remaining 8 patients, the histopathologic findings demonstrated diffuse chronic sialoadenitis. The 16 patients had had symptoms of chronic parotitis for 6 months–10 years and 8 had prior hospitalizations for severe parotid sialoadenitis. The clinical response to parotidectomy resulted in the total resolution of recurrent painful swelling of the parotid gland in 14 patients. Two patients with previously undiagnosed Sjögren's syndrome required a bilateral total parotidectomy. Complications occurred infrequently; however, some facial nerve weakness was observed in 26% of the patients. No cases of total permanent paralysis resulted from the procedure.

Implications.—These findings indicate that total parotidectomy with facial nerve dissection works well to completely eliminate the chronic infections of the parotid glands in these patients. The risk of harming the facial nerve, both in this series of patients and in the literature, appears to be small.

Pilocarpine Treatment of Salivary Gland Hypofunction and Dry Mouth (Xerostomia)

Fox PC, Atkinson JC, Macynski AA, Wolff A, Kung DS, Valdez IH, Jackson W, Delapenha RA, Shiroky J, Baum BJ (Natl Inst of Health, Bethesda, Md; Columbia Univ)

Arch Intern Med 151:1149–1152, 1991 15–4

Background.—The common problem of xerostomia has many side effects that have a negative effect on the patient's quality of life. None of the current methods of treatment for salivary gland hypofunction and xerostomia are accepted and effective. The parasympathomimetic agent pilocarpine has been shown to be effective in the short term in patients who have functioning salivary tissue. The safety and efficacy of this agent for long-term use were determined.

Methods.—The subjects were 39 patients, 29 females and 10 males with an average age of 55.4 years. All patients complained of xerostomia for at least 1 year. Patients received a 5 mg capsule of pilocarpine hydrochloride, 3 times daily for 5 months and a placebo in a randomly assigned month. Each month, objective measures of major salivary gland output and subjective impressions of oral moisture, treatment-related side effects, and physiologic measures were assessed. A total of 31 patients completed the protocol.

Results.—Salivary output was significantly increased by pilocarpine in 21 of 31 patients (Fig 15–2). Twenty-seven patients reported significant

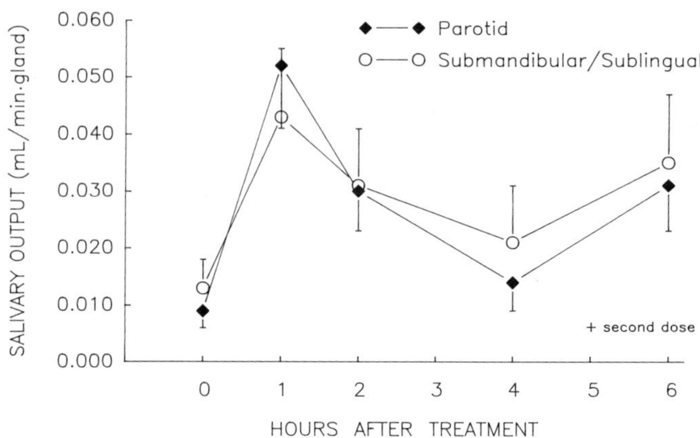

Fig 15–2.—Parotid (*solid diamonds*) and submandibular/sublingual (*open circles*) gland salivary output of 31 patients after administration of pilocarpine. Values are the mean of 6 collections after pilocarpine from each individual obtained during 5 months of active drug therapy. (Courtesy of Fox PC, Atkinson JC, Macynski AA, et al: *Arch Intern Med* 151:1149–1152, 1991.)

improvement in the feeling of oral dryness, speaking, chewing, and swallowing. Side effects were common, but they were generally mild and tolerable. Cardiovascular and other physiologic measures were not significantly altered.

Conclusions.—Pilocarpine appears to be a safe and effective treatment for salivary gland hypofunction and xerostomia in some patients. Some patients may have improvements in subjective but not objective responses. Further studies are needed to find a dose that will optimize effectiveness and minimize side effects.

► Managing patients with chronic parotitis is challenging, and several approaches have been proposed. Experience has led physicians to discard the use of radiation therapy and autogenous vaccination. Tympanic neurectomy and ligation of Stensen's duct may be helpful in some patients; however, the long-term results indicate that many patients resume a pattern of recurrent infections. Although concern about injury to the facial nerve has been expressed by those who criticize parotidectomy, this series (Abstract 15–3) joins others in documenting the relative safety of gland excision. In fact, earlier performance of superficial parotidectomy may be a larger factor in limiting the risk of parotidectomy in this patient group.

Xerostomia is a common complaint, particularly in its milder and transient forms. When this problem results from radiation therapy or Sjögren's disease, there may be extreme dryness that impairs chewing and swallowing as well as pain, dental caries, and frequent oral cavity infection. Pilocarpine was safe and effective in increasing salivary flow in most of the patients studied, and the parasympathetic side effects were tolerable at the dosage level of 15 mg per day.—B.J. Bailey, M.D., F.A.C.S.

Hyperbaric Oxygen Therapy for Necrotizing Fasciitis Reduces Mortality and the Need for Debridements

Riseman JA, Zamboni WA, Curtis A, Graham DR, Konrad HR, Ross DS
(Southern Illinois University School of Medicine, Springfield, Ill)
Surgery 108:847–850, 1990 15–5

Background.—The overall mortality of necrotizing fasciitis remains high despite improvements in antimicrobial therapy and surgical technique. An experience with 29 patients was reviewed to compare the results of treatment with and without adjuvant hyperbaric oxygen (HBO) therapy.

Methods.—Group 1 comprised 12 patients treated before HBO therapy was available, whereas group 2 comprised 17 patients whose treatment included HBO. The group 1 patients received surgical debridement and antibiotics only; group 2 patients received an average of 7.4 90-minute HBO treatments at 2.5 standard atmosphere in addition to surgery and antibiotics. The patient and clinical characteristics were reviewed to compare the 2 groups.

Results.—Of the group 2 patients, 53% had perineal involvement, compared with 12% of group 1; affected body surface was similar. In group 1, admitting conditions were diabetes in 33%, white blood cell count greater than 12,000 in 50%, and shock in 8%. In group 2, 47% had diabetes, 59% had elevated white blood cell count, and 29% were in shock. Despite the fact that they were more seriously ill, the patients in group 2 had a mortality of 23%, compared with 66% in group 1. Group 2 required 1.2 debridements per patient to achieve wound control compared with 3.3 in group 1 (table). In group 2, nonclostridial infections were associated with a lower mortality.

Conclusions.—Hyperbaric oxygen therapy used in addition to surgical and antimicrobial treatment significantly reduces mortality and wound morbidity in patients with necrotizing fasciitis. More specific antibiotic therapy and earlier recognition and treatment may improve results. Hy-

Outcome of Patients With Necrotizing Fasciitis

	Group 1 (n = 12)	*Group 2 (n = 17)*	p
Deaths (mortality rate)	8 (67%)	4 (23%)	<0.025
Total debridements among patients that lived	13	14	
Mean debridements per patient	3.25	1.16	<0.03

(Courtesy of Riseman JA, Zomboni WA, Curtis A, et al: *Surgery* 108:847–850, 1990.)

perbaric oxygen therapy should be a routine part of treatment for these patients.

Necrotizing Tracheobronchitis: Complication of Mechanical Ventilation in an Adult

Chechani V, Vasudevan VP, Kamholz SL (Woodhull Med and Mental Health Ctr, Brooklyn, NY; State Univ of New York Health Science Ctr, Brooklyn; Univ of Missouri-Columbia School of Medicine/Harry S Truman Mem Veterans Hosp, Columbia, Mo)

South Med J 84:271–273, 1991 15–6

Objective.—Necrotizing tracheobronchitis (NTB) is a complication of mechanical ventilation that has been well described in pediatric patients. Although it was described as "hemorrhagic tracheitis" in 2 adults treated with high-frequency jet ventilation, NTB has not been previously reported in adults treated with mechanical ventilation.

Case Report.—Woman, 51, had localized interstitial pneumonia that rapidly progressed to involve all lung fields. After 9 days of mechanical ventilation a right pneumothorax was observed. Bronchoscopy and endobronchial biopsies revealed NTB involving the tracheal mucosa distal to the tip of the endotrachial tube. The right main bronchus was totally occluded by a bloody, crusted, hard exudate. Subsequent bronchoscopy (20 days later) revealed that the proximal tracheal mucosa and larynx were normal. High peak airway pressures persisted after the evacuation of the pneumothorax and decreased to normal with the resolution of NTB at subsequent bronchoscopy. The patient died after reintubation for respiratory failure. No infectious cause was identified on cultures of bronchoalveolar lavage fluid and open lung biopsy tissue.

Conclusion.—Necrotizing tracheobronchitis should be suspected in adult patients who have had mechanical ventilation and who are experiencing ventilatory difficulties despite treatment or the exclusion of routine problems.

▶ Necrotizing fasciitis (NF) is an uncommon problem, with about 1,000 cases occurring in the United States each year; however, mortality rates of approximately 40% are reported in most series. Abstract 15–5 joins several previous reports in documenting the effectiveness of HBO in reducing the mortality and morbidity from NF. Mortality was reduced from 67% in the group that did not receive HBO to 23% in the population treated with HBO. The authors emphasize the importance of a multidisciplinary approach that also includes wide surgical debridement and aggressive, broad-spectrum antibiotic therapy.

Necrotizing tracheobronchitis is recognized as a complication of mechanical ventilation of neonates. Sometimes described as "hemorrhagic tracheitis", it has been reported as an autopsy finding that ranges in frequency from

4% to 44%. The condition appears to require more than 3 hours of assisted ventilation, and it is usually associated with sloughing of the respiratory epithelium (which may produce airway occlusion).

In spite of the obvious logistical problems and risks of using HBO in neonates, there may be a role for HBO in the management and salvage of some newborn infants in whom NTB is diagnosed.—B.J. Bailey, M.D., F.A.C.S.

The Prevalence of Mycoplasma Pneumoniae in Ambulatory Patients With Nonstreptococcal Sore Throat

Williams WC, Williamson HA Jr, LeFevre ML (Bowman Gray School of Medicine; Univ of Missouri-Columbia)

Fam Med 23:117–121, 1991 15–7

Objective.—The role of *Mycoplasma pneumoniae* in nonstreptococcal pharyngitis has been a topic of interest. The prevalance of *M. pneumoniae* infection in family practice patients with sore throats was determined, and patient characteristics that may be predictive of mycoplasmal infection were identified.

Study Design.—During a 4-month period, *M. pneumoniae* throat cultures were obtained from 419 patients aged 5 years and older who had a chief complaint of sore throat.

Results.—The overall prevalance of *M. pneumoniae* infection was 12.7%. Stepwise logistic regression identified hoarseness and absence of postnasal drip as symptoms predictive of mycoplasmal infection. When compared with patients with positive streptococcal tests, the patients with mycoplasma infection exhibited a markedly dissimilar disease presentation. Patients with *M. pneumoniae* infection tended to be older and less ill. They also had less evidence of pharyngitis and more evidence of tracheobronchitis. The presence of pharyngitis was not predictive of mycoplasmal infection.

Conclusion.—A notable percentage of nonstreptococcal sore throats seen in a family practice setting is associated with *M. pneumoniae.* Mycoplasmal infection is a rather nondescript upper respiratory illness that is distinguishable only by its contrast to streptococcal pharyngitis and its tendency to involve the lower portions of the airway. The development of rapid office-based diagnostic tests for *M. pneumoniae* allows timely diagnosis of this common and formerly elusive pathogen.

A Simple Sore Throat?: Retropharyngeal Emphysema Secondary to Free-Basing Cocaine

Riccio JC, Abbott J (Salem Hosp, Salem, Mass; Univ Health Sciences Ctr, Denver)

J Emerg Med 8:709–712, 1990 15–8

Introduction.—Retropharyngeal emphysema (in association with pneumomediastinum) has been associated with marijuana smoking, heroin injection, and free-basing cocaine. An experience with a healthy young woman with retropharyngeal emphysema secondary to drug use who complained of a sore throat was reviewed.

Case Report.—Woman, 19, had a 1-week history of mild sore throat with a marked increase in the severity of pain during the prior 8 hours. She also complained of right ear pain and odynophagia. The patient had no history of neck trauma, sharp object ingestion, other toxic exposure, or recent dental procedures. Her vital signs were normal. The patient exhibited a minimally injected pharynx, and palpitation lateral to the right side of the thyroid cartilage elicited tenderness. No abnormalities appeared on visualization of the epiglottis, and the lungs were clear to ausculation and percussion. Laboratory data revealed a white blood cell count of 18,300/mm^3. A lateral neck roentgenogram demonstrated retropharyngeal air, a widened retropharyngeal space, and kyphosis of the cervical spine without abnormal calcification. The patient admitted that she had been free-basing cocaine just before the onset of her sore throat and again just before her increased pain. The patient was given 100% oxygen and admitted to the hospital. Her vital signs remained normal and the white blood cell count was 8,600/mm^3 after 24 hours. The patient became asymptomatic and was discharged.

Discussion.—In cases of uncomplicated cervical emphysema or pneumomediastinum associated with substance abuse, extensive workups are almost always negative and may be unnecessary. Conservative treatment (including use of 100% oxygen and observation) can be used in the absence of infection or respiratory compromise.

▶ The frequency with which *M. pneumoniae* (Abstract 15–7) is responsible for clinical pharyngitis is of interest to primary physicians and otolaryngologists. Although it was previously identified as the etiologic agent in only 3% to 4% of patients, this careful study noted a prevalence of 13% in a general population. The likelihood that a patient has a mycoplasma pharyngitis is greater when the patient appears to be less ill, has less pain, and does not complain of postnasal drainage. In addition, mycoplasma patients often come from within a relatively "closed population", complain of hoarseness more frequently, or are older.

The report by Riccio and Abbott alerts us to a new clinical entity to add to our differential diagnosis list for "sore throat". Retropharyngeal abscess may result from foreign bodies, trauma, or infection. This report of abscess plus cervical emphysema (Abstract 15–8) discusses free-basing with cocaine. Previous publications have described pneumomediastinum occurring after drug use and have documented the appropriateness of conservative management in most instances.—B.J. Bailey, M.D., F.A.C.S.

Helping Your Patients Who Smoke Quit for Good: A Quick and Easy Approach

Kraner SE, Graham KE (Maricopa Area Health Education Ctr, Phoenix, Arizona)
Postgrad Med 90:233–248, 1991 15–9

Background.—Cigarette smoking is an important contributor to illness, disability, and death. By using appropriate techniques, physicians can help patients quit smoking, even when office visits are limited. An approach for helping patients quit smoking was outlined.

First Stage of Smoking Cessation.—The "differential diagnosis approach" is based on the stage theory of behavior change. In stage 1 the patient has not yet considered quitting. Although patients are rarely ignorant of the major effects of smoking on health, they often deny the seriousness of the consequences of smoking, doubt personal susceptibility to these consequences, and lack confidence in their ability to successfully quit smoking. The management of patients in this stage includes personalizing both the dangers of smoking and the benefits of quitting, dispelling myths to increase the patient's sense of susceptibility, building the patient's sense of self-efficacy in the ability to quit, reinforcing other positive behaviors, and stating plainly that you are willing to help them when they are ready to quit.

Second Stage of Smoking Cessation.—Patients in stage 2 are thinking of quitting. Most smokers are in this stage. Patient awareness of smoking behavior may be increased by having patients list the personal reasons for smoking and for wanting to quit. They should also monitor smoking habits and change their consumption patterns. Patients should then ask for support from family and friends and set a date for quitting.

Third Stage of Smoking Cessation.—The patients in stage 3 are initiating change, and they need to be warned about withdrawal and other physical symptoms. Coping strategies include identifying a buddy; identifying difficult situations and planning avoidance maneuvers; and throwing away cigarettes, matches, lighters, and ashtrays on the date set for quitting. Patients should invest in becoming a nonsmoker. They should remove smoking contaminants from the body by exercising; consuming more fiber, fruit juice, and water; reducing caffeine intake; and having their teeth cleaned. They also should find a hobby, frequent places where smoking is not permitted, and clean smoking contaminants from their homes. They should also reward themselves for becoming nonsmokers.

Fourth Stage of Smoking Cessation.—Stage 4 patients have successfully quit smoking for more than 2 weeks. Physicians should reinforce nonsmoking behavior through follow-up phone calls or office visits. They should also reinforce the patient's sense of the importance of not smoking, reinforce coping strategies, and emphasize that a lapse is not an insurmountable failure. When lapses occur, physicians should encourage early reassessment and remotivation.

Conclusions.—Physicians who use this approach to help their patients quit smoking have more confidence in their ability to effect changes in smoking behaviors. They therefore have a significant impact on the large number of smokers who seek medical attention each year.

Clinical and Pharmacokinetic Properties of a Transdermal Nicotine Patch

Mulligan SC, Masterson JG, Devane JG, Kelly JG (Elan Corp; Inst of Biopharmaceutics, Monksland, Athlone, Ireland)

Clin Pharmacol Ther 47:331–337, 1990 15–10

Background.—The use of a transdermal nicotine patch for nicotine replacement therapy has recently been described. The pharmacokinetics of a patch containing 30 mg of nicotine was investigated, and its efficacy in smoking cessation was evaluated in a double-blind study of 80 smokers.

Methods.—An inpatient unblinded pharmacokinetic study was done in 24 healthy men who smoked. The men had a nicotine patch applied to the forearm every day for 7 days. Venous blood specimens were obtained periodically throughout the study period, and urine was collected for 24 hours on days 1 and 7. The nicotine and cotinine concentrations were estimated by gas liquid chromatography. In the clinical study, smokers were randomly assigned to active-patch and placebo-patch groups. The subjects recorded the number of cigarettes smoked per week, and carbon monoxide analysis in expired breath was used as an

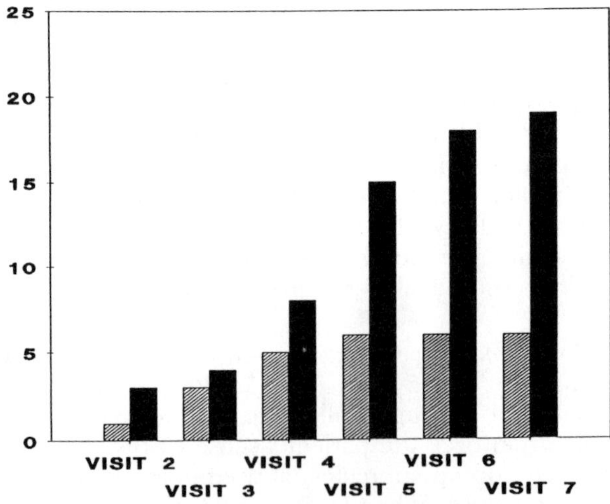

Fig 15–3.—Quit rate based on subjects who quit and remained abstinent for the remainder of the study. *Solid bars* indicate nicotine; *hatched bars,* placebo. (Courtesy of Mulligan SC, Masterson JG, Devane JG, et al: *Clin Pharmacol Ther* 47:331–337, 1990.)

independent assessment of smoking. The men received counseling and participated in a behavioral modification program.

Results.—In the pharmacokinetic study, significant nicotine concentrations appeared quite quickly; the highest mean plasma concentration was 12.09 ng/mL at 8 hours. The apparent elimination half-life was 11.71 hours, which probably reflected continuing absorption. The cotinine concentrations tended to increase during the study period, slowing after day 4. On day 7, the average peak nicotine concentration was 17.02 ng/mL at 8.96 hours and the apparent half-life was 5.6 hours. Absorption of nicotine from the patch was about 75%; at steady state, nearly 11% of the dose was recovered in urine.

In the clinical study, 50% of the patients in the nicotine group claimed to have quit smoking, compared with 17.5% of the placebo group. These findings were consistent with carbon monoxide concentrations. Most subjects who quit smoking in a particular week had not resumed at subsequent visits (Fig 15–3). Nonspecific local effects were equally divided between the 2 groups; erythema was the most common consequence of nicotine application, and it disappeared after patch removal.

Conclusions.—Application of a 30-mg transdermal nicotine patch produces sustained plasma concentrations of nicotine and results in significant smoking cessation or reduction. Studies to assess the cessation rates in larger populations are underway.

▶ Efforts to reduce the incidence of tobacco use in the United States continue because of the desire to reduce the high mortality rates associated with smoking. Kraner and Graham (Abstract 15–9) provide a step-by-step guide for physicians to use with their patients. They describe the 4 practical steps at which patients are seen and the specific strategies that are most likely to succeed at each stage. Nicotine gum has been an effective adjunctive agent because it allows patients to deal with the pharmacological and psychological addictions separately. This struggle can be won on the basis of further educational efforts directed at the young and by attempting patient-by-patient intervention with established smokers. Physicians must acknowledge the power they possess to influence the behavior of their patients.

The new player in the arena of smoking cessation therapy is the transdermal nicotine patch. The product described in Abstract 15–10 is a 1-day patch worn on the arm. It delivers blood levels comparable to those occurring when patients smoke or chew nicotine gum. In this study, the patch was found to be safe and effective, suggesting that it will be an important addition to the anti-smoking armamentarium.—B.J. Bailey, M.D., F.A.C.S.

Access to Health Care in the United States

Bailey BJ

Arch Otolaryngol Head Neck Surg 117:481–483, 1991 15–11

Background.—The basic issues in the health care controversy are access, quality, and cost, with access taking on the greatest importance in proposals that will shape the future of health care. It is estimated that 33 million Americans do not have access to the high-quality, advanced medicine available in the United States. The issues related to health care access are reviewed.

Discussion.—The United States has a philanthropic tradition of caring for the needs of the poor and underprivileged; however, these efforts now make only a modest dent in an enormous problem. Many state medical associations have taken the lead in improving access to existing programs, creating new programs, and increasing physician participation in the provision of care to the poor. These efforts still fail to meet the health needs of all citizens. Although the problem is often concentrated in urban areas, rural patients are sometimes more likely to live in poverty and have limited access to health care. It is widely thought that the problem of access can only be addressed by national legislative programs. Insurers and corporations are lobbying vigorously for universal health insurance with federal financial support. The American Medical Association (AMA) is directing its attention to a comprehensive and specific program to meet the challenges of health care access. Each physician should be familiar with the Association's "Health Across America" initiative. This initiative addresses major reform of Medicare, including measures to prevent bankruptcy of the program; employer provision of health insurance; risk pools for people without insurance; and expansion of private sector coverage. It supports professional liability reform to reduce health care costs, development of professional practice parameters, changes in tax treatment of employee health care benefits, and encouragement of cost-conscious decisions by patients. Innovative approaches to insurance underwriting, expanded federal support by medical education and research, health promotion by physicians and patients, amendment of the Employee Retirement Income Security Act, and repeal of state-mandated benefit laws are among the other measures advocated by the AMA.

Conclusions.—The challenge of increasing access to health care is difficult, and every physician should become involved.

▶ Events continue to unfold in the process that could be termed "the reformation of the health care system" in the United States. Media attention to the problems associated with the public's access to health care and endless reports of high-tech medical "miracles" have created the distorted perception of a system that is in total disarray and that tends to fuel unrealistic expectations. The day-to-day performance of physicians and other health care professionals is a story of achievement without parallel in the rest of the world. We have embarked upon a decade of predictable change in medicine; however, the nature of those changes has not yet become clear. Clearly, the impact of societal problems such as AIDS, drugs, violence, and teenage parents will stress the system further. Until we solve the problems of patient access to basic care, we run the risk of imposing solutions that could result in a significant decline in the quality of care already provided.—B.J. Bailey, M.D., F.A.C.S.

Endolaryngeal Jet Ventilation: A 10-Year Review

Shikowitz MJ, Abramson AL, Liberatore L (Long Island Jewish Med Ctr; Schneider Children's Hosp, New Hyde Park, NY)

Laryngoscope 101:455–461, 1991 15–12

Background.—Venturi jet ventilation for microsurgery of the larynx allows an unobstructed view of the larynx and eliminates the hazard of accidental endotracheal tube ignition. A 10-year experience with this technique is reviewed to evaluate its safety and efficacy.

Methods.—A total of 942 patients, ranging in age from 7 days to 90 years, was reviewed. The equipment used was a specially modified laryngoscope with multiple ports, into which a 14- or 16-gauge ventilation needle could be advanced just distal to the vocal cords. Fentanyl was generally used in children, but it was largely replaced by Sufenta or Alfenta in adults. All drugs were titrated to the patient, with muscle relaxation monitored by nerve stimulation.

Results.—All cases were successful. The average duration of anesthesia was 30 minutes. No laser ignitions in the trachea or surrounding tissue

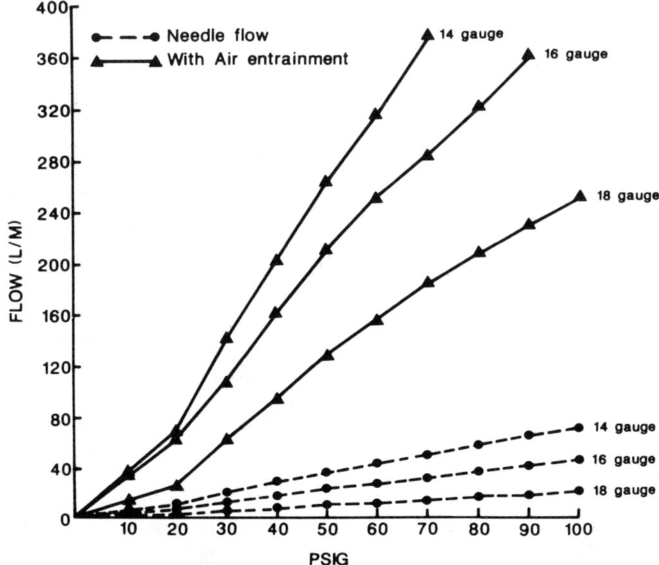

Fig 15–4.—The oxygen flow through the jet ventilating needle, demonstrating the venturi effect. (Courtesy of Shikowitz MJ, Abramson AL, Liberatore L: *Laryngoscope* 101:455–461, 1991.)

occurred, and all postoperative chest radiographs were normal except in 4 infants with pneumothoraces, for a complication rate of .42%. There was a .96% rate of arrhythmia (which resolved spontaneously during continued ventilation) and a .32% incidence of gastric distention.

Conclusions.—Anesthesia for microlaryngeal surgery may be delivered safely, and often preferably, by endolaryngeal jet ventilation. Experimental findings showing a linear relationship between rate of jet flow vs. driving pressure and the subsequent venturi effect with air entrainment have carried over into the clinical setting (Fig 15–4). The team approach is most important in the use of this technique.

▶ The authors evaluate an extensive series of patients who underwent jet ventilation anesthesia for laryngeal microsurgery. The results were excellent, with a very low complication rate. It is important to note that, because the ventilation needle is placed distal to the vocal cords, care must be taken to assure that there is adequate space for the escape of the anesthetic gases from the lungs. The presence of laryngeal narrowing from scar tissue, tumor, or other pathologic changes greatly increases the risk of gas entrapment (which could lead to pneumothorax).—B.J. Bailey, M.D., F.A.C.S.

Proximal Esophageal pH-Metry in Patients With "Reflux Laryngitis"

Jacob P, Kahrilas PJ, Herzon G (Northwestern Univ Med School, Chicago; VA Lakeside Med Ctr, Chicago)

Gastroenterology 100:305–310, 1991 15–13

Objective.—Posterior laryngitis has been related to gastroesophageal reflux; however, most affected individuals lack overt esophagitis. Fiberoptic laryngoscopy was performed in 40 patients who had reflux; 25 of the patients also had persistent laryngeal symptoms such as dysphonia, cough, and frequent clearing of the throat. Fifteen patients with reflux lacked laryngeal symptoms.

Observations.—The distal esophagus was exposed to acid significantly longer than the proximal esophagus in all groups of patients, although reflux sometimes acidified the entire organ. Most acid exposure occurred during the day. Exposure of the proximal esophagus to acid was significantly greater in symptomatic patients than in asymptomatic patients, whether laryngoscopy showed changes of reflex laryngitis or not. More than half of the symptomatic patients and none of those without symptoms had significantly increased exposure of the proximal esophagus to acid.

Discussion.—The presence of acid-induced laryngitis is associated with increased proximal esophageal exposure to gastric acid in patients with gastroesophageal reflux. Posterior laryngitis is much less frequent in patients with reflux who lack laryngeal symptoms and significant esophageal exposure to acid.

▶ Patients who present with sensation, chronic scratchy throat, hoarseness, or chronic cough should be evaluated for possible gastroesophageal reflux. This disorder is now being diagnosed more frequently because of the introduction of flexible fiberoptic endoscopes into many more otolaryngologists' offices. Although the authors of this study recommend ambulatory dual-site pH recordings to evaluate these patients, they emphasize that the study has technical problems and that there is a lack of relevant normative data to rely upon, especially in the instance of marginal findings.—B.J. Bailey, M.D., F.A.C.S.

Percutaneous Tracheostomy: Ready or Not?

Pelausa EO (Natl Defence Med Centre, Ottawa, Canada)

J Otolaryngol 20:88–92, 1991 15–14

Background.—Percutaneous tracheostomy procedures, which are based on the Seldinger guidewire technique, have given promising early results. Reports claim that the procedure is faster and easier than conventional methods and that it is easily learned. The approach was attempted in 4 patients, and its usefulness was evaluated.

Procedure.—The Schachner-Ovil kit was obtained (Fig 15–5). The procedure was learned using the printed instructions and videotaped demonstrations that were provided. The procedure includes a 1-cm transverse incision, insertion of

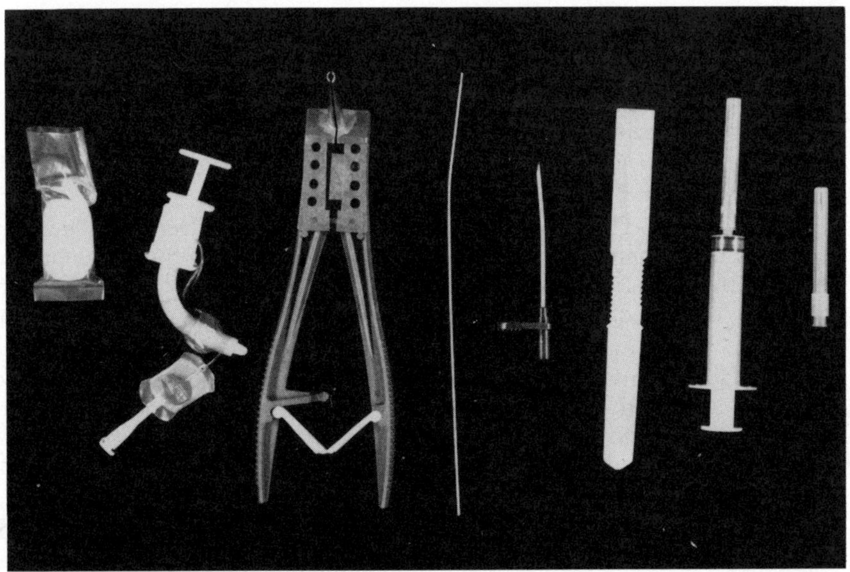

Fig 15–5.—Rapitrac sterile disposable percutaneous tracheostomy kit. (Courtesy of Pelausa EO: *J Otolaryngol* 20:88–92, 1991.)

the guidewire through a 12-gauge needle, insertion of a percutaneous tracheostomy tool, and insertion of a Portex tracheostomy tool.

Results.—Several unexpected difficulties were encountered. Proper patient selection was essential because the kit is applicable only to lean patients with supple necks and prominent cervical landmarks. The penetrator was too short for use in 2 of the 4 patients. In addition, the Portex tube was small for adults and vulnerable to blockage from crusting. The fastest procedure lasted 10 minutes. In one case, a traditional open tracheostomy was required to stem bleeding. Although it was recognized that any new procedure requires sufficient learning time, the use of the kit was discontinued because of its evident deficiencies.

Conclusions.—Percutaneous tracheostomy has not yet been perfected. The kit described may need to be modified, or the success of the serial-dilatation technique may help to fulfill its promise.

▶ The search continues for a safe and relatively easier tracheotomy technique. There have been numerous kits and instruments proposed during the past 3 decades; however, none has proven to be a lasting alternative to surgical tracheotomy. This study concludes that the Schachner-Ovil kit has limited clinical versatility and is associated with numerous problems. It is reasonable to expect that there will eventually be refinements of this product. Products of greater value may also be introduced because of the continuing need for a device that is useful when a surgeon is not immediately available.—B.J. Bailey, M.D., F.A.C.S.

Infiltration of Epinephrine in Tonsillectomy: A Randomized, Prospective, Double-Blind Study

Rasgon BM, Cruz RM, Hilsinger RL Jr, Korol HW, Callan E, Wolgat RA, Selby JV (Kaiser Permanente Med Ctr, Oakland, Calif)

Laryngoscope 101:114–118, 1991 15–15

Introduction.—The most common cause of death after tonsillectomy is postoperative hemorrhage. The effect of a direct injection of epinephrine into the tonsil was studied and evaluated for blood loss during surgery, time of dissection, cardiac manifestations, and bleeding postoperatively.

Methods.—Before tonsillectomy, normal saline solution was injected in 1 tonsil and epinephrine was injected in the other tonsil of 92 patients in a randomized, prospective, double-blind fashion. The patients were their own controls. Blood loss from the right and left tonsils and the adenoids was collected separately.

Results.—Blood loss on the injected side was significantly decreased, averaging about one third less than that on the side injected with normal saline. Dissection time was also significantly decreased on the epinephrine side, primarily because of less visual obstruction from loss of blood;

this resulted in easier identification and cautery of the blood vessels. The cardiac manifestations were minimal and short-lived. Whether surgeons were right- or left-handed demonstrated no significant difference.

Discussion.—Epinephrine has been used during general anesthesia in otolaryngologic procedures for hemostasis purposes. In this study, no significant differences were found in the rate of postoperative hemmorhage between epinephrine and saline solution tonsils. Injectable epinephrine pretonsillectomy appears to effectively reduce intraoperative bleeding and dissection time.

▶ The authors conclude that blood loss is "significantly" reduced when epinephrine is injected before tonsillectomy. It is important to remember that it is possible to achieve improvements that are statistically significant but not clinically important. The ability to reduce blood loss by 30 cc and decrease operative time by 5 minutes is desirable; however, it must be weighed against the added risks of cardiac arrhythmias. Given these results, one would be hard pressed to conclude that there is an important clinical advantage associated with the injection of epinephrine.—B.J. Bailey, M.D., F.A.C.S.

Removal of Blunt Foreign Bodies From the Esophagus

Hawkins DB (Univ of Southern California)

Ann Otol Rhinol Laryngol 99:935–940, 1990 15–16

Introduction.—Blunt objects are commonly swallowed by children, and the usual technique for their removal has been via esophagoscopy with the patient under general endotracheal anesthesia. Recent alternative procedures that have been used to remove a foreign body include extraction with a Foley catheter under fluoroscopy and pushing the object into the stomach with a bougie. The complication rate for the removal of only blunt foreign bodies by using esophagoscopy was assessed during a 19-year period at the university medical center.

Methods.—A total of 246 esophagoscopies was performed to remove blunt foreign bodies from the esophagi of 231 pediatric patients between January 1, 1971, and March 1, 1990. Coins comprised 80% of all the objects removed. Of the 196 patients who swallowed coins, 74% were younger than 3 years of age and 25% were younger than 1 year of age. The usual location for a swallowed coin was in the cervical esophagus just below the cricopharyngeus muscle. The records of 157 patients noted the time between swallowing the foreign body and its removal, and they showed that 86 patients (55%) were treated within the first 24 hours. Fifty esophagoscopies were performed to remove blunt objects other than coins; the most common of these objects was meat, which was usually caught above a stricture.

Results.—In 187 patients, an esophagoscope was used to remove the coin. In 9 patients, the coin had passed into the stomach because of the muscle relaxation induced by general anesthesia. Esophageal injury secondary to the foreign body (including edema, erosion, and granulation tissue) was found in 47 patients (27%); mucosal erosions were observed in 39% of the patients younger than 1 year of age and in 90% of those with the coin in the esophagus for more than a week. Multiple foreign bodies were removed in 10 of the 196 patients. No deaths, perforations, or cases of mediastinitis occurred in this population. Fourteen patients experienced respiratory complications caused by the length of time the foreign body remained in place, preexisting disease, or general anesthesia. Three additional patients experienced adverse effects of general anesthesia. Overall, 80% of the children left the hospital within 24 hours. No deaths, perforations, or instances of mediastinitis occurred in the patients who had foreign bodies other than coins removed. However, 1 patient, aged 9 months, did have an infection and complications that required a 19-day hospital stay.

Conclusions.—Esophagoscopy appears to be relatively safe in the removal of blunt foreign bodies, particularly when performed by skilled endoscopists and anesthesiologists. From the standpoint of safety, there does not seem to be a need for alternative techniques involving blind removal.

▶ The author presents his experience removing foreign bodies via esophagoscopy with the patient under general anesthesia. His results are useful in countering the proponents of other methods, who emphasize the risk of esophagoscopy. An important element of this study is the survey questionnaire designed to collect responses concerning complications associated with foreign body removal via esophagoscopy or alternative methods, such as Foley catheter extraction. The survey results may provide enlightenment regarding this controversy.—B.J. Bailey, M.D., F.A.C.S.

The Effects of Relaxation/Imagery Training on Recurrent Aphthous Stomatitis: A Preliminary Study

Andrews VH, Hall HR (Pennsylvania State Univ, University Park; Case Western Reserve Univ)

Psychosom Med 52:526–535, 1990 15–17

Introduction.—Recurrent aphthous stomatitis (RAS), a common disease of the oral mucosa, has an unknown etiology that has been linked to emotional and psychological factors. Although no effective treatment has been found for RAS, research and clinical literature now suggest that immunological factors may be involved in the disorder. The effects of relaxation/imagery training on RAS were assessed.

Methods.—Two men and 5 women (age range, 16–166 years) participated in a study that assessed daily diary self-reports, dental ratings, and pyschological measures—the Symptom Checklist-90 Revised (SCL-90R) and the Stanford Hypnotic Susceptibility Scale, Form C (Stanford C). The study had a single-case, multiple-baseline design.

Technique.—Each relaxation and imagery session lasted 30 minutes and was administered by the same individual. After relaxation induction and deeper relaxation, the participants were asked to visualize "immune system imagery", such as imaging their white blood cells helping to heal their mouth ulcers; visualization lasted approximately 5 minutes. The subjects were also given postinduction suggestions that their immune systems would continue to work against the ulcers even though they were not actively imaging this. The patients were trained in home use of these methods, using written instructions.

Results.—Complete data was collected from the 5 subjects who completed 12 relaxation sessions; 1 subject completed 7 sessions and 1 completed 5 sessions. The overall results demonstrate significant decreases in the percentage of days with ulcers from baseline to the treatment phase. The mean percentage of improvement for the 5 patients who completed 12 sessions was 35.5%; for the 2 patients who completed 7 and 5 sessions, it was 33.2%. Although some subjects experienced severe outbreaks of ulcers during treatment, they managed to significantly reduce their overall mean number of ulcers during this time. Of the 7 patients, 6 demonstrated a decrease in their overall level of psychological distress.

Implications.—These results suggest that the 12-session treatment protocol was associated with a significant reduction in the frequency of ulcer recurrence. Although the treatment did not appear to reduce pain itself, it did decrease overall pain because of the reduction in the number of ulcers. The decrease in ulcers in the patient who had only 5 sessions indicates that positive significant results may be possible with less than 12 treatment sessions.

▶ This interesting article explores the use of "alternative medicine" strategies in the treatment of a disorder that usually persists after conventional medical therapy. The successful results suggest that we should acknowledge the probability that emotional, psychological, and immunological factors are interwoven in a way that clinicians can exploit. We often require control groups in clinical studies because of the need to document the "placebo effect" (which is another recognition of the healing power of the mind). There are 2 drawbacks to this study: (1) the sample size is small, and (2) the study lacks a control group that did not receive relaxation/imagery training. Both of these issues are important because of the tendency of the disorder to wax and wane. Nevertheless, the results of this study demand our serious consideration, and the implications of a new, safe, and effective form of therapy are intriguing.—B.J. Bailey, M.D., F.A.C.S.

Otolaryngology Problems in the Immune Compromised Patient: An Evolving Natural History

Corey JP, Seligman I (Univ of Chicago)

Otolaryngol Head Neck Surg 104:196–203, 1991 15–18

Introduction.—In patients with immunodeficiency states, the role of the otolaryngologist-head and neck surgeon is to diagnose the prodromal or early stages of the disease and to act as a consultant to patients with mid-to-late disease involving the head and neck. The diagnosis and treatment of the most commonly encountered immunodeficiency diseases in the head and neck were reviewed.

Discussion.—Newer, earlier patterns of disease become apparent as HIV is detected in increasing numbers of asymptomatic individuals who are at risk. The findings of cranial and cervical herpes zoster, oral hairy leukoplakia, and oral candidiasis link viral disease and other disease to the development of AIDS (Fig 15–6). It is now recognized that patients with AIDS and patients with other immunosuppressed conditions have many similarities. Lymphomas and squamous cell cancers, in addition to Kaposi's sarcoma, may be seen as immunosuppressed patients survive longer. In these patients, the otolaryngologist can learn to identify and treat otitis and sinusitis; to identify early predictive signs; and to diagnose and treat Kaposi's sarcoma of the head and neck, lymphomas, squamous cell cancers, and opportunistic infections. Any suspected infection should be treated early and aggressively. The suspected areas should be

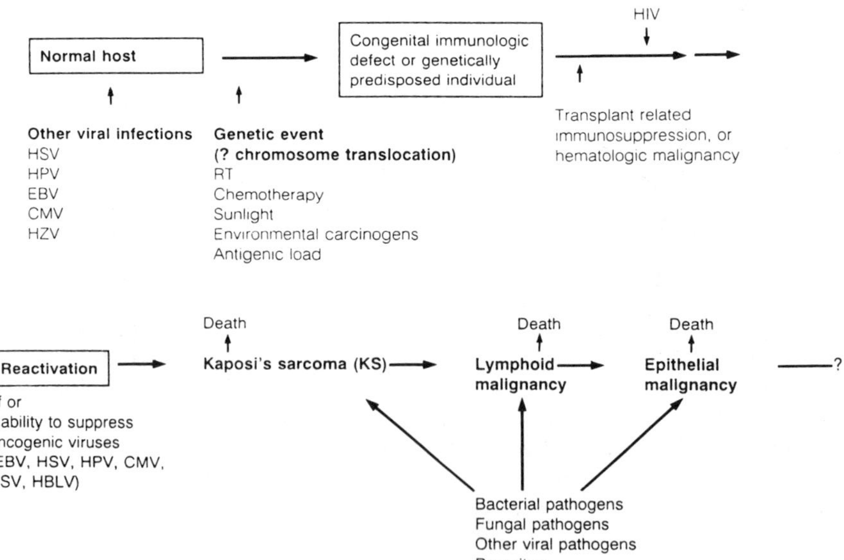

Fig 15–6.—Proposed pathogenesis of cancer in immunodeficient individuals. (Courtesy of Corey JP, Seligman I: *Otolaryngol Head Neck Surg* 104:196–203, 1991.)

cultured. Antibiotic prophylaxis should be considered for patients at risk or patients who have a history of ear, nose, or throat disease. Biopsy specimens should be obtained from all available areas, which should be re-examined carefully for suspicious lesions. Noninvasive studies such as CT and MRI are particularly useful in disease detection and staging. Airway management should be used as necessary.

Conclusion.—Recommendations for management of such patients are included, as are typical case reports of immunosuppressed adult and pediatric patients with head and neck complaints.

▶ Otolaryngologists have a key role to play in the diagnosis and management of HIV-immunocompromised patients. A high index of suspicion is important when unusual symptoms and/or findings are encountered.—B.J. Bailey, M.D., F.A.C.S.

Diagnostic Usefulness of Nasal Biopsy in Wegener's Granulomatosis

Del Buono EA, Flint A (Univ of Michigan)

Hum Pathol 22:107–110, 1991 15–19

Introduction.—Wegener's granulomatosis (WG) is an aggressive systemic disease that may be lethal if left untreated. Immunosuppressive and cytotoxic chemotherapy can significantly alter the course of the disease; however, treatment is associated with potentially severe side effects. Because WG often involves the upper respiratory tract, a nasal mucosal biopsy specimen is usually used initially for histological confirmation of the clinical diagnosis before starting therapy. The pathologic manifestations of nasal mucosal involvement in WG, and the diagnostic value of nasal biopsy in this disease were evaluated.

Patients.—A total of 30 nasal and paranasal sinus biopsy specimens from 17 patients (aged 17–77 years) with documented WG were reviewed. Sixteen patients had initially sought medical attention because of signs or symptoms of upper respiratory tract disorders. Of the 17 patients, 16 were treated with steroids and cytotoxic agents. One patient also received radiation therapy to the nasal lesion. The clinical follow-up ranged from 1 month to 24 years. Fifteen patients had a favorable response or complete remission, 1 patient died of sepsis during the first month of therapy, and 1 patient was lost to follow-up.

Findings.—The biopsy specimens from 4 patients showed active granulomatous vasculitis. An additional 3 patients had evidence of active nongranulomatous vasculitis. The remaining 10 patients had no evidence of vasculitis, although the specimens from 2 of these patients had foci of extravascular fibrinoid necrosis. Four patients with evidence of vasculitis also had extravascular foci of necrosis. A sample size that was larger than 5 mm in at least 1 dimension was significantly correlated with the presence of active vasculitis and foci of fibrinoid necrosis.

Conclusion.—Nasal biopsy is of somewhat limited usefulness when only granulomatous vasculitis is considered diagnostic of WG. The diagnostic efficacy of nasal biopsy is enhanced when extravascular foci of necrosis are also regarded as being diagnostic of WG. The usefulness of nasal biopsy can be maximized by obtaining samples larger than 5 mm in diameter from areas away from the ulcerated sites.

▶ The authors describe the contemporary views on biopsy diagnosis of WG. They point out that extravascular foci of necrosis are identifiable in a high percentage of patients. In some instances, such foci are present even when vasculitis cannot be confirmed. Early clarification is important in WG because there is evidence that treatment is more effective when it is begun early.—B.J. Bailey, M.D., F.A.C.S.

The Normal and Diseased Retropharyngeal and Prevertebral Spaces

Davis WL, Smoker WRK, Harnsberger HR (Univ of Utah, Salt Lake City)

Semin Ultrasound CT MR 11:520–533, 1990 15–20

Introduction.—The retropharyngeal space (RPS) and prevertebral space (PVS) are distinct midline spaces of the extracranial head and neck that form an integral part of the suprahyoid neck (Fig 15–7). Lymph nodes and fat are found in the RPS, whereas muscles, vertebral artery, clivus, and cervical vertebrae are found in the PVS. The disease processes in these spaces are relatively uncommon; however, these spaces are radiologically important because of their proximity to the airway and the inability to examine them clinically.

Discussion.—The RPS extends from the skull base to the level of the third thoracic vertebrae, where the middle and deep layers of the deep cervical fascia fuse. Therefore, the RPS serves as a potential conduit for the spread of infection or tumor between the neck and mediastinum. The most common lesions in the RPS are inflammatory lesions and metastases from squamous cell carcinoma, seen with either a nodal or nonnodal pattern of disease. Nodal masses enlarge the RPS in an asymmetric pattern sparing the midline, whereas the nonnodal disease is seen with a horizontal, rectangular, or oval mass in the posterior midline. In both patterns, the mass flattens and remains anterior to the prevertebral musculature. Other lesions in the RPS include lipoma, hemangioma, pseudotumors (e.g., tortuous carotid artery and edema fluid), and lesions secondary to trauma. The most common abnormalities in the PVS are malignant tumors and inflammatory disease. These lesions displace the paravertebral muscles anteriorly, thus distinguishing a PVS mass from a RPS process. The most common malignant tumors of the PVS include metastatic disease to the vertebral body or posterior elements, lymphoma or leukemia, and direct invasion by squamous cell carcinoma. Metastases from other organs are typically seen as expansile lesions with

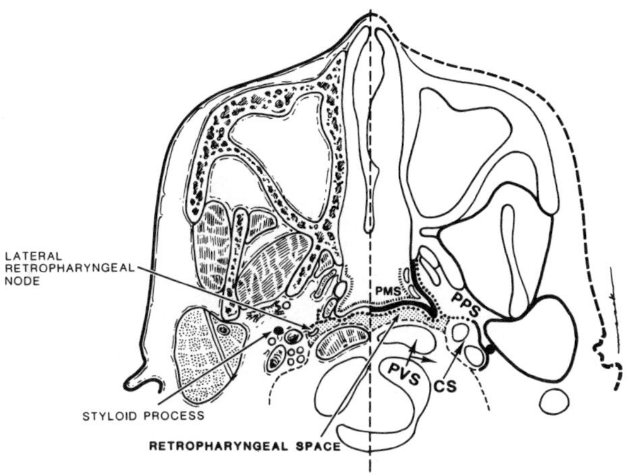

Fig 15–7.—Axial drawing through the level of the nasopharynx demonstrates the normal shape of the retropharyngeal space (*shaded area*); *dotted line,* middle layer of the deep cervical fascia; *broken line,* deep layer of the deep cervical fascia. (Courtesy of Davis WL, Smoker WRK, Harnsberger HR: *Semin Ultrasound CT MR* 11:520–533, 1990.)

destruction of the vertebral body. Other lesions in the PVS include chordomas, benign primary bone tumors, and psuedotumors. Inflammatory lesions are common and may occur as vertebral body osteomyelitis, diskitis, or PVS abscess.

▶ This article is 1 in a series of radiographic correlations with both normal anatomical features and a variety of pathological conditions. The authors emphasize that once an abnormality is identified in radiographs of this region, a discrete differential diagnostic list must be considered. Inflammatory processes and metastatic squamous cell carcinoma are the most common diagnoses, and the features of these and other diseases are reviewed.—B.J. Bailey, M.D., F.A.C.S.

Subject Index

A

B

C

D

E

F

M

N

P

R

S

T

V

W

X

Author Index

L

M

N

O

P

R

S

T

U

V

W

Y

Z